D0100155

LANCHESTER LIBRARY

WITHDRAWN

LANCHESTER LIBRARY

Gosford Street, Coventry C

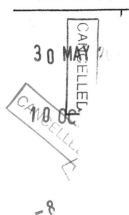

3 0 MAY

CANCELLED

10 OC

CANCELLED

-8

NUTRITIONAL HEALTH

NUTRITION ◊ AND ◊ HEALTH
Adrianne Bendich, Series Editor

Fatty Acids: Physiological and Behavioral Functions, edited by
David I. Mostofsky, Shlomo Yehuda, and Norman Salem, Jr., 2001

Preventive Nutrition: The Comprehensive Guide for Health Professionals,
SECOND EDITION, edited by **Adrianne Bendich and Richard J. Deckelbaum,** 2001

Nutritional Health: Strategies for Disease Prevention, edited by **Ted Wilson and Norman J. Temple,** 2001

Clinical Nutrition of the Essential Trace Elements and Minerals: The Guide for Health Professionals, edited by **John D. Bogden and Leslie M. Klevey,** 2000

Primary and Secondary Preventive Nutrition, edited by **Adrianne Bendich and Richard J. Deckelbaum,** 2000

The Management of Eating Disorders and Obesity, edited by **David J. Goldstein,** 1999

Vitamin D: Physiology, Molecular Biology, and Clinical Applications, edited by **Michael F. Holick,** 1999

Preventive Nutrition: The Comprehensive Guide for Health Professionals, edited by **Adrianne Bendich and Richard J. Deckelbaum,** 1997

NUTRITIONAL HEALTH

STRATEGIES FOR DISEASE PREVENTION

Edited by

TED WILSON, PhD

Departments of Exercise and Sport Science/Health Education, University of Wisconsin-La Crosse, La Crosse, WI

and

NORMAN J. TEMPLE, PhD

Centre for Science, Athabasca University, Athabasca, Alberta, Canada

Foreword by

ERIC B. RIMM, ScD

 HUMANA PRESS
TOTOWA, NEW JERSEY

© 2001 Humana Press Inc.
999 Riverview Drive, Suite 208
Totowa, New Jersey 07512

All rights reserved. No part of this book may be reproduced, stored in a retrieval system, or transmitted in any form or by any means, electronic, mechanical, photocopying, microfilming, recording, or otherwise without written permission from the Publisher.

All authored papers, comments, opinions, conclusions, or recommendations are those of the author(s), and do not necessarily reflect the views of the publisher.

Cover design by Patricia F. Cleary.
Production Editor: Jessica Jannicelli

For additional copies, pricing for bulk purchases, and/or information about other Humana titles, contact Humana at the above address or at any of the following numbers: Tel.: 973-256-1699; Fax: 973-256-8341; E-mail: humana@humanapr.com or visit our website at http://humanapress.com

This publication is printed on acid-free paper. ∞
ANSI Z39.48-1984 (American National Standards Institute) Permanence of Paper for Printed Library Materials.

Photocopy Authorization Policy:
Authorization to photocopy items for internal or personal use, or the internal or personal use of specific clients, is granted by Humana Press Inc., provided that the base fee of US $10.00 per copy, plus US $00.25 per page, is paid directly to the Copyright Clearance Center at 222 Rosewood Drive, Danvers, MA 01923. For those organizations that have been granted a photocopy license from the CCC, a separate system of payment has been arranged and is acceptable to Humana Press Inc. The fee code for users of the Transactional Reporting Service is: [0-89603-864-5/01 $10.00 + $00.25].

Printed in the United States of America.   10 9 8 7 6 5 4 3 2 1

Library of Congress Cataloging-in-Publication Data

Nutritional Health : strategies for disease prevention / edited by Ted Wilson and
Norman J. Temple.
      p. ; cm. -- (Nutrition and health)
   Includes bibliographical references and index.
   ISBN 0-89603-864-5 (alk. paper)
    1. Diet in disease. 2. Diet therapy. 3. Medicine, Preventive. I. Wilson, Ted. II. Temple,
   Norman J. III. Nutrition and health (Totowa, N.J.)
   [DNLM: 1. Nutrition. 2. Chronic Disease. 3. Diabetes Mellitus--prevention & control.
   4. Heart Diseases--prevention & control. 5. Hypertension--prevention & control. 6.
   Neoplasms--prevention & control. WB 400 f935 2001]
   RM216 .F89 2001
   615.8'54--dc21
                                                                      00-057513

Coventry University

DEDICATION

To Ed and Sue, thanks for the genes and the dreams.
A special thanks to Loki, thanks for the great advice.

—Ted

To Luciana, my wife, with love.

—Norman

SERIES INTRODUCTION

The *Nutrition and Health* series of books provide health professionals with texts that are essential for professional development because each includes: (1) a synthesis of the state of the science, (2) timely, in-depth reviews by the leading researchers in their respective fields, (3) extensive, up-to-date fully annotated reference lists, (4) a detailed index, (5) relevant tables and figures, (6) identification of paradigm shifts and their consequences, (7) virtually no overlap of information between chapters, but targeted, interchapter referrals, (8) suggestions of areas for future research, and (9) balanced, data-driven answers to patient questions that are based upon the totality of evidence rather than the findings of any single study.

The series volumes are not the outcome of a symposium. Rather, the editors have the potential to examine a chosen area with a broad perspective, both in subject matter and in the choice of chapter authors. The international perspective, especially with regard to public health initiatives, is emphasized where appropriate. The editors, whose trainings are both research- and practice- oriented, have the opportunity to develop a primary objective for their book; define the scope and focus, and then invite the leading authorities from around the world to be part of their initiative. The authors are encouraged to provide an overview of the field, discuss their own research, and relate the research findings to potential human health consequences. Because each book is developed *de novo*, the chapters can be coordinated so that the resulting volume imparts greater knowledge than the sum of the information contained in the individual chapters.

Nutritional Health: Strategies for Disease Prevention, edited by Ted Wilson and Norman Temple clearly adheres to the mission of the *Nutrition and Health* series. Drs. Wilson and Temple provide the reader with a number of chapters with unique and compelling perspectives concerning the importance of the essential and currently characterized, nonessential components of the diet and their potential roles in reaching optimal health. The critical role of nutrition, from fetal life to senior years, in chronic diseases, especially osteoporosis, cancer, diabetes, and cardiovascular disease, is reviewed in depth in a number of key chapters. Requirements and functions for dietary components such as antioxidants, soy isoflavones, and long-chain polyunsaturated fatty acids are discussed in light of their importance in primary as well as secondary prevention of specific disease conditions. By including chapters on the role of biotechnology in the development of the food supply, nutritional epidemiology, as well as nutrition for exercise/sport applications, the editors have made this volume more appealing to a wider audience than most basic nutrition texts. Moreover, *Nutritional Health: Strategies for Disease Prevention* is especially unique in the inclusion of a chapter by Michael Jacobson of the Centers for Science in the Public Interest on the role of the private versus public sector in nutrition advocacy. Other provocative chapters include two coauthored by Norman Temple: one, coauthored with Marion Nestle, that addresses the role of government in nutrition policy and a final chapter coauthored with Ted Wilson that projects the potential consequences of nutrition policies on health in the 21st century. Readers will also gain timely information about the role of the Internet in nutrition communications and resource availability. Thus, *Nutritional Health: Strategies for Disease Prevention* represents a comprehensive, up-to-date resource for undergraduate, graduate, and medical students, nutrition and public health educators, practicing physicians, and other health care providers as well as policy makers.

Adrianne Bendich, PhD, FACN
GlaxoSmithKline, Parsippany, NJ

FOREWORD

The role of nutrition in the prevention of chronic diseases has gained greater awareness among funding agencies and food producers, and in national dietary guidelines. Over the last 20 years, the explosive growth of the field of nutritional epidemiology has helped guide this transition. The earliest cross-cultural studies provided an inexpensive method for examining associations between food and nutrient intake and chronic disease. Since then, metabolic studies and large-scaled prospective cohort studies and clinical trials have provided detailed insight into the importance of specific nutrients in the prevention of chronic disease. With the refinement of scientific tools to study nutrition, we have become more focused and narrow in the topics we study. Scientifically, this allows us to understand the complex biological processes that form the basis for associations between nutrients and disease. However, from a public health perspective, we cannot lose sight of our larger goals of understanding how foods and food groups affect a multitude of health conditions. *Nutritional Health: Strategies for Disease Prevention* addresses this issue by putting into a public health context the most recent scientific evidence for the health effects of vitamins, minerals, functional foods, and other classes of foods.

Nutritional Health: Strategies for Disease Prevention fills a gap appparent in other publications. First, it provides readers with updated and detailed reviews of the literature in several new areas of nutritional research. Importantly, each chapter also emphasizes how the specific food components may affect a wide range of health conditions. Second, several chapters address more global issues related to the importance of preventive nutrition for food advocacy groups, for government agencies, and for shaping nutritional research for the new century.

One important concept that we should always keep in mind when reading new scientific publications is that conclusive evidence documenting an association between food and chronic disease can sometimes take decades to complete. Therefore, our understanding that fruits and vegetables lower the risk of cancer or cardiovascular disease is based on much more substantial evidence than more recent research findings on the health benefits of soy isoflavones or nutraceuticals. The editors in *Nutritional Health: Strategies for Disease Prevention* appropriately describe the current state of knowledge in each of the areas highlighting those topics where research is definitive and others where it is promising or speculative.

Medical educators of the future will need to incorporate the concept of preventive nutrition into their training programs, and health providers will need to incorporate sound clinical advice on nutrition habits. This book can serve as an important guide to help us all weave through the growing body of literature that suggests nutritional interventions are essential in reducing risk of chronic disease.

Eric B. Rimm, ScD
Harvard School of Public Health
Boston, MA

PREFACE

During the last century of continuous nutritional advancement, we have frequently been faced with great opportunities that were brilliantly disguised as insoluble problems. Perhaps we are biased, but in our eyes, the apparently unsolvable problems associated with nutrition are among the most exciting of those in the life sciences. How many other branches of the life sciences offer the promise of slashing the burden of human disease by one third or more?

With a scattering of brilliant exceptions, until the 1970s, few gave serious consideration to the notion that our diet plays an important role in such chronic problems as heart disease and cancer. Today, we have a vastly improved understanding of the role of diet in disease; we know, for example, how fats, fruits, and vegetables affect cancer and heart disease, how salts and calcium affect blood pressure and osteoporosis. Now, at the dawn of the 21st century, our vastly improved nutritional knowledge affords us the capability of preventing a sizable fraction of the chronic diseases that afflict the people of our world, but only if we can fully inform its populace about these discoveries.

Ironically, despite overwhelming evidence that nutrition has such enormous potential to improve human well-being, the field still fails to receive the resources it merits. Growth in funding for nutrition research and education remains stunted. By contrast, countless millions of dollars are spent on the glamour areas of biomedical research, such as genetic engineering and gene therapy. But we already know that our genes can only explain a fraction of our disease burden. Even if gene therapy reaches its full potential, it seems most improbable that it will ever achieve a quarter of what nutrition can do for us today.

In the words of Confucius: "The essence of knowledge is that, having acquired it, one must apply it." But a major barrier is that nutrition information often fails to reach the health professionals who most need to apply it. This is illustrated by a recent survey of physicians in Canada (1) conducted by one of us. This study revealed mixed results on the depth and breadth of nutrition knowlege. For example, barely half of those surveyed knew that potassium is protective against hypertension or that hydrogenated fats contain *trans* fatty acids.

How can our exciting discoveries in nutrition be applied when much of this information has not filtered through to the people who most need it, namely, the physicians, dietitians, and nurses who represent the frontline workers in health care? How do we bring this information to others who also need it, such as the professors of nutrition who lack the time to read more than a tiny portion of the literature outside of their main area of interest?

Nutritional Health: Strategies for Disease Prevention endeavors to address the needs of those who would most benefit from up-to-date information on recent advances in the field. Accordingly, our book contains a series of chapters by well-established experts across a diverse range of nutritional areas. Our aim is not so much to cover all the leading edges of nutrition, as it is to discuss recent thinking and discoveries that have the greatest capacity to improve human health and nutritional implementation.

Some readers may disagree with the opinions presented, but in nutrition, differences of opinion are often unavoidable. Owing to the constant changes in our diet, nutrition is by nature in constant dynamic flow, as are our opinions of what constitutes the best nutritional habits. The views expressed in *Nutritional Health: Strategies for Disease Prevention* are in many cases particular interpretations by the authors of each chapter on their areas of specialization.

Ted Wilson, PhD
Norman J. Temple, PhD

1. Temple NJ. Survey of nutrition knowledge of Canadian physicians. J Am Coll Nutr 1999; 18:26–29.

CONTENTS

CONTRIBUTORS

DAVID J. P. BARKER, MD, PHD, FRS • *Medical Research Council Environmental Epidemiology Unit, University of Southampton, Southampton, UK*

DONALD C. BEITZ, MS, PHD • *Departments of Animal Science and of Biochemistry, Biophysics and Molecular Biology, Iowa State University, Ames, IA*

GEORGE A. BRAY, PHD • *Pennington Biomedical Research Center, Louisiana State University, Baton Rouge, LA*

ROBERT CLARKE, MD, MRCP • *Clinical Trial Service Unit, Radcliffe Infirmary, Oxford, UK*

CAROLYN K. CLIFFORD, PHD • *Division of Cancer Prevention, National Cancer Institute, National Institutes of Health, Bethesda, MD*

WINSTON J. CRAIG, PHD, RD • *Department of Nutrition, Andrews University, Berrien Springs, MI*

EMILE A. M. DE DECKERE, PHD • *Unilever Health Institute, Unilever Research Vlaardingen, Vlaardingen, Netherlands*

MARION J. FRANZ, MS, RD, LD, CDE • *International Diabetes Center, Minneapolis, MN*

CHRIS FROST, MSC • *Medical Statistics Unit, London School of Hygiene and Tropical Medicine, London, UK*

KEITH M. GODFREY, BM, PHD, FRCP • *Medical Research Council Environmental Epidemiology Unit, University of Southampton, Southampton, UK*

ROBERT P. HEANEY, MD, FACP, FAIN • *Osteoporosis Research Center, Creighton University, Omaha, NE*

TONY HELMAN, MB, BS, MAST MED, GRD HUM NUTR, D OBST RCOG, MRACGP • *International Primary Care Nutrition Network, Sydney, Australia*

MICHAEL F. JACOBSON, PHD • *Center for Science in the Public Interest, Washington, DC*

RICHARD B. KREIDER, PHD, FACSM • *Exercise and Sports Nutrition Laboratory, Department of Human Movement Sciences and Education, University of Memphis, Memphis, TN*

BRAIN LEUTHOLZ, PHD, FACSM • *Department of Exercise Science, Physical Education, and Recreation, Old Dominion University, Norfolk, VA*

ARTUR MACHNER, BS • *Edmonton, Alberta, Canada*

BARRIE M. MARGETTS, MSC, PHD, RPHNUTR, FRSH • *Institute of Human Nutrition, University of Southampton, Southampton, UK*

xv

SHARON S. MCDONALD, MS • *The Scientific Consulting Group, Gaithersburg, MD*

PATRICIA A. MURPHY, PHD • *Department of Food Science and Human Nutrition, Iowa State University, Ames, IA*

MARION NESTLE, PHD, MPH • *Department of Nutrition and Food Studies, New York University, New York, NY*

SAHASPORN PAERATAKUL, PHD • *Pennington Biomedical Research Center, Louisiana State University, Baton Rouge, LA*

BARRY M. POPKIN, PHD • *Department of Nutrition, University of North Carolina at Chapel Hill, Chapel Hill, NC*

MARIE K. RICHARDS, PHD • *Department of Nutrition, University of North Carolina at Chapel Hill, Chapel Hill, NC*

ERIC B. RIMM, SCD • *Harvard School of Public Health, Boston, MA*

NORMAN J. TEMPLE, PHD • *Centre for Science, Athabasca University, Athabasca, Alberta, Canada*

MYRON H. WEINBERGER, MD • *Hypertension Research Center, Indiana University School of Medicine, Indianapolis, IN*

TED WILSON, PHD • *Departments of Exercise and Sport Science/Health Education, University of Wisconsin, La Crosse, WI*

JAYNE V. WOODSIDE, BA, PHD • *Department of Surgery, Royal Free and University College Medical School, London, UK*

IAN S. YOUNG, MD, FRCP, FRCPATH • *Department of Clinical Biochemistry, Institute of Clinical Science, Belfast, Northern Ireland*

1 Nutrition Advocacy for Better Health

Michael F. Jacobson

1. INTRODUCTION

As other chapters in this book make clear, the broad outlines of good nutrition are well known: eat more foods rich in vitamins, minerals, fiber, and phytochemicals (fruits, vegetables, whole grains, and low-fat animal products), and fewer foods rich in saturated and trans fats, cholesterol, refined sugars, and salt (meat, cheese, hydrogenated shortening, egg yolks, soft drinks, sweet baked goods, and salty processed foods).

The challenge to health officials and nutrition educators is to make that healthy diet the preferred diet of the nation. Working against good nutrition is everything from consumers' taste buds to the corporations that market pathogenic foods. The soft drink, fast food, meat, egg, and other marketers not only advertise their products heavily and distribute them widely, but they use every opportunity to influence legislators and government officials. With government being heavily pressured by industry, advocacy groups like the Center for Science in the Public Interest (CSPI) seek to represent the public interest in influencing both public opinion and public policies. This chapter uses several case studies to indicate how CSPI and other consumer-advocacy groups function.

CSPI is a nonprofit organization that was founded in 1971 by three scientists who wanted to apply their expertise to solving social problems. In general terms, CSPI investigates whether corporate practices and government policies are consistent with scientific research and, if not, seeks to bring about greater consistency. The organization has received some funding from foundations and the sale of publications, but most of its funding has come from subscribers to its *Nutrition Action Healthletter*. CSPI, unlike many nonprofit organizations, does not accept funding from industry or government.

From: *Nutritional Health: Strategies for Disease Prevention*
Edited by: T. Wilson and N. J. Temple © Humana Press Inc., Totowa, NJ

Since its founding, CSPI has been concerned with, among other issues, nutrition and food safety. Nutrition has been a priority because of diet's great impact on health. According to US government estimates, poor diet (coupled with a sedentary lifestyle) causes between 310,000 and 580,000 deaths per year *(1)*. Just four diet-related health problems—heart disease, cancer, diabetes, and stroke—are responsible for at least $71 billion in direct and indirect costs annually *(2)*. On the food-safety side, food poisoning is estimated to cause about 5000 deaths and 76 million illnesses annually. In addition, food additives may cause illnesses or deaths due to allergic reactions, congestive heart failure, cancer, and other health problems. Government health agencies have the primary responsibility for reducing those tolls. However, in practice, government is often limited by political considerations deriving from the power of the agricultural, food-processing, supermarket, restaurant, and advertising industries. Consumer groups like CSPI attempt to balance that power by encouraging government to act more aggressively in the public interest.

2. EDUCATION

Public education is the bedrock of CSPI's activities. Not only does education directly assist consumers who are seeking to improve their diets and health, but it also serves as a foundation for activism on the policy front. CSPI provides information by means of such traditional methods as newsletters, books, pamphlets, media interviews, and, more recently, the Internet (www.cspinet.org). It also holds press conferences to draw media attention to timely issues and new reports. And occasionally it sponsors paid mass-media ads (newspapers, television, radio).

CSPI's first educational campaign was grassroots-oriented. In April of 1975, 1976, and 1977, CSPI sponsored the national Food Day. The annual event spurred activities in thousands of classrooms and communities around the United States. It encouraged improved diets, greater support for anti-hunger programs in the United States and abroad, and discussion of problems caused by agribusiness. The local efforts were reinforced and stimulated by a handbook *(3)* and national publicity in newspapers and on television. Food Day introduced millions of people both to concerns about nutrition and to the fledgling activist organization.

Currently, CSPI's major educational medium is its own newsletter, *Nutrition Action Healthletter*, which has more than 800,000 subscribers in the United States and Canada. That newsletter has articles on nutrition research, the nutritional quality of natural and processed foods, and other consumer information. It also supports CSPI's policy initiatives by encouraging readers to write to or call government and industry officials.

Information in the form of occasional articles and media appearances only has limited power to influence the national diet, especially when one voice, such as CSPI's, is only one of hundreds of voices vying for the public ear. CSPI has long advocated that government should mount much more aggressive educational campaigns to improve the public's diet. Opponents of such campaigns have contended that nutrition education is a waste of public funds because it has little impact. Thus, in the late 1990s, CSPI sought to develop a model for an effective community-wide dietary-change campaign.

For people who do not smoke tobacco, saturated fat is one of the leading cause of heart disease. Milk is the third largest source of saturated fat for adults *(4)* and the largest source for children *(5)*. In 1994, CSPI staff scientist Margo Wootan developed a campaign—1% Or Less—designed to switch entire communities from higher-fat (whole, 2%) to lower-fat (1%, fat-free) milk.

We focused on milk because of its importance to health. Although consumers are slowly moving toward lower-fat milks, whole and 2% milk still make up 70% of national beverage milk sales *(6)*. Simply changing the kind of milk consumed can make a big difference to a person's overall diet. We have estimated that if the average American who consumes the average quantities of saturated fat, calories, and milk switched from drinking whole milk to fat-free milk, his or her saturated-fat intake would decrease from 12% of calories to 10%, *(7)* the level recommended by the Dietary Guidelines for Americans.

CSPI's strategy differed markedly from most previous nutrition campaigns. Its core feature was *paid* broadcast advertising. CSPI developed two 30-s television and two 60-s radio messages and placed them during times of large audiences over a 6-wk period. By comparison, most other campaigns that used the broadcast media depended on public-service announcements (PSAs) that stations played for free, but infrequently and at times that reached few people. Moreover, stations are unlikely to broadcast PSAs that may offend major industries—and major advertisers—such as the dairy industry. The messages noted that a glass of whole milk contains as much saturated fat as five strips of bacon and urged viewers and listeners simply to switch from fattier milk to "1% Or Less" *(8)*.

Although educators usually consider the costs of advertising prohibitively expensive, CSPI found that the costs, at least in small cities, were relatively economical compared to the costs of hiring nutritionists to convey messages by more traditional means. We found that local personnel and program costs for the pilot 1% Or Less campaign were higher than the advertising costs *(7)*. Together, the community education components cost approx $36,000 compared with $24,000 for the placement costs of the advertising.

In most 1% Or Less campaigns, the TV and radio spots were reinforced by occasional paid print ads and a variety of public-relation activities to generate news coverage. The campaigns were announced at news conferences designed to attract free publicity. Several times during the campaign, spokespersons appeared on news and talk shows, and a series of guest columns were published in local newspapers. Halfway through the campaigns, cardiologists and pediatricians held press conferences to highlight the health reasons for switching to lower-fat milk.

Local grocery stores played key roles in several 1% Or Less campaigns by providing campaign organizers with data on sales on the various types of milk. That was crucial for evaluating the effectiveness of campaigns. However, effectiveness was also measured by telephone surveys of people in test and control cities before and after campaigns.

The campaigns proved to be highly effective in influencing milk-buying habits. In the first campaign, in Clarksburg and Bridgeport, West Virginia, the market share of 1% and fat-free milk sold in supermarkets doubled, from 18 to 41% of all milk sold *(7)*. In fact, the campaign was so successful that stores frequently ran out of 1% milk. One year after the campaign ended, milk sales data showed that the change largely persisted.

That first campaign was conducted jointly with West Virginia University. Additional campaigns have been conducted in collaboration with health departments and universities in West Virginia, California, New York, Pennsylvania, Maine, and elsewhere.

We compared the cost and effectiveness of a 1% Or Less campaign that included community-based educational programs and public relations (PR) activities (to generate free news coverage) *(9)* to a campaign that used paid advertising and PR (in the absence of any other programs) *(10)*. The ads-plus-PR campaign had a slightly smaller budget of $43,000, yet it resulted in 34% of high-fat milk drinkers switching to low-fat milk compared with approx 20% in the community-program-plus-PR campaign, which had a $51,000 budget. In terms of the number of people exposed to the campaign message, the community-programs-plus-PR campaign cost approx 22 times that of the ads-plus-PR campaign ($2.28 per person reached compared to 10¢ per person).

Paid advertising and news coverage can reach more people than can community programs. We worked very hard in the community-programs-plus-PR campaign and had good community involvement, yet reached less than 20% of the population. In contrast, the ads and news coverage reached 80–95% of the population, according to telephone surveys. In addition, advertising provides more message reinforcement than do community programs. The ads aired several times a day for six weeks. The community programs were a one-time interaction.

CSPI's 1% Or Less campaigns proved that focused, intensive, economical, educational campaigns can improve the public's diet on a community-wide basis. The same approach could be used to encourage diets higher in whole grains, fruits, and vegetables, and lower in meat, cheese, and soft drinks. However, a small group like CSPI cannot fund such campaigns nationally. Hence, CSPI has encouraged the federal government to invest tens of millions of dollars annually in those dietary-change campaigns. Currently, the largest US campaign for the general public is 5-A-Day for Better Health, which is sponsored by the National Cancer Institute to encourage greater fruit and vegetable consumption. Unfortunately, the NCI spends only about $1 million per year on communications, an amount that pales in comparison with the tens or even hundreds of millions of dollars that companies spend to advertise their candy bars and french fries. We have suggested that one way to finance health campaigns is to tax soft drinks, candy, and other low-nutrition foods. More than a dozen states in the United States, as well as Canada, tax some of these foods, but they do not use the revenues to promote health (11).

3. ADVOCACY

Education is a long slow process and, with competing messages from diverse sources, is often not sufficient to attain health goals. Consequently, CSPI has always complemented educational activities with advocacy efforts. Such efforts seek to encourage companies to market more healthful products or to eliminate illusive advertising and encourage government agencies to ban unsafe additives, stop deceptive advertising campaigns, undertake educational campaigns, or provide better labeling.

3.1. Nutrition Labeling

One of the most powerful educational media is the food label, and some of CSPI's most important activities have sought to persuade Congress, the US Food and Drug Administration (FDA), and the US Department of Agriculture (USDA) to require labeling that provides clear, useful information. The first nutrition-labeling requirements were issued by the FDA in 1973. Although that labeling represented an advance, it had severe limitations. First, it was voluntary, except when a company made a nutrition claim, such as "low salt," on the label. Thus, even after 20 yr, only about half the foods in supermarkets carried nutrition information. Second, labels were not required to provide information about nutrients that represented clear health concerns, including saturated fat, cholesterol, refined sugars, and dietary fiber. Third, even when information about a macronutrient was provided, that often had little meaning to the consumer. A label might state 10 g of fat, but consumers had no way of knowing if 10 g was a lot or a little. Finally, the typeface used was small, rendering the labels difficult to use.

In the mid-1980s, CSPI began to call attention to deceptive labels. Some products labeled as "Light" were only light in color, not in calories or other nutrients. Some "Low Cholesterol" products were high in saturated fat. Even *Business Week* magazine, in a 1989 cover story, proclaimed "Can corn flakes cure cancer? Of course not, but health claims for foods are becoming ridiculous" *(12)*. Initially, CSPI petitioned the FDA to stop those deceptive claims, but the FDA was slow to act. CSPI then sought support from influential members of Congress, several of whom, at widely publicized press conferences, expressed their outrage at deceptively labeled foods. Finally, those members of Congress concluded that the only way to obtain real progress was not to expect after-the-fact enforcement actions by the FDA to stop deceptions, but the passage of new laws to ensure that labels were more honest and informative.

CSPI legal director, Bruce Silverglade, organized a coalition of health organizations—including the American Cancer Society, the American Dietetic Association, and the American Heart Association—to work with Congress to develop a comprehensive nutrition-labeling bill. The legislation had two main goals: provide comprehensive, easy-to-understand nutrition labels on all foods and ensure that health claims (for instance, "helps prevent cancer") and nutrition claims (for instance, "low sodium") were honest. Congressman Henry Waxman and Senator Howard Metzenbaum were key sponsors. They held hearings on the problems with current labels and participated in press conferences with CSPI and other health organizations to draw public attention to the issue.

Introduction of the legislation in 1989 spurred the FDA to develop its own proposals, but by then Congress recognized that any FDA action could be blocked by the food industry so it was vital to pass new legislation. The Nutrition Labeling and Education Act (NLEA) was signed into law by President George Bush in 1990. Although the "education" component of the act has been virtually nonexistent, the labeling portion gave the United States the best nutrition labels in the world (of course, many less-developed nations had much less need of labels, because they relied far more on traditional, natural foods and very little on processed foods). It took the FDA another 2 yr to write an extraordinarily complex set of regulations to implement the law.

The law took effect in 1994, and consumers rapidly took advantage of the valuable information that was provided on the clear and conspicuous labels (*see* Fig. 1). Having nutrition information on labels enabled consumers to compare the nutrition profiles of different foods and of different brands of a given food. Companies began to compete, to a certain extent, on the basis of nutritional quality and introduced an unprecedented number of new low- and reduced-fat foods.

Surveys sponsored by the FDA and the food industry show that about two-thirds of Americans check the nutrition label the first time they buy a product, and about one-third of those consumers have stopped buying a food because of the label. A survey sponsored by the National Cancer Institute showed that consumers who read nutrition labels consume diets containing about five percentage

Nutrition Facts

Serving Size 1 cup (228 g)

Amount Per Serving

Calories 260	Calories from Fat 120

	% Daily Value*
Total Fat 13 g	**20%**
Saturated Fat 5 g	**25%**
Cholesterol 30 mg	**10%**
Sodium 660 mg	**28%**
Total Carbohydrate 31g	**10%**
Dietary Fiber 0 g	**0%**
Sugars 15 g	
Protein 5 g	

Vitamin A 4% • Vitamin C 2%

Calcium 15% • Iron 4%

*Percent daily values are based on a 2,000 calorie diet. Your daily values may be higher or lower depending on your calorie needs:

	Calories	2,000	2,500
Total Fat	Less than	65 g	80 g
Sat Fat	Less than	20 g	25 g
Cholesterol	Less than	300 mg	300 mg
Sodium	Less than	2,400 mg	2,400 mg
Total Carbohydrate		300 g	375 g
Dietary Fiber		25 g	30 g

Calories per gram:

Fat 9 • Carbohydrate 4 • Protein 4

Fig. 1. The "Nutrition Facts" label was developed by the US Food and Drug Administration pursuant to the 1990 Nutrition Labeling and Education Act.

points fewer calories from fat than consumers who do not. It is hoped that nutrition labeling will lead to actual decreases in the incidence of heart disease and other chronic diseases as the FDA predicted after enactment of the labeling law.

3.2. Labeling of Trans Fat

In the several years since NLEA was implemented CSPI has sought to improve it. For one thing, when the FDA was writing its regulations, little was known about the atherogenicity of *trans* fat, a monounsaturated fat produced when vegetable oil is partially hydrogenated. Hence, the label did not require that *trans* fat be listed, only that it *not* be included in with monounsaturated fat, if the different types of fat voluntarily were listed. Shortly after the regulations were published, several studies demonstrated convincingly that *trans* fat was about as atherogenic as saturated fat *(13,14)*.

That research impelled CSPI in 1994 to file a petition calling on the FDA to require that the amount of *trans* fat be included on food labels. As with many other CSPI actions, that petition was supported by several leading nutrition researchers. CSPI announced its petition at a press conference and followed up with articles in its newsletter, analyses of the *trans*-fat content of various packaged and restaurant foods, and a letter-writing campaign from health-conscious consumers. As the biomedical research in support of the petition accumulated, the FDA ultimately decided to require *trans*-fat labeling. In November 1999, the FDA proposed that *trans* fat be listed on food labels *(15)*. Improved labels should appear on store shelves a year or two after a regulation is finalized.

3.3. Labeling of Fresh Meat

Another problem with the NLEA is that it does not require nutrition labels on fresh meat and poultry, because those products are regulated by the USDA, not the FDA. That means that some of the biggest dietary sources of saturated fat and cholesterol usually lack "Nutrition Facts" labels, though some supermarket chains voluntarily provide them. Therefore, in 1997, CSPI again petitioned the USDA to require nutrition labeling on ground beef (which contributes about 60% of the saturated fat Americans get from beef *[4]*) and all other cuts of fresh meat and poultry. In 2000, USDA officials said that they planned to propose a regulation to require nutrition labeling of ground beef.

3.4. Labeling of Refined Sugars

A third labeling initiative followed from CSPI's concern about increasing consumption of refined sugars. The amount of refined sugars (beet and cane sucrose, and dextrose, corn syrup, and high-fructose corn syrup) used in the United States increased by 28% between 1983 and 1998, with no sign that that increase would stop *(16)*. In 1994–1996, the average American obtained 16% of calories from refined sugars, and the average teenager 20%, with many people consuming upwards of one-third of their calories from that source.

Excessive refined-sugars consumption, aside from contributing to dental caries, appears to increase triglyceride levels and the risk of heart disease in insulin-resistant individuals *(17,18)*. Perhaps more importantly, heavy consumption of calorie-dense foods, such as those high in refined sugars and fat, may increase the risk of obesity *(19)* or displace more nutritious foods from the diet. The USDA has found that people who consume high levels of refined sugars are likely to consume less protein; dietary fiber; vitamins A, riboflavin, niacin, B_6, B_{12}, C, E, and folate; calcium; iron; zinc; and magnesium *(20)*. The leading contributor to increased refined-sugars consumption is soft drinks, which provide one-third of all refined sugars. A particular concern about soft drinks is that they are likely to replace more nutritious beverages. For instance, in 1977–1978, American teenagers consumed almost twice as much milk as soft drinks; in 1994–1996, they consumed twice as much soft drinks as milk *(21)*. That reversal may portend increased rates of osteoporosis several decades from now. As a means of educating the public and arousing nutritionists, CSPI published a report, *Liquid Candy*, that detailed the increase in soft-drink consumption.

To help consumers ascertain their own intake of refined sugars, and to reduce those levels when appropriate, CSPI again sought to build upon the nutrition label. Currently, labels do not distinguish between the sugars that occur naturally in fruits, vegetables, and dairy products and the refined sugars that are added to foods. Chemically, of course, those sugars are identical. But naturally occurring sugars are accompanied by vitamins, minerals, and other nutrients, whereas refined sugars are, by definition, pure "empty" calories. CSPI has been concerned about refined sugars because so many Americans consume such huge quantities of those sugars.

In 1999, CSPI, again with support from nutrition scientists and health organizations, including the American Public Health Association and 40 others, petitioned the FDA to take two actions to provide more information to consumers. First, CSPI asked the FDA to separate added sugars from total sugars and list the number of grams per serving of each on the label. Second, CSPI asked the FDA to establish a "Daily Value" for added sugars. The Daily Value is a recommended maximum daily intake; food labels indicate the percentage of the Daily Value a serving of food provides for nutrients such as saturated fat and sodium. The FDA did not, and could not, set a Daily Value for total sugars, because consumers should be eating *more* foods with naturally occurring sugars, but *fewer* foods with refined sugars. CSPI urged the FDA to set a Daily Value for refined sugars of 40 g per day, the amount that USDA nutritionists have estimated would fit into a nutritious 2000-calorie diet *(22,23)*. The FDA was considering the petition as this book went to press.

4. PUBLICITY

A small consumer group like CSPI lacks many of the tools that major corporations have at their disposal to convey their messages to the public and to influence policy makers: high-powered lobbyists, political-campaign contributions, influential stockholders, large advertising budgets, and thousands of employees who can be asked to write to legislators. Compensating for those deficiencies is the public recognition that consumer groups are acting more in the public interest than in the self-interest—plus their credibility and motivated staff members. Consumer groups use those positive attributes to magnify their voices in the mass media.

CSPI regularly issues press releases and holds press conferences to deliver its messages to the general public. That free publicity, although not as focused as advertising, can be highly effective in informing the public and generating political support. The critical ingredient to reaching the public through the mass media is credibility and accuracy. An organization or individual whose information is not accurate quickly loses respect and attention from journalists.

In addition to the previous examples related to 1% Or Less and nutrition labeling, a good example of how CSPI has used publicity is a campaign to restrict the use of a dangerous preservative. In 1982, the FDA proposed that sulfite preservatives—which had been widely used in wine, packaged foods, and restaurant salads—be affirmed as Generally Recognized As Safe food ingredients. CSPI conducted a literature review and discovered studies demonstrating that sulfites could cause severe anaphylaxis in sensitive individuals, usually asthmatics. CSPI petitioned the FDA to ban sulfites, issuing a news release that generated substantial publicity. CSPI announced a clearinghouse to which sulfite victims could write and gradually accumulated reports of more than a dozen deaths. Submitting those case reports to the FDA generated even more public attention, including reports on some of the most-watched national television shows. Ultimately, a congressional committee held a hearing, at which parents told how their daughter died due to anaphylaxis caused by a sulfite-treated salad, that exposed the FDA's failure to restrict the use of that preservative. Finally, the FDA banned the use of sulfites on restaurant salad ingredients and required labeling on any product that contained 10 ppm or more of added sulfites. In the decade since then, no deaths have been reported. Without the media publicity, it would have been difficult to generate the public and congressional pressure that ultimately brought about the new policies.

5. CONCLUSION

The food industry has almost limitless funds to advertise its products, hire professors to do research and serve as consultants, and lobby legislative and regulatory authorities. In contrast, only a very few comparatively small non-profit organizations have the expertise and resources to represent the public interest in government proceedings on selected nutrition issues and to challenge inappropriate corporate practices. Over the years, CSPI and other such organizations, with assistance from academic scientists, have effectively promoted the public's health by educating the public, pressing industry to improve its products, and persuading government to improve its policies.

REFERENCES

1. McGinnis JM, Foege WH. Actual causes of death in the United States. JAMA 1993; 270: 2207–2212.
2. Department of Agriculture (U.S.), Economic Research Service, Food and Rural Economics Division. America's Eating Habits: changes and consequences. Agriculture Information Bulletin No. 750, 1999.
3. Lerza C, Jacobson M (eds.) Food for People, Not for Profit. Ballantine Books, New York, 1975.
4. Subar AF, Krebs-Smith SM, Cook A, Kahle LL. Dietary sources of nutrients among US adults, 1989–1991. J Am Diet Assoc 1998; 98: 537–547.
5. Subar AF, Krebs-Smith SM, Cook A, Kahle LL. Dietary sources of nutrients among U.S. children, 1989–1991. Pediatrics 1998: 102: 913–23.
6. Department of Agriculture (U.S.), Economic Research Service. Food Consumption, Prices, and Expenditures, 1970–1997. Statistical Bulletin No. 965. USDA, Washington, DC, 1999.
7. Reger B, Wootan MG, Booth-Butterfield S, Smith H. 1% Or Less: a community-based nutrition campaign. Public Health Rep 1998; 113: 410–419.
8. CSPI's "1% Or Less Handbook" provides complete instructions for conducting a community-wide campaign. For more information, contact CSPI-1% Or Less, 1875 Connecticut Ave. NW, Suite 300, Washington, DC 20009.
9. Reger B, Wootan MG, Booth-Butterfield S. A comparison of different approaches to promote community-wide dietary change. Am J Prev Med 2000; 18: 271–275.
10. Reger B, Wootan MG, Booth-Butterfield S. Using mass media to promote healthy eating: a community-based demonstration project. Prev Med 1999; 29: 414–421.
11. Jacobson MF, Brownell KD. Small taxes on soft drinks and snack foods to promote health. Am J Public Health 2000; 90: 854–857.
12. Business Week. Oct. 9, 1989.
13. Judd JT, Clevidence BA, Muesing RA, et al. Dietary trans fatty acids: effect on plasma lipids and lipoproteins of healthy men and women. Am J Clin Nutr 1994; 59: 861–868.
14. Troisi R, Willett WC, Weiss ST. *Trans* fatty-acid intake in relation to serum lipid concentrations in adult men. Am J Clin Nutr 1992; 56: 1019–1024.
15. U.S. Food and Drug Administration (Nov. 12, 1999 news release) FDA proposes new rules for trans fatty acids in nutrition labeling, nutrient content claims, and health claims.
16. Department of Agriculture (U.S.), Economic Research Service (1999) Food Consumption, Prices, and Expenditures, 1970–1997; p.76. Department of Agriculture (U.S.), Economic Research Service (May 1999) Sugar and Sweetener. Publication SSS-225; p.87 (Table 59).
17. Grundy, SM. Hypertriglyceridemia, insulin resistance, and the metabolic syndrome. Am J Cardiology 1999; 83: 25F–29F.
18. Hollenbeck, C. B. Dietary fructose effects on lipoprotein metabolism and risk for coronary artery disease. Am J Clin Nutr 1993; 58: 800S.
19. Roberts SB, et al. Physiology of fat replacement and fat reduction: effects of dietary fat and fat substitutes on energy regulation. Nutr Rev 1998; 56: S29–S41.
20. Bowman S. Diets of individuals based on energy intakes from added sugars. Fam Econ Nutr Rev 1999; 12: 31–38.
21. U.S. Department of Agriculture. Nationwide Food Consumption Survey, 1977–78. Tables A1.2-1; 1.7-1 and -2. U.S. Department of Agriculture, Continuing Survey of Food Intakes of Individuals (CSFII), 1994–96. Data Tables 9.4, 9.7, 10.4, 10.7.
22. U.S. Department of Agriculture. Center for Nutrition Policy and Promotion (April, 1992; revised Oct., 1996), USDA's Food Guide Pyramid.
23. U.S. Department of Agriculture. Human Nutrition Information Service (Sept. 1993) USDA's Food Guide: background and development. Misc. Pub. No. 1514. 14.

2 Population Nutrition, Health Promotion, and Government Policy

Norman J. Temple and Marion Nestle

1. INTRODUCTION

It is now generally accepted that lifestyle—diet, tobacco use, exercise—has a major impact on health, especially Western diseases. However, there is a world of difference between awareness of these facts and their translation into preventive action.

This chapter not only focuses on nutrition in relation to health promotion, it also examines other areas, especially smoking and exercise. This is necessary because most health promotion campaigns take a broad lifestyle approach and simultaneously tackle nutrition, exercise, and smoking.

Trends toward a healthier lifestyle over the last 20 yr have been inconsistent. In the United States, deaths from coronary heart disease (CHD) have fallen by half since their peak in the late 1960s. Contrariwise, from 1976–1980 and 1988–1994 about 7% of American adults became newly obese (1). A rising prevalence of obesity has also been reported from other Western countries (2).

In the United States, per capita intake of fruit and vegetables increased by about 20% from 1970 to 1994 (3). Nevertheless, only about two Americans in five consume the recommended five or more servings per day of these vital foods (4). Moreover, half of Americans eat no fruit on any given day (5).

This poor rate of progress in the area of diet should be seen as part of a more general problem that large sections of the population give a low priority to a healthy lifestyle. For instance, the proportion of middle-aged adults in England engaged in at least moderate exercise, such as a brisk walk for at least 30 min 5 or more days each week, is no more than one half of men and one quarter of women (6). In the United States about one third of adults achieve this level of exercise (7), and another one third report no leisure time physical activity (8).

There has been an impressive fall by about half in smoking rates in men in many Western countries over the last 30 yr. The percentage of American men

From: *Nutritional Health: Strategies for Disease Prevention*
Edited by: T. Wilson and N. J. Temple © Humana Press Inc., Totowa, NJ

who smoke dropped from 44 to 28% between 1970 and 1993 *(9)*. However, recent trends indicate that smoking rates have been creeping up in recent years, especially in young people. For instance, 37% of American students in grade 10 are smokers *(4)*.

2. HEALTH PROMOTION CAMPAIGNS

During the 1970s, the intimate connection between lifestyle and health became increasingly apparent. As a result, many people assumed that the next step was to disseminate this information to the public and exhort lifestyle changes, action deemed sufficient to bring about the necessary changes. However, a review of 24 evaluations of the effectiveness of using the mass media across a range of health topics found little evidence of behavior change as a result of education alone *(10)*. Here, we look at various types of health promotion campaigns, most of them focused on risk factors for cardiovascular disease.

2.1. Campaigns in Communities

A number of community interventions have used the mass media combined with various other methods to reach the target population. Three major projects were carried out in the United States during the 1980s. Their aims were to lower elevated levels of blood cholesterol, blood pressure, and weight, to cut smoking rates, and to persuade more people to exercise. Each program lasted 5–8 yr and succeeded in implementing its intervention on a broad scale, involving large numbers of programs and participants. In the Stanford Five-City Project, conducted by Farquhar and colleagues *(11)* in California, two intervention cities received health education via TV, radio, newspapers, other mass-distributed print media, direct education, and schools. On average each adult was exposed to 26 h of education, achieved at the remarkably low per capita cost of $4 per year (i.e., about 800 times less than total health-care costs). A similar project was the Minnesota Heart Health Program, which included three intervention cities and three control cities in the upper Midwest *(12)*. A third project was the Pawtucket Heart Health Program in which the population of Pawtucket, RI, received intensive education at the grass roots level: schools, local government, community organizations, supermarkets, and so forth, but without involving the media *(13)*.

A recent analysis combined the results of the three studies so as to increase the sample size to 12 cities *(14)*. Improvements in blood pressure, blood cholesterol, body-mass index (BMI), and smoking were of very low magnitude and were not statistically significant; the estimated risk of CHD mortality was unchanged. These results are mirrored by two additional community projects: the Heart To Heart Project in Florence, South Carolina *(15)*, and the Bootheel Heart Health Project in Missouri also showed little success *(16)*.

One factor contributing to the lack of effect may have been that the projects took place at a time when American lifestyles were becoming generally more healthy and CHD rates were falling. This suggests that when a population starts receiving health education, even if little more than reports in the mass media and government policy pronouncements, large numbers of people will be induced to make changes in lifestyle. A health promotion campaign superimposed on such secular trends may have little *additional* benefit. However, we cannot discount the possibility that different types of intervention might be successful where those just described were not.

Fortunately, we have some examples of reasonably successful community projects for heart disease prevention. One of the earliest and most informative such projects was conducted in North Karelia, a region of eastern Finland with an exceptionally high rate of the disease *(17)*. The intervention began in 1972 before much health information had reached the population. Nutrition education was an important component of the intervention. Over the next few years, CHD rates in North Karelia fell sharply. Later, an intensive educational campaign spread to the rest of the country leading to a national drop in CHD rates *(18)*.

Two other European studies also achieved some success. Positive results were seen in the German Cardiovascular Prevention Study *(19)*, which took place from about 1985–1992, when there was no particular favorable trend in risk factors for the population as a whole. It was carried out in six regions of the former West Germany using a wide-ranging approach similar to that used in the American community studies. The intervention caused a small decrease in blood pressure and serum cholesterol (about 2%) and a 7% fall in smoking, but had no effect on weight. Action Heart was a community-based health promotion campaign conducted in Rotherham, England *(20)*. After 4 yr, 7% fewer people smoked and 9% more drank low-fat milk, but there was no change in exercise habits, obesity, or consumption of wholemeal bread.

Recent American and Australian community campaigns are of particular interest because each was narrowly focused on changing only one aspect of lifestyle and used paid advertising as a major intervention strategy. The 1% Or Less campaign aimed to persuade the population of two cities in West Virginia to switch from whole milk to low-fat milk (1% or less) *(21)*. The campaign is further described in Chapter 1 by Jacobson. Advertising in the media was a major component of the intervention (at a cost of slightly less than a dollar per person) together with supermarket campaigns (taste tests and display signs), education in schools, as well as other community education activities. Low-fat milk sales, as a proportion of total milk sales, increased from 18 to 41% within just a few weeks. The intervention campaign was repeated in another city in West Virginia; this time only paid advertising was used *(21a)*. Low-fat milk sales increased from 29 to 46% of total milk sales. An Australian intervention campaign also used paid advertising as a major component *(22)*. The campaign ran in the State of Victoria from 1992–1995 and aimed to increase consumption of fruit and vegetables. Significant increases in consumption of these foods was reported (fruit by 11% and vegetables by 17%).

Taken together, the community intervention studies indicate that small changes in cardiovascular risk factors can be made by the methods used to date. The evidence is suggestive that interventions focusing on a small number of changes and using paid advertising can be more successful.

2.2. Worksite Health Promotion

As an alternative to health promotion using a community intervention approach, other interventions have focused on the worksite. A pioneering project of this type, which started in 1976, was carried out in Europe by the World Health Organization. The project was conducted over 6 yr in 80 factories in Belgium, Italy, Poland, and the UK with the aim of preventing CHD (23,24). The trial achieved modest risk factor reductions (1.2% for plasma cholesterol, 9% for smoking, 2% for systolic blood pressure, and 0.4% for weight); these were associated with a 10% reduction in CHD.

At around the same time, "Live for Life" was carried out by the Johnson & Johnson company in the United States. This comprehensive intervention was started in 1979 and lasted 2 yr. Employees exposed to the program showed significant improvements in smoking behavior, weight, aerobic capacity, incidence of hypertension, days of sickness, and health-care expenses (25).

Another worksite project took place in New England (26). Employees were encouraged to increase their intake of fiber and to reduce their fat intake. Compared with the control sites, the program had no effect on fiber intake, but fat intake fell by about 3%. A few years later, the research team reported that they succeeded in increasing employees' intake of fruit and vegetables by 19% (half a serving per day) using an approach that targeted employees and their families (27). A similar project in Minnesota offered employees weight control and smoking cessation programs (28). The program had no effect on weight, but the prevalence of smoking was reduced by 2% more than occured in the control worksites.

2.3. Health Promotion in the Physician's Office

In 1994, two British studies reported the effects of intervention carried out by nurses in the offices of family physicians. The aim was to improve cardiovascular risk factors. Each study was a randomized trial aimed at cardiovascular screening and lifestyle intervention. Both studies achieved only modest changes despite intensive intervention. The OXCHECK study reported no significant effect on smoking or excessive alcohol intake but did observe small significant improvements in exercise participation, weight, dietary intake of saturated fat, and serum cholesterol (29,30). The Family Heart Study achieved a 12% lowering of risk of CHD (based on a risk factor score) (31). These results are consistent with the results of a meta-analysis of 17 randomized controlled intervention trials where dietary advice was given to healthy adults (32). Changes over 9–18 mo included small decreases in serum cholesterol and blood pressure, leading to a 14% fall in the estimated risk of CHD.

A variation of the foregoing trials is the targeting of patients at high risk of CHD, probably the most cost-effective form of intervention *(33)*. A study from Sweden exemplifies this approach. Subjects at relatively high risk of cardiovascular disease received either simple advice from their physician or intensive advice (five 90-min sessions plus an all-day session) *(34)*. The intensive advice had a modest impact; it reduced the risk of CHD by approx 6%.

The major deficiency of the high-risk approach, as Rose *(35)* has pointed out, is that it only affects a minority of future cases: the 15% of men at "high risk" of CHD account for only 32% of future cases. Therefore, to achieve a major effect on CHD, it is necessary to target the entire population. This logic also applies to other diseases related to diet and lifestyle practices such as stroke and cancer.

2.4. Health Promotion and the Individual

What the foregoing projects teach us is that appealing to individuals to change their lifestyles will be effective in some instances but not in others and can therefore be frustratingly difficult. Although some projects have achieved a moderate degree of success, typically progress has amounted to no more than a few percentage points. This might be expected to reduce the risk of CHD by about 5–15%. Although this is certainly beneficial, it will not affect the majority of people at risk, however. Thus, exhortations to the individual, whether via the media, in the community, at the worksite, or in the physician's office, are most unlikely to turn the tide of Western diseases.

Myriad factors influence people's lifestyle behavior besides concerns about how to protect health. Social factors, such as housing, employment, and income also shape people's attitudes, as does education. Advertising directly affects what people want and prices determine whether they can afford it. We are also creatures of habit and custom; resistance may therefore be expected when lifestyle modification demands changes in longstanding behavior and goes against fashion or peer pressure. We must also bear in mind that individuals have little control over many aspects of their physical environment, such as pollution and food contamination. It is probably naïve, therefore, to expect dramatic results from interventions that merely exhort the individual to lead a healthier lifestyle. Indeed, this has sometimes been characterized as "victim blaming."

This in no way dismisses interventions aimed at encouraging people to improve their lifestyle. Quite the contrary. Minor changes can make valuable contributions to public health that more than justify the expense and effort involved. For instance, Jeffery and associates *(28)* concluded that a smoking cessation program at a worksite costs about $100 to $200 per smoker who quits, whereas the cost to the employer for each employee who smokes is far greater.

Similarly, Action Heart estimated that the cost per year of life gained was a mere 31 (British) pounds *(20)*. Each reduction in blood cholesterol of 1% yields a 2% decrease in coronary risk, and reductions of risk in the range 10–15% would have a huge beneficial impact if achieved in entire populations.

Health promotion, therefore, can be a cost-effective way to improve lifestyles and thereby improve the health of large numbers of people. This is emphasized by the fact that in the United States poor dietary practices cost an estimated $71 billion per year in lost productivity, premature deaths, and medical costs *(36)*. More research is required to determine why different health promotion projects have achieved such varying levels of success. Would campaigns be more successful if the focus was on one lifestyle change rather than many? Is paid advertising the best means to utilize scarce resources?

3. GOVERNMENT POLICY

Effective interventions may need to tackle the factors that determine how people make food choices. Such interventions require the implementation of policies, especially by governments. In the words of Davey Smith and Ebrahim *(37)*: "…even with the substantial resources given to changing people's diets the resulting reductions in cholesterol concentrations is disappointing. [Health promotion programs] are of limited effectiveness. Health protection—through legislative and fiscal means—is likely to be a better investment."

Governments have a variety of powers at their disposal that can be put into service. One approach, which relies entirely on voluntary cooperation, is to issue statements of policy. However, these can easily amount to no more than hollow declarations as is illustrated by government policies on tobacco in many countries. On the other hand, policy statements can serve as a clarion call to action. For instance, British and American government policy on diet and disease, in conjunction with the media and medical science, helped change the climate of opinion so that it is now widely accepted that diets should preferably be much lower in fat and richer in fiber.

3.1. The Effect of Price on Sales

Prominent among available government powers are legislation and the use of taxation and subsidies. Action on tobacco control most graphically illustrates the necessity for placing these powers as a tool of health promotion. Educational efforts over the last three decades have been enormously important in persuading millions of people to quit smoking. Nevertheless, smoking rates are still well over half of their level of 30 yr ago. There is convincing evidence that price hikes are an effective means to reduce smoking rates (i.e., there is price elasticity) *(38)*. It has been estimated that a 10% increase in price reduces tobacco consumption by about 5%, especially among the lower socioeconomic groups *(39)*. The Canadian experience is particularly illuminating. The prevalence of smoking in young Canadians fell by half during the 1980s in tandem with a doubling of the price. This trend was reversed in the early 1990s when the price was slashed in an attempt to reduce smuggling from the United States *(40)*. Price increases appear to be a far more effective means of tobacco control than education or media campaigns *(41)*.

Alcohol intake shows a similar price elasticity to tobacco intake: a price rise of 10% causes a decrease in consumption by 3–8% *(42)*. Studies in Eastern Europe, especially Poland and the former USSR, have demonstrated that pricing, sometimes in combination with rationing, sharply reduces consumption and associated mortality *(43)*.

The lesson we learn from tobacco and alcohol is, first and foremost, that price increases are an effective vehicle to lower consumption.

What applies to cigarettes and alcohol no doubt also applies to food. By means of taxes and subsidies fruit, vegetables, and whole-grain cereals might become more attractively priced in comparison with less healthy choices. This would most likely induce many people to shift their diets in a healthier direction. Recommendations along these lines in the area of food and nutrition policy were advocated by the World Health Organization *(44)* at the Adelaide Conference in 1988. The policy recommendation given was: "Taxation and subsidies should discriminate in favor of easy access for all to healthy food and improved diet."

Jeffery and colleagues in the United States carried out a series of studies that have demonstrated the potential of policy interventions, especially of low prices, to increase the consumption of healthy food choices. In one study, the price of low-fat snacks sold in worksite vending machines was halved. Purchases of these foods increased from 26% of total sales before intervention to 46% after *(45)*. In a worksite cafeteria, the range of fruit and salad ingredients was increased at the same time as the price was halved. As a result, purchases tripled *(46)*. In a similar study conducted in a high school cafeteria, prices for fruit, carrots, and salads was halved. This led to a fourfold increase in sales of fruit, a twofold increase for carrots, and a slight increase for salads *(47)*.

3.2. Advertising, Marketing, and Labeling of Food

Another area where policy interventions could positively affect food choices concerns food advertising. The annual advertising budget for Coca-Cola Classic alone is over $130 million a year, and the budget for McDonalds is over $600 million *(48)*. In stark contrast, the education component of the National Cancer Institute-sponsored 5-A-Day campaign to promote fruit and vegetable consumption receives well under 1 million. The extent to which these huge imbalances in advertising budgets affect people's actual diets is not known, but is almost certainly significant *(49)*. Common sense dictates that if advertising did not work, the advertisers would not be wasting their money.

A particular issue is food advertising on children's TV. A study of advertisements appearing on Saturday morning TV in the United States found that 44% were for fats, oils, and sugar, 23% were for highly sugared cereals, and 11% were for fast food restaurants *(50)*. None were for fruit and vegetables. The authors concluded that: "The diet that is presented on Saturday morning television is the antithesis of what is recommended for healthful eating for children." Similar findings were reported for Canadian TV *(51)*.

Advertising is but one part of the wider production and marketing strategy of the food industry. James and Ralph *(52)* pointed out that in response to demand, manufacturers sell foods with less fat, but the missing fat often reappears in "added value" foods, which may be little more than concoctions of fat, sugar, and salt. James *(53)* made the compelling point that the food industry promotes high-fat food because it is so profitable, while at the same time, food labeling is "completely confusing" (with particular reference to Britain). The system is, in theory, based on "consumer choice" but, in reality, choices become largely uninformed decisions.

3.3. Government Policy and Food

The foregoing discussion suggests that government policies concerning food prices and, to a lesser extent, food advertising and labeling may be an effective means to induce desirable changes in eating patterns.

Here, we offer some specific suggestions as to how existing government policies could be modified along the foregoing lines so as to encourage diets higher in fruit and vegetables and lower in fat *(54)*.

1. Subsidies paid to milk producers could be changed to favor low-fat milk. Similarly, by the use of such means as subsidies, grading regulations, and labeling, and perhaps even taxation, the sale of low-fat meat could be encouraged over high-fat varieties.
2. There is always scope for improved food labels to facilitate purchase of foods with a low content of fat, especially saturated fat. In addition, labeling and nutrition information should be extended to areas presently outside the system, especially restaurant menus, soft drinks, snack foods, and fresh meat.
3. By means of regulations and rewards, schools could be encouraged to sell meals of superior health value while restricting the sale of junk food. Similar policies could be applied to other institutions under government control, such as the military, prisons, and cafeterias in government offices.
4. Television advertising could be regulated so as to control the content, duration, and frequency of commercials for unhealthy food products, especially when the target audience is children.

Jeffery *(55)* argued that this approach be used as a strategy against obesity: "I believe that it is time to think about alternatives to the traditional individual-focused strategies for obesity control. I believe we should also view our food supply as a potential environmental hazard that promotes obesity and to consider public health policy strategies for improving it." He suggested that perhaps calorie-dense products should be packaged in small serving sizes and that taxation should be based on the fat and sugar content of food. James *(53)* also made proposals for how policies could be used to help combat obesity.

The approach discussed above was well put by Blackburn *(56)*:

...even the newer community-based lifestyle strategies continue to assign much of the burden of change to the individual. A shift of focus to reducing, by policy change, many widespread practices that are life-threatening, while enhancing life-supportive practices, should redirect the currently misplaced emphasis on achieving "responsible" behavior and its purported difficulty. For example, local communities may more appropriately be considered to have a "youth tobacco access problem," approachable in part by regulation, than a "youth smoking problem," approachable mainly by education. Policy interventions may also be designed to .... make preventive practice more economical, as well as to encourage the development of more healthy products by industry. They may be a partial answer to another major paradox: while unhealthy personal behavior is medically discouraged for individuals, the whole of society legalizes, tolerates, and even encourages the same practices in the population.

Schmid et al. *(57)* summed up the approach discussed here:

Health departments that support disincentives for high-fat foods, tax breaks for cafeterias that offer healthy food choices, policies that require zoning ordinances to include sidewalks, or school facilities open to the public might be labeled radical or experimental today; tomorrow, however, they may be considered prudent stewards of the public health.

The problem of lead pollution is an excellent illustration of what can be achieved by governmental action. In the 1970s, regulations implemented by the American government forced major reductions or removal of lead from gasoline, paint, water, and consumer products. As a result, the blood lead level of the average American child is now less than one quarter of what it had been in the late 1970s *(58,59)*.

3.4. Barriers Against Public Health Policies

Although many might consider the policies discussed here to be worthy of implementation, it must be appreciated that barriers exist. In particular, industry profits enormously from the sale of highly processed food and has often shown itself to be resistant to change. In this regard, industry often secures government support.

The history of attempts to enact legislative control over tobacco illustrate how effective an industry can be when it utilizes a large budget in attempts to delay, dilute, or stop laws. There is clear evidence as to the likely reason why the US Congress has been so lethargic when it comes to antismoking legislation. In 1991 and 1992, the average senator received $11,600 per year from the tobacco industry *(60)*. In the opinion of the researchers who carried out this study: "The money that the tobacco industry donates to members of Congress ensures that the tobacco industry will retain its strong influence in the federal tobacco policy process." Similarly, researchers looked at the California legislature and concluded: "Legislative behavior is following tobacco money rather than reflecting constituents' prohealth attitudes on tobacco control" *(61)*.

If the tobacco industry can achieve so many successes, then it will likely be much easier for the food industry to thwart interventions that threaten its profits. This is because the relationship between diet and disease is far less clear than is the case with tobacco. Indeed, there is ample evidence that governments are sympathetic to the wishes of the agricultural and food industries. Typically, although the health arm of governments encourages people to eat less fat, the departments responsible for the agricultural and food industries are largely concerned with maintaining high sales. James and Ralph *(52)* asserted that: "Analysis of different policies suggest that health issues are readily squeezed out of discussion by economic and vested interests."

There is considerable evidence of how industry has successfully pressured governments to bow to their wishes on questions of nutrition policy. As discussed by Nestle *(62,63)*, the meat industry has been particularly effective in rewriting dietary guidelines. In the late 1970s, the goal was "eat less meat." This then became "choose lean meat." By 1992, people were encouraged to consume at least two or three servings daily. There is also evidence that the 1992 version of Canada's Food Guide was similarly modified under pressure from the food industry *(64)*.

Discussing the question of salt, Goodlee *(65)*, assistant editor of the British Medical Journal, put it as follows:

> *...some of the world's major food manufacturers have adopted desperate measures to try to stop governments from recommending salt reduction. Rather than reformulate their products, manufacturers have lobbied governments, refused to cooperate with expert working parties, encouraged misinformation campaigns, and tried to discredit the evidence...The tactics over salt are much the same as those used by other sectors of industry. The Sugar Association in the United States and the Sugar Bureau in Britain have waged fierce campaigns against links between sugar and obesity and dental caries.*

3.5. National Nutrition Policies: Examples

One pioneering project was the Norwegian Nutrition and Food Policy *(66)*. Implemented in 1976, it recognized the need to integrate agricultural, economic, and health policy. The policy included consumer and price subsidies, marketing measures, consumer information, and nutrition education in schools. Unfortunately, the policy clashed with policies aiming to stimulate agriculture. As a result, subsidies went to pork, butter, and margarine rather than to potatoes, vegetables, and fruit. Despite these setbacks, the policy has achieved some success in moving the national diet in the intended direction *(67)*.

Another noteworthy effort which implemented several of the policies discussed here was Heartbeat Wales *(68)*. This project was carried out in Wales with the aim of preventing CHD. Specific measures included better food labeling, price incentives, and greater availability of healthier food. The active support was enlisted of catering departments and a food retailer. Unfortunately, little information appears to be available as to the degree of success of this policy.

3.6. Are Nutrition Policies Acceptable to the Public?

An important question concerns the extent to which the public would accept the suggested policies. The issues of seat belt use and drunk driving illustrate that when legislation is implemented and the public is educated as to their importance, there is a high degree of acceptance. A study by Jeffery and colleagues *(69)* in the upper midwest of the United States indicated widespread support for regulatory controls in the areas of alcohol, tobacco and, to a lesser extent, high-fat foods, especially with respect to children and youths. If such policies are acceptable to Americans, then they are also likely to be acceptable in other countries.

4. SOCIOECONOMIC STATUS AND HEALTH

One area of importance is the relationship between socioeconomic status (SES) and health. Low SES is strongly and consistently associated with a raised mortality rate. This applies to total mortality, as well as to death from CHD and cancer. The risk ratios are in the range 1.5–4, clearly making SES a major determinant of health. Various measures of SES have been examined—income, social status of job, being unemployed, area of residence, and education—and each seems to manifest a similar relationship to mortality *(70–75)*. Another important finding is that the degree of inequality within a country predicts morbidity and mortality. In other words, the key factor predicting health and life expectancy of a country is not average income or average level of education, but the gap between the rich and poor *(76)*.

Various studies have investigated why SES is associated with increased mortality. In general, lower SES is associated with higher rates of smoking and a diet of lower nutritional quality. Is SES merely a proxy measure of lifestyle? Or does SES affect health by a more direct mechanism? This question is of much more than mere theoretical importance and has a bearing on health strategies. If people of low SES are unhealthy because they lead an unhealthy lifestyle, then the solution lies in encouraging changes in their lifestyles. But, if a low SES is intrinsically unhealthy, then the solution lies elsewhere.

Our best evidence is that both possibilities are partially correct. After correcting for confounding variables, especially smoking, exercise, blood cholesterol, blood pressure, and weight, most studies have found that the strength of the association between SES and mortality is reduced by about a quarter or a half *(70,73,77,78)*. This indicates that people with lower SES tend to lead a less healthy lifestyle and this partly explains their poorer health.

But this still leaves half to three-quarters of the association between SES and mortality unexplained. None of the studies we cited examined diet in relation to SES. If people of low SES tend to eat a less nutritious diet, this would help explain why such conditions as hypercholesterolemia, hypertension, and overweight are associated with low SES. Nevertheless, it appears that much of the association between SES and mortality cannot be explained by lifestyle and must therefore be a more direct consequence of low SES.

Psychological factors appear to play an important role in explaining the association between SES and mortality *(74,79)*. The psychological factor most closely associated with risk of poor health is lack of control at work *(79–81)*. We can speculate that other psychological factors, such as resentment, frustration, and a feeling of disempowerment, all contribute to poor health among low-income groups. Whatever the precise mechanisms, there is little doubt that structural elements of inequality within Western societies—economic, educational, social status—lead to reduced health.

What should be done about this? An effective strategy to deal with the challenge of low SES may have to include efforts to reduce socioeconomic inequalities. If people of lower SES could be persuaded to adopt the same lifestyle, including diet, as those of higher SES, perhaps as much as half of the problem would likely disappear. Therefore, dietary advice is still worth the effort.

5. CONCLUSIONS

Based on the close association between income inequalities in a society and health, an essential component of enhancing a population's health must be government measures to make societies more egalitarian. Unfortunately, the legacy of Thatcherism and Reagonomics means that many governments are ideologically opposed to taking such action. At the same time, governments have been even more business friendly and non-interventionist than ever.

This was well put by James *(53)* with specific regard to obesity:

The needed transformation in thinking on transport, environment, work facilities, education, health and food policies, and perhaps in social and economic policies is unlikely when governments are wedded to individualism, but with-

out these changes to enhance physical activity and alter food quality, societies are doomed to escalating obesity rates.

This viewpoint applies to the relationship between nutrition and all diseases related to it. The primary force driving government policy is economics rather than a desire to improve the national health. However, the weight of evidence strongly suggests that until governments reorientate their nutrition policies so that national health becomes the first priority, we will be losing great opportunities for the prevention of such diseases as cancer and CHD.

The philosophy discussed here need not stop at nutrition: what applies to nutrition certainly applies to other areas of lifestyle, especially to smoking. Exercise also lends itself to policy initiatives. What is the point in telling people to exercise if there is a lack of appropriate facilities? What is the point in telling people to cycle if the roads are too dangerous for bikes? What is needed is a comprehensive view of human health that takes all such factors into consideration.

In the 21st century, no doubt, people will look back with incredulity on today's world where narrow commercial interests and government laissez-faire predominate while the national health founders.

ACKNOWLEDGMENT

The work in this chapter done by NT was carried out at the CDL Programme, Medical Research Council, Cape Town, South Africa.

REFERENCES

1. Flegal, KM, Carroll MD, Kuczmarski RJ, Johnson CL. Overweight and obesity in the United States: prevalence and trends, 1960–1994. Int J Obes 1998; 22:39–47.
2. Siedell JC. Obesity in Europe: scaling an epidemic. Int J Obes 1995; 19(Suppl. 3): S1–S4.
3. Krebs-Smith SM. Progress in improving diet to reduce cancer risk. Cancer 1998; 83:1425–1432.
4. US Department of Health and Human Services. Healthy People 2010 Objectives: Draft for Public Comment. Government Printing Office, Washington DC, September 15, 1998.
5. Tippett KS, Cleveland LE. In: Frazao E., ed. America's Eating Habits: Changes and Consequences. Washington DC: USDA/ERS, April 1999. Agricultural Information Bulletin Number 750:51–70.
6. Activity and Health Research. Allied Dunbar National Fitness Survey, a Report on Activity Patterns and Fitness Levels: Main Findings. London: Sports Council and Health Education Authority, 1992.
7. Jones DA, Ainsworth BE, Croft JB, Macera CA, Lloyd EE, Yusuf HR. Moderate leisure-time physical activity: who is meeting the public health recommendations? A national cross-sectional study. Arch Fam Med 1998; 7:285–289.
8. Anon. Self-reported physical inactivity by degree of urbanization – United States, 1996. MMWR Morbidity Mortality Weekly Report 1998; 47:1097–1100.
9. World Health Organization. Tobacco or Health. A Global Status Report. World Health Organization, Geneva, 1997.
10. Redman S, Spencer EA, Sanson-Fisher R. The role of the mass media in changing health-related behavior: a critical appraisal of two models. Health Prom Int 1990; 5:85–101.

11. Farquhar JW, Fortmann SP, Flora JA, Taylor CB, Haskell WL, Williams PT, et al. Effects of communitywide education on cardiovascular disease risk factors. The Stanford Five-City Project. JAMA 1990; 264:359–365.
12. Luepker RV, Murray DM, Jacobs DR, Mittelmark MB, Bracht N, Carlaw R, et al. Community education for cardiovascular disease prevention: risk factor changes in the Minnesota Heart Health Program. Am J Public Health 1994; 84:1383–1393.
13. Carleton RA, Lasater TM, Assaf AR, Feldman HA, McKinlay S, for the Pawtucket Heart Health Program Writing Group. The Pawtucket Heart Health Program: community changes in cardiovascular risk factors and projected disease risk. Am J Public Health 1995; 85:777–785.
14. Winkleby MA, Feldman HA, Murray DM. Joint analysis of three U.S. community intervention trials for reduction of cardiovascular risk. J Clin Epidemiol 1997; 50:645–658.
15. Goodman RM, Wheeler FC, Lee PR. Evaluation of the Heart To Heart Project: lessons from a community-based chronic disease prevention project. Am J Health Promot 1995; 9:443–455.
16. Brownson RC, Smith CA, Pratt M, Mack NE, Jackson-Thompson J, Dean CG, et al. Preventing cardiovascular disease through community-based risk reduction: the Bootheel Heart Health Project. Am J Public Health 1996; 86:206–213.
17. Puska P, Nissinen A, Tuomilehto J, Salonen JT, Koskela K, McAlister A, et al. The community based strategy to prevent coronary heart disease: conclusions from the ten years of North Karelia project. Ann Rev Public Health 1985; 6:147–193.
18. Valkonen T. Trends in regional and socio-economic mortality differentials in Finland. Int J Health Sci 1992; 3:157–166.
19. Hoffmeister H, Mensink GB, Stolzenberg H, Hoeltz J, Kreuter H, Laaser U, et al. Reduction of coronary heart disease risk factors in the German Cardiovascular Prevention study. Prev Med 1996; 25:135–145.
20. Baxter T, Milner P, Wilson K, Leaf M, Nicholl J, Freeman J, Cooper N. A cost effective, community based heart health promotion project in England: prospective comparative study. Br Med J 1997; 315:582–585.
21. Reger B, Wootan MG, Booth-Butterfield S, Smith H. 1% Or Less: a community-based nutrition campaign. Public Health Rep 1998; 113:410–419.
21a. Reger B, Wootan MG, Booth-Butterfield S. Using mass media to promote healthy eating: a community-based demonstration project. Prev Med 1999; 29:414–421.
22. Dixon H, Boland R, Segan C, Stafford H, Sindall C. Public reaction to Victoria's "2 Fruit 'n' 5 Veg Day" campaign and reported consumption of fruit and vegetables. Prev Med 1998; 27:572–582.
23. World Health Organization European Collaborative Group. Multifactorial trial in the prevention of coronary heart disease. Eur Heart J 1983; 4:141–147.
24. World Health Organization European Collaborative Group. European collaborative trial of multifactorial prevention of coronary heart disease: final report on the 6-year results. Lancet 1986; i:869–872.
25. Breslow L, Fielding J, Herrman AA, Wilbur CS. Worksite health promotion: its evolution and the Johnson & Johnson experience. Prev Med 1990; 19:13–21.
26. Sorensen G, Morris DM, Hunt MK, Hebert JR, Harris DR, Stoddard A, Ockene JK. Work-site nutrition intervention and employees' dietary habits: the Treatwell program. Am J Public Health 1992; 82:877–880.
27. Sorensen G, Stoddard A, Peterson K, Cohen N, Hunt MK, Stein E, Palombo R, Lederman R. Increasing fruit and vegetable consumption through worksites and families in the Treatwell 5-a-Day Study. Am J Public Health 1999; 89:54–60.
28. Jeffery RW, Forster JL, French SA, Kelder SH, Lando HA, McGovern PG, et al. The Healthy Worker Project: a work-site intervention for weight control and smoking cessation. Am J Public Health 1993; 83:395–401.

29. Imperial Cancer Research Fund OXCHECK Study Group. Effectiveness of health checks conducted by nurses in primary care: results of the OXCHECK study after one year. Br Med J 1994; 308:308-312.

30. Imperial Cancer Research Fund OXCHECK Study Group. Effectiveness of health checks conducted by nurses in primary care: final results of the OXCHECK study. Br Med J 1995; 310:1099-1104.

31. Family Heart Study Group. Randomized controlled trial evaluating cardiovascular screening and intervention in general practice: principal results of British Family Heart Study. Br Med J 1994; 308:313-320.

32. Brunner E, White I, Thorogood M, Bristow A, Curle D, Marmot M. Can dietary interventions change diet and cardiovascular risk factors? A meta-analysis of randomized controlled trials. Am J Public Health 1997; 87:1415-1422.

33. Field K, Thorogood M, Silagy C, Normand C, O'Neill C, Muir J. Strategies for reducing coronary risk factors in primary care: which is most cost effective? Br Med J 1995; 310:1109-1112.

34. Lindholm LH, Ekbom T, Dash C, Eriksson M, Tibblin G, Schersten B. The impact of health care advice given in primary care on cardiovascular risk. Br Med J 1995; 310:1105-1109.

35. Rose G. The Strategy of Preventive Medicine. Oxford University Press, Oxford, UK, 1992.

36. Frazao E. High costs of poor eating patterns. In: Frazao E., ed. America's Eating Habits: Changes and Consequences. Washington, DC: USDA/ERS, April 1999. Agricultural Information Bulletin Number 750:5-32.

37. Davey Smith G, Ebrahim S. Dietary change, cholesterol reduction, and the public health—what does meta-analysis add? Br Med J 1998; 316:1220.

38. Meier KJ, Licari MJ. The effect of cigarette taxes on cigarette consumption, 1955 through 1994. Am J Public Health 1997; 87:1126-1130.

39. Townsend J. Price and consumption of tobacco. Br Med Bull 1996; 52:132-142.

40. Stephens T, Pedersen LL, Koval JJ, Kim C. The relationship of cigarette prices and no-smoking bylaws to the prevalence of smoking in Canada. Am J Public Health 1997; 87:1519-1521.

41. Townsend J, Roderick P, Cooper J. Cigarette smoking by socioeconomic group, sex, and age: effects of price income, and health publicity. Br Med J 1994; 309:923-927.

42. Anderson P, Lehto G. Prevention policies. Br Med Bull 1994; 50:171-185.

43. Zatonski W. Alcohol and health: what is good for the French may not be good for the Russians. J Epidemiol Commun Health 1998; 52:766-767.

44. World Health Organization Regional Office for Europe. The Adelaide Recommendations: Healthy Public Policy Regional Office for Europe. World Health Organization, Geneva, 1988.

45. French SA, Jeffery RW, Story M, Hannan P, Snyder P. A pricing strategy to promote low-fat snack choices through vending machines. Am J Public Health 1997; 87:849-851.

46. Jeffery RW, French SA, Raether C, Baxter JE. An environmental intervention to increase fruit and salad purchases in a cafeteria. Prev Med 1994; 23:788-792.

47. French SA, Story M, Jeffery RW, Snyder P, Eisenberg M, Sidebottom A, Murray D. Pricing strategy to promote fruit and vegetable purchase in high school cafeterias. J Am Diet Assoc 1997; 97:1008-1010.

48. Advertising Age. 100 leading national advertisers: 43rd annual report. 1998 (September 28): S3-S50.

49. Nestle M, Wing R, Birch L, DiSogra A, Drewnowski A, Middleton S, et al. Behavioral and social influence on food choice. Nutr Rev 1998; 56:S50-S64.

50. Kotz K, Story M. Food advertisements during children's Saturday morning television programming: Are they consistent with dietary recommendations? J Am Diet Assoc 1994; 94:1296-1300.

51. Ostbye T, Pomerleau J, White M, Coolich M, McWhinney J. Food and nutrition in Canadian "prime time" television commercials. Can J Public Health 1993; 84:370-374.

52. James WPT, Ralph A. National strategies for dietary change, In: Marmot M, Elliott P, eds. Coronary Heart Disease. From Aetiology to Public Health. Oxford University Press, Oxford, 1992; 525–540.

53. James WPT. A public health approach to the problem of obesity. Int J Obes 1995; 19 (Suppl. 3):S37–S45.

54. Nestle M. Toward more healthful dietary patterns-a matter of policy. Public Health Rep 1998; 113:420–423.

55. Jeffery RW. Population perspectives on the prevention and treatment of obesity in minority populations. Am J Clin Nutr 1991; 53:1621S–1624S.

56. Blackburn H. Community programmes in coronary heart disease prevention health promotion: changing community behaviour. In: Marmot M, Elliott P, eds. Coronary Heart Disease. From Aetiology to Public Health. Oxford University Press, Oxford,1992; 495–514.

57. Schmid TL, Pratt M, Howze E. Policy as intervention: environmental and policy approaches to the prevention of cardiovascular disease. Am J Public Health 1995; 85:1207–1211.

58. Pirkle JL, Brody DJ, Gunter EW, Kramer RA, Paschal DC, Flegal KM, Matte TD. The decline in blood lead levels in the United States. JAMA 1994; 272:284–291.

59. Brody DJ, Pirkle JL, Kramer RA, Flegal KM, Matte TD, Gunter EW, Paschal DC. Blood lead levels in the US population. JAMA 1994; 272:277–283.

60. Moore S, Wolfe SM, Lindes D, Douglas CE. Epidemiology of failed tobacco control legislation. JAMA 1994; 272:1171–1175.

61. Glantz SA, Begay ME. Tobacco industry campaign contributions are affecting tobacco control policymaking in California. JAMA 1994; 272:1176–1182.

62. Nestle M. Food lobbies, the food pyramid and U.S. Nutrition policy. Int J Health Serv 1993; 23:483–496.

63. Nestle M. The politics of dietary guidance—a new opportunity. Am J Public Health 1994; 84:713–715.

64. Anon. Industry forced changes to food guide, papers show. Toronto Star, 1993 (January 15):A2.

65. Goodlee F. The food industry fights for salt. Br Med J 1996; 312:1239–1240.

66. Klepp K, Forster JL. The Norwegian Nutrition and Food Policy: an integrated approach to a public health problem. J Public Health Policy 1985; 6:447–463.

67. Norum KR, Johansson L, Botten G, Bjornboe G-EA, Oshaug A. Nutrition and food policy in Norway: effects on reduction of coronary heart disease. Nutr Rev 1997; 55:S32–S39.

68. Corson J. Heartbeat Wales: a challenge for change. World Health Forum 1990;11:405–411.

69. Jeffery RW, Forster JL, Schmid TL, McBride CM, Rooney BL, Pirie PL. Community attitudes toward public policies to control alcohol, tobacco, and high-fat food consumption. Am J Prev Med 1990; 6:12–19.

70. Bucher HC, Ragland DR. Socioeconomic indicators and mortality from coronary heart disease and cancer: a 22-year follow-up of middle-aged men. Am J Public Health 1995; 85:1231–1236.

71. Lin RJ, Shah CP, Svoboda TJ. The impact of unemployment on health: a review. Can Med Assoc J 1995; 153:529–540.

72. Sorlie PD, Backlund E, Keller JB. US mortality by economic, demographic, and social characteristics: The National Longitudinal Mortality Study. Am J Public Health 1995; 85:949–956.

73. Davey Smith G, Neaton JD, Wentworth D, Stamler R, Stamler J. Socioeconomic differentials in mortality risk among men screened for the Multiple Risk Factor Intervention Trial: I. White men. Am J Public Health 1996; 86:486–496.

74. Lynch JW, Kaplan GA, Cohen RD, Tuomilehto J, Salonen JT. Do cardiovascular risk factors explain the relation between socioeconomic status, risk of all-cause mortality, cardiovascular mortality, and acute myocardial infarction? Am J Epidemiol 1996; 144:934–942.

75. Morris JN, Blane DB, White IR. Levels of mortality, education, and social conditions in the 107 local education authority areas of England. J Epidemiol Commun Hlth 1996; 50:15–17.

76. Mackenbach JP, Kunst AE, Cavelaars AEJM, Groenhof F, Geurts JJM. Socioeconomic inequalities in morbidity and mortality in western Europe. Lancet 1997; 349:1655–1659.

77. Morris JK, Cook DG, Shaper AG. Loss of employment and mortality. Br Med J 1994; 308:1135–1139.

78. Pekkanen J, Tuomilehto J, Uutela A, Vartiainen E, Nissinen A. Social class, health behaviour, and mortality among men and women in eastern Finland. Br Med J 1995; 311:589–593.

79. Marmot MG, Bosma H, Brunner E, Stansfield S. Contribution of job control and other risk factors to social variations in coronary heart disease incidence. Lancet 1997; 350:235–239.

80. North FM, Syme SL, Feeney A, Shipley M, Marmot M. Psychosocial work environment and sickness absence among British civil servants: The Whitehall II Study. Am J Public Health 1996; 86:332–340.

81. Johnson JV, Stewart W, Hall EM, Fredlund P, Theorell T. Long-term psychosocial work environment and cardiovascular mortality and among Swedish men. Am J Public Health 1996; 86:324–331.

3 Calcium Intake and the Prevention of Chronic Disease

From Osteoporosis to Premenstrual Syndrome

Robert P. Heaney

1. INTRODUCTION

Calcium is the principal cation of bone. The human body at birth contains 25–30 g calcium (6.25–7.5 mol), and at maturity, 1000–1500 g (25–37.5 mol). All of this postnatal increase must come in by way of the diet. It is not surprising, therefore, that deficiency of bony tissue was linked to a low calcium intake approx 100 yr ago when the major bone diseases were being sorted out. Appreciation of the importance of calcium for bone health has waxed and waned over the ensuing century; nevertheless, the connection between calcium and bone is intuitive and reasonable. Moreover, evidence establishing the importance of an adequate calcium intake for skeletal health has now accumulated to the point that is incontrovertible.

In the past 25 yr, other studies were reported showing an association between calcium intake and certain nonskeletal disorders, first hypertension and colon cancer, and more recently preeclampsia, renolithiasis, obesity, premenstrual syndrome (PMS), and polycystic ovary syndrome (PCO). This diversity of effects was initially puzzling, it not being clear how these seemingly unrelated disorders could have a common dietary basis. Gradually, however, some understanding of the underlying mechanisms has emerged. The explanation ultimately goes back to paleolithic times, i.e., to the conditions that prevailed during hominid evolution, to the physiological adaptations that evolved (or failed to evolve) in response to those conditions, and to ecologic changes that have occurred since the agricultural revolution, roughly 10,000 yr ago.

This background is described, both physiological and ecological, and then the mechanisms by which low calcium intake produces these diverse effects are

From: *Nutritional Health: Strategies for Disease Prevention*
Edited by: T. Wilson and N. J. Temple © Humana Press Inc., Totowa, NJ

reviewed, as well as the evidence with respect to those chronic diseases for which there is today a reasonably solid evidential base. Finally, these observations are integrated and conclusions for calcium nutritional policy derived.

2. PHYSIOLOGICAL BACKGROUND

It is widely recognized that the calcium ion plays an essential role as an intracellular second messenger and that it mediates processes as diverse as muscle contraction, interneuronal synaptic signal transmission, glandular secretion, cell division, and blood clotting. These biochemical functions of calcium are exceedingly well protected, first by a combination of intracellular calcium stores and an immense extracellular nutrient reserve (the skeleton), and second by an elaborate endocrine control system (the parathyroid hormone–vitamin D axis and calcitonin) that maintains blood calcium concentration. As a consequence of these protections, a low calcium intake virtually never compromises, or even threatens, the essential biochemical functions of the mineral. Instead, chronic low calcium intakes result in (1) depletion of the reserve; (2) a continuous homeostatic adaptive response in the attempt to compensate for low intake; and (3) diminution of the physical chemical effects associated with high calcium levels in the intestinal lumen. It is in connection with these secondary phenomena that calcium nutritional deficiency manifestations arise.

2.1. Regulation of Extracellular Fluid Calcium Concentration

A central feature of the calcium economy of all mammals is the tight control of calcium in extracellular fluid (ECF). This comes about by adjusting both the renal calcium threshold and the flows of calcium into and out of the ECF. These processes, in turn, are regulated by parathyroid hormone (PTH), 1,25-dihydroxyvitamin D [1,25(OH)$_2$D], and calcitonin. PTH acts to correct a fall in calcium concentration by a complex set of interacting effects. These actions include, in the probable order of the appearance of their effects, (1) decreased renal tubular reabsorption of blood inorganic phosphate, (2) increased resorptive efficiency of osteoclasts already working on bone surfaces, (3) increased renal 1-α-hydroxylation of circulating 25(OH)vitamin D to produce the chemically most active form of vitamin D, (4) increased renal tubular reabsorption of calcium, and (5) activation of new bone remodeling loci. These effects interact and reinforce one another in important ways. For example, the reduced ECF phosphate caused by the immediate fall in tubular reabsorption of phosphate is itself a potent stimulus to the synthesis of 1,25(OH)$_2$D, and it also increases the resorptive efficiency of osteoclasts already in place and working in bone, and thereby augments their release of calcium from the bony reserves. The 1,25(OH)$_2$D directly increases intestinal absorption of both calcium ingested in food or supplement form and the endogenous calcium contained in the digestive secretions; it also is necessary for the full expression of PTH effects in bone, particularly the maturation of cells in the myelomonocytic line that produce new osteoclasts.

Although a great deal more complicated in detail, these actions amount to three effects: reduced losses through the kidneys, improved utilization of dietary calcium, and withdrawal of calcium from the bony reserves. The aggregate effect of all three is to prevent or reverse a fall in ECF [Ca^{2+}] and, at a whole body level, to conserve calcium in the face of an environmental shortage. However, the first of these takes priority, i.e., the maintenance of ECF [Ca^{2+}] occurs at the expense of the skeletal reserve.

A key feature of the triple end organ response to the calcium-conserving action of PTH is the balance between the three responses, and particularly the relative sensitivity of the internal (bone) and the external (gut, kidney) effector organs. In blacks, for example, the bony effects are relatively resistant to PTH (1–3). In order to maintain ECF [Ca^{2+}], Blacks must secrete more PTH and 1,25(OH)$_2$D, which produce a correspondingly greater absorptive response at the gut and a greater calcium-conserving response at the kidney. This explains why, despite lower mean calcium intakes, blacks nevertheless develop and maintain skeletons approx 10% more dense than Caucasians or Asians. A similar, although smaller, difference exists between pre- and postmenopausal women. In the presence of estrogen, bone is slightly more resistant to PTH (4), which explains why the calcium requirement for skeletal maintenance rises after menopause.

2.2. Inputs, Outputs, and the Requirement

On the input side, gross intestinal absorption in adults, at prevailing intakes, averages about 30%; and because substantial quantities of calcium enter the digestive tract with gastrointestinal secretions, net absorption is generally only 10–15% (5,6). These calcium movements are depicted schematically in Fig. 1, which illustrates the relationship of gross and net absorption for an intake of 800 mg (20 mmol) and approx 32% absorption efficiency.

On the output side, many dietary components interfere with renal calcium conservation, notably sodium (7), net acid production (8,9), and sulfur-containing amino acids (10). These agencies create a floor below which urinary calcium cannot be reduced, despite the effect of PTH on increasing renal tubular calcium reabsorption. Finally, resting dermal losses (i.e., without sweating) are in the range of 1.5 mmol (60 mg)/d (11), and copious sweating can cause losses 5–10× larger (12).

The net result of all these excretory forces is that total obligatory calcium losses in sedentary adults on typical diets are generally in the range of 4–6 mmol (160–240 mg)/d. To stay in balance, i.e., to maintain skeletal integrity, adults must absorb at least this much calcium from ingested food. At typical absorptive

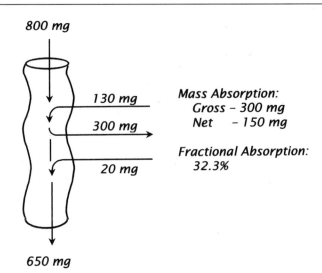

Fig. 1. Schematic illustration of the fluxes of calcium into and out of the intestine for a hypothetical intake of 800 mg (20 mmol) and an absorption efficiency of approx 32%. Calcium entering the gut from endogenous sources is continuous along the GI tract, but is depicted here in two components, one proximal to most of the absorbing surface and one distal, the values for which are based on measurements in adult humans. (Copyright Robert P. Heaney, 1999. Reproduced with permission.)

efficiencies, net absorption of 160–240 mg requires a total intake of at least 1000–1500 mg/d (25–37.5 mmol/d).

Because absorptive extraction is low, even low calcium diets might seem to be adequate, since, in theory, much more calcium *could* be absorbed. Awareness of this potential may explain why nutritional scientists had been slow to accept the lifelong importance of a high calcium intake for contemporary humans. If the calcium was in the diet and the body was not fully accessing it, then—it was argued—the body did not really need it.

That conclusion proved to be wrong, as was definitively shown on publication of several randomized, controlled trials (e.g., refs. *13–15*) that demonstrated that the body would indeed use extra calcium and improve calcium balance if the mineral were provided by a high enough intake. Failure to retain calcium at low intakes reflected not absence of need but the fact that human absorption and conservation efficiencies for calcium are simply not up to the challenge of a low intake, particularly when the bony reserves are so accessible. As noted in the following section, there was no evolutionary need for hominids to develop the type of absorptive and excretory conservation that today's diets demand, when then-available foods provided a surplus of calcium. In brief: although our diets are modern, our physiologies are paleolithic.

3. PALEOLITHIC CONDITIONS

Calcium is the fifth most abundant element in the environment in which life evolved, and was present in high concentrations in the foods consumed by evolving hominids and hunter–gatherer humans *(7)*. During the evolution of human physiology, calcium intake would have averaged approx 0.8 mmol (32 mg)/kg body weight/d. When adequate food was available, the gut would have served as a nearly continuous source of calcium. Despite low absorption efficiency, such a diet provided sufficient calcium to offset obligatory losses (*see* previous section), and to adjust to day-to-day variability in intake and excretion. The mechanisms for dealing with a fall in ECF [Ca^{2+}], described earlier, would have been called into play only infrequently, i.e., at times of food shortage or for long intervals between meals. Thus, PTH secretion is basically an emergency measure. Intermittent utilization of the reserve would not have resulted in lasting effects under primitive conditions. In fact, the diet was so calcium dense that human physiology has been optimized to prevent calcium intoxication, rather than to deal with chronic shortages. This is the reason intestinal calcium absorption efficiency is low, renal conservation is weak, and dermal losses are completely unregulated. (Contrast this behavior with that of sodium, a scarce mineral in the primitive environment: sodium is absorbed at nearly 100% efficiency and, in trained individuals, both urinary and sweat losses can be reduced nearly to zero.)

By contrast, under contemporary conditions, adult diets often contain less than 0.2 mmol (8 mg) Ca/kg body weight/d. The reason for the fall in the calcium content of the human diet from paleolithic to historic times is that cereal grains and legumes, which constitute more than half the total food intake of agriculture-based populations, are typically poor sources of calcium. Neither food group was prominent in preagricultural diets. Hence, the shift from a hunter-gatherer to an agricultural base for the feeding of humans produced a marked decline in calcium density of the food supply.

The much lower calcium intake of contemporary diets requires that adaptive mechanisms be invoked frequently, and in some individuals, constantly. The ability to adapt to low intake or high loss varies, and depends upon genetics, life stage, and environmental factors. As already noted, blacks adapt with high efficiency. Similarly, most young individuals can increase absorptive efficiency sufficiently to permit building a skeleton during growth. However, even in the young, adaptation is often not fully optimal, i.e., bone mass probably does not reach its full genetic potential on prevailing calcium intakes. Moreover, this ability to get by on low intakes declines with age. Various policymaking bodies have recently recognized this decline by recommending higher calcium intakes for the elderly *(16,17)*. But beyond simply recognizing a special need in the elderly, there is a sense in which the requirement in the elderly uncovers the true requirement for all ages, that is, it reveals the intake that protects the skeleton without requiring constant adaptation. It is the spectrum of responses to this constant adaptation that constitutes the basis for the role of low calcium intakes in nonskeletal disorders.

4. MECHANISMS OF CALCIUM DEFICIENCY DISEASE

In regulating ECF $[Ca^{2+}]$, and specifically in adapting to low calcium intake, effects occur not just for bone health but for nonskeletal systems such as blood pressure and body fat regulation. Adaptation, although obviously a necessary capacity, may nevertheless exert undesirable effects when constantly invoked. In addition to sustaining ECF $[Ca^{2+}]$ by withdrawing calcium from the reserve, PTH elicits responses in extraskeletal tissues that may be inappropriate. Medical science is familiar with this phenomenon in the case of stress—with its high adrenergic hormone levels and high secretion of adrenal glucocorticoids. Less well understood, but gradually becoming clearer, are the counterpart effects following from constant high secretion of PTH with its cascade of mechanisms. First is an increase in the parathyroid cell mass itself (18). Associated with this phenomenon is an age-specific increase in incidence of hyperparathyroidism among postmenopausal women (19). Whether the two phenomena are causally related is not settled, but it is true for other organ systems that constant stimulation promotes neoplasia, and it would be surprising if this relationship were not true for the parathyroid glands as well.

All of the disorders currently linked to calcium relate either to decrease in the size of the calcium reserve, to decrease in residual calcium in the intestinal contents as they reach the lower bowel, or to nonskeletal responses to the hormones mediating adaptation to low calcium intake. The principal disorders linked to low calcium intake are classified on this mechanistic basis in Table 1.

Osteoporosis is the disorder that results when the size of the calcium reserve (the skeleton) is depleted for nutritional reasons. (As described briefly below, osteoporosis has other causes as well.) The hormonal responses regulating ECF $[Ca^{2+}]$ succeed in maintaining that critical value, but they do so by depleting the nutrient reserve (bone mass). The risk of both colon cancer and kidney stones rises as the calcium content of the diet residue falls, both for the same basic reason: failure to complex potentially harmful chemicals in the food residue. The best available explanation for the remaining disorders lies in the fact that, in addition to its classical effects regulating ECF $[Ca^{2+}]$, PTH and/or $1,25(OH)_2D$ elevate cytosolic calcium ion concentrations in many tissues, thereby altering their basal level of functional activity. Hyperparathyroidism, listed as a consequence of the adaptive mechanism, is placed in parentheses because the evidence linking this disorder to low calcium intake is less clear than for the other disorders.

Table 1
Classification of Disorders Related to Low Calcium Intake

As a result of		
Decreased Ca nutrient reserve	Decreased food residue Ca in chyme	Adaptive mechanisms maintaining ECF $[Ca^{2+}]$
Osteoporosis	Colon cancer	Hypertension
	Renolithiasis	Preeclampsia
		Premenstrual syndrome
		Obesity
		Polycystic Ovary Syndrome
		(Hyperparathyroidism)

The first two mechanisms are straightforward, related directly to reduction in calcium mass—either the total body mass difference between calcium absorption and calcium excretion or to the mass of calcium in the intestine left over from the diet. Both are inescapable aspects of low intake. The mechanisms for the other disorders are more subtle and are set forth schematically in Fig. 2. In addition to the effect of PTH on cytosolic calcium concentration, expression of these disorders almost certainly requires other defects. The constant high blood PTH level and the consequent high blood $1,25(OH)_2D$ level stress the system beyond the reserve capacity of sensitive individuals. In this sense, such response to chronically high PTH levels is analogous to the hemolytic anemia that develops, for example, on exposure to certain drugs or to fava beans in individuals with glucose-6-phosphate dehydrogenase deficiency. In the absence of a stressor agent, little or no clinical evidence of anemia is present. Presumably, the disorders that follow on a hypersensitivity to PTH and/or $1,25(OH)_2D$ manifest themselves in individuals who lack sufficient redundancy in the cell control mechanisms to compensate for the unsignalled elevation in cytosolic calcium ion concentration.

At the same time, it must also be emphasized that all of the disorders in all three categories are, in their own right, multifactorial. For example, there are many ways to have a reduced skeletal mass in addition to inadequate nutrient intake, and there are many ways to have elevated blood pressure in addition to high endogenous PTH levels. Thus, low calcium intake is only one factor in the genesis of these disorders, and if one could optimize calcium intake in the entire population, it is certain that none of the diseases concerned would be totally eradicated. Nevertheless, altering calcium intake will reduce the total disease burden for all of these disorders. Furthermore, doing so is a cost-effective intervention within society's grasp, and one that therefore demands attention.

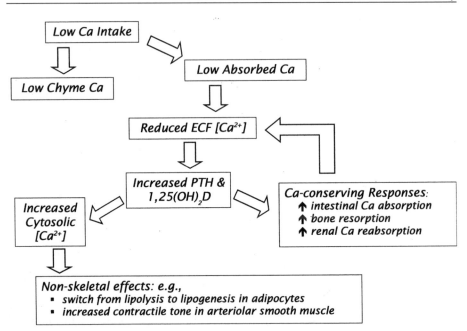

Fig. 2. Schematic depiction of the consequences of low levels of ingested and/or absorbed calcium. The primary hormonal response (i.e., increased PTH secretion) initiates not only the well described calcium-conserving responses that are a part of the negative feedback loop regulating ECF [Ca^{2+}], but also elevates cytosolic [Ca^{2+}] in certain tissues, thereby falsely signaling responses in cells that are not a part of the calcium homeostatic control loop. (Copyright Robert P. Heaney, 1999. Reproduced with permission.)

5. CALCIUM DEFICIENCY DISORDERS

5.1. Reduction in the Size of the Nutrient Reserve

As noted earlier, bone is the body's calcium reserve, and mechanisms designed to protect ECF [Ca^{2+}] tear down bone to scavenge its calcium when excretory and dermal losses exceed absorbed dietary intake. In providing the calcium needed to maintain critical body fluid concentrations, the reserve is functioning precisely as it should. But sooner or later there has to be payback, or the reserve becomes depleted, with an inescapable weakening of skeletal structures. During growth, on any but the most severely restricted of intakes, some bony accumulation does occur, but the result is usually failure to achieve the full genetic potential for bone mass. Later in life, the result is failure to maintain the mass achieved. As also noted earlier, both osteoporotic fractures and low bone mass have many causes other than low calcium intake. Nevertheless, under prevailing conditions in the industrialized nations at high latitudes, the effect size for calcium is large. Calcium supplemented trials, even of short duration, have resulted in 30+% reductions in fractures in the elderly *(13,15)*.

In addition to the effect size's being large, the evidence for calcium's role is itself very strong. There have been roughly 50 published reports of investigator-controlled increases in calcium intake with skeletal endpoints, most of them randomized controlled trials and most of them published since 1990 *(20)*. All but two demonstrated either greater bone mass gain during growth, reduced bone loss with age, and/or reduced osteoporotic fractures. The sole exceptions among these studies were a supplementation trial in men in which the calcium intake of the control group was itself already high (nearly 1200 mg/d) *(21)*, and a study confined to early postmenopausal women in whom bone loss is known to be predominantly due to estrogen deficiency *(22)*.

Complementing this primary evidence are roughly 80 observational studies testing the association of calcium intake with bone mass, bone loss, or fracture *(20)*. It has been shown elsewhere *(23)* that such observational studies are inherently weak, not only for the generally recognized reason that uncontrolled or unrecognized factors may produce or obscure associations between the variables of interest, but because the principal variable in this case, lifetime calcium intake, cannot be directly measured and must be estimated by dietary recall methods. The errors of such estimates are immense and have been abundantly documented *(24,25)*. Their effect is to bias all such investigations toward the null. Nevertheless, more than three-fourths of these observational studies reported a significant calcium benefit. Given the insensitivity of the method, the fact that most of these reports are positive emphasizes the strength of the association; at the same time, it provides reassurance that the effects achievable in the artificial context of a clinical trial can be observed in real world settings as well.

Calcium is a unique nutrient in several respects. It is the only nutrient for which the reserve has required an important function in its own right. We use the reserve for structural support, i.e., we literally walk on our calcium nutrient reserve. Calcium is unique also in that our bodies cannot store a surplus, unlike, for example, energy or the fat-soluble vitamins. Calcium is stored not as such but as bone tissue, and regulation of bone mass is cell mediated, with the responsible bone cellular apparatus controlled through a feedback loop regulated by mechanical forces. In brief, given an adequate calcium intake, we have only as much bone as we need for the loads we currently sustain.

These features are the basis for the designation of calcium as a threshold nutrient with respect to skeletal status, a term that means that calcium retention rises as intake rises, up to some threshold value that provides optimal bone strength; then, above that level, increased calcium intake produces no further retention and is simply excreted. This threshold intake is the lowest intake at which retention is maximal, i.e., it is the minimum daily requirement (MDR) for skeletal health. The MDR varies with age, and is currently estimated to be about 20–25 mmol (800–1000 mg)/d during childhood, 30–40 mmol (1200–1600 mg)/d during adolescence, approx 25 mmol (1000 mg)/d during the mature adult years, and 35–40 mmol (1400–1600 mg)/d in the elderly *(16,17,26)*. As previously noted, the rise in the requirement in old age reflects a corresponding decline in ability to adapt, i.e., to respond to low intakes with improved absorption and retention.

At the same time, as already noted, osteoporosis is a distinctly multifactorial disorder, both in the sense that many factors contribute to bone loss and fracture risk, and also in the sense that yet other factors influence the body's handling of calcium. Of most importance in the latter respect are dietary factors such as caffeine, which reduces calcium absorption very slightly, and protein and sodium, both of which increase urinary calcium loss. The urinary effects are the larger, but for all three nutrients, the impact on the calcium economy disappears at high calcium intakes (40 mmol/d or above). As already noted, such intakes, although high by today's standards, are typical of the paleolithic intake.

The behavior of the calcium homeostatic system in response to a challenge such as sodium- or protein-induced hypercalciuria illustrates beautifully how the fine tuning of the calcium economy presumes a high intake. A provoked increase in urinary calcium loss, if not offset, leads to a fall in ECF [Ca^{2+}], which evokes an increase in PTH and in $1,25(OH)_2D$ levels. These hormones act on bone as well as on the gut, and it is the combined response of both effector organs that offsets the drop in ECF [Ca^{2+}]. However, the balance between the bone and dietary components of this response depends entirely on the calcium content of the diet. For example, the increase in $1,25 OH)_2D$ evoked by a 1 mmol/d additional loss of calcium leads to an increase in absorption efficiency of 1.5–2.0 absorption percentage points. At an intake of 50 mmol/d, that absorptive increase is entirely adequate to compensate for the additional urinary loss. On the other hand, at intakes such as those at the bottom quartile in NHANES-III (National Health and Nutrition Examination Survey), the absorptive increase offsets less than one-eighth of the urinary calcium loss. The rest must come from bone.

Of the factors that influence bone more directly (rather than by way of the calcium economy), one can list smoking, alcohol abuse, hormonal status, body weight, and exercise. Smoking and alcohol abuse exert slow, cumulative effects by uncertain mechanisms that result in reduced bone mass and increased fracture risk. Low estrogen status and hyperthyroidism produce similar net effects, although probably by very different mechanisms. Bone mass rises directly with body weight, again by uncertain mechanisms. Exercise, particularly impact loading, is osteotrophic and is important both for building optimal bone mass during growth and for maintaining it during maturity and senescence.

In a sense, bone health is like a three-legged stool; one leg is nutrition, another is hormones, and the third is lifestyle. All three legs must be strong if the stool (or the skeleton) is to support us. Strengthening of one leg will not compensate for weakness of another.

5.2. Reduction of Residual Calcium in the Chyme

An inevitable consequence of reduced calcium intake is a reduction of calcium in the food residue delivered to the ileum, cecum, and colon. This is both because less calcium is ingested and because fractional absorption rises as intake drops. The quantitative features of the relationship between diet and fecal calcium are illustrated in Fig. 3, which is based on over 500 calcium balance studies performed by the author in middle-aged women. With the primitive diet, net calcium absorption would have been approx 10%, and fecal calcium would thus have been nearly as high as dietary intake. The upshot of low intakes is that there is less calcium available to form complexes with other food residue substances that may be harmful in some individuals. The two conditions for which this effect is best established are colon cancer and renolithiasis. The potentially harmful chyme substances are free fatty acids and bile acids for colon cancer, and oxalic acid for renolithiasis.

There is no good chemical theory for a mixture as complex as the chyme at any location through the gastrointestinal tract, let alone in its distal segments. Nevertheless, a few observations concerning the quantities of reactants required to complex possibly noxious substances in the chyme may be useful.

Fat absorption is highly efficient; nevertheless from 1–5% of ingested fat normally escapes absorption in the small bowel and is delivered to the cecum as free fatty acids. For a typical North American diet with 35% of calories from fat, that translates to 3–15 mmol of unabsorbed fatty acid, plus a smaller quantity of unreabsorbed bile acid. If there were no other ligands for the calcium in the chyme, this quantity of fatty acid would require, for its full neutralization, the presence in the mixture of 1.5–15 mmol (60–600 mg) of calcium [depending on the mixture of $Ca(FA)^+$ and $Ca(FA)_2$]. As the relationship in Fig. 3 shows, it would require a diet containing up to 680 mg calcium to achieve that level. This is slightly above the median for U.S. women.

But fatty acids are not the only ligand competing for calcium. Phosphate, oxalate, phytate, and various organic acids produced by bacterial fermentation of colonic contents are also present in varying abundance. Unabsorbed phosphate from a typical diet alone amounts to 10–15 mmol, and would be expected to bind with an equivalent quantity of calcium (forming $CaHPO_4$). Thus, it can be estimated that chyme calcium levels of more than 30 mmol/d are required to neutralize the potentially noxious products of digestion left in the food residue. As the relationship of Fig. 3 indicates, that level in the chyme requires an intake of at least 34 mmol (1360 mg) Ca/d. This value should be taken as a lower estimate, as the efficiency of ligand binding and the respective binding constants in a medium such as chyme are unknown.

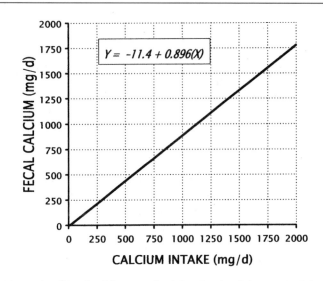

Fig. 3. The regression line (and its equation) for fecal calcium on calcium intake from over 500 balance studies in healthy middle-aged women. (Copyright Robert P. Heaney, 1999. Reproduced with permission.)

5.2.1. COLON CANCER

As just described, unabsorbed dietary calcium forms complexes with unabsorbed fatty acids and bile acids that would otherwise serve as mucosal irritants (and hence cancer promoters). Such complexation effectively renders these irritants harmless, thereby breaking one of the chains of potential colon cancer development.

Early epidemiological studies noted a strong inverse relationship between calcium intake and colon cancer risk, with several studies indicating that the risk was minimal at intakes in the range of 45 mmol (1800 mg)/d or higher *(27–29)*. As with observational studies in most disorders, the evidence implicating calcium intake is mixed, and even when positive, the results could not by themselves be used to establish a causal connection. However, animal carcinogenesis studies followed the observational data, showing that unabsorbed fatty acids and bile acids serve as cancer promoters in systems using potent carcinogens, and that a high calcium intake complexed (and hence effectively neutralized) both types of promoter. More importantly, calcium reduced the numbers of cancers that developed *(30,31)*. Similarly, studies in humans with a familial cancer tendency showed lower levels of cellular atypia and reduced mitotic indices in those whose calcium intakes were high *(32,33)*. At least two randomized trials of calcium supplementation have been recently reported. Neither used actual cancer as the endpoint, but in one, adenoma recurrence was significantly reduced in calcium-supplemented individuals *(34)*, and in the other, various indices of mucosal hyperplasia were significantly reduced *(35)*.

Thus, although the bulk of the evidence points to protection, final proof is still not available. This may be because sample size requirements for a cancer endpoint are large, and no controlled trials to date have involved the requisite number of subject-years of observation.

In summary, the epidemiological data, the animal models, the chemistry of the chyme, and the still limited clinical trials are all concordant, pointing to a protective effect of high calcium intakes for colon cancer risk.

5.2.2. RENOLITHIASIS

Renal stones develop primarily in individuals who, for whatever reason, lack a solution stabilizer in their urine. In such individuals, solute concentration, calcium loads, and oxalate load are some of the risk factors for oxalate stone formation (the most common variety in North America today). Normally, 75–85% of the renal oxalate burden comes from endogenous (i.e., metabolic) sources, and the remainder is dietary in origin, coming mainly from vegetable sources and from bacterial fermentation of food residues in the distal bowel. Chyme calcium complexes this oxalate in the intestine before it can be absorbed, thereby reducing the renal oxalate burden. Renal oxalate load is a more powerful risk factor for stone formation than is the renal calcium load, which explains the seemingly paradoxical effect of calcium intake on calcium stone risk. It should be noted that this is not a new observation. Therapeutic nutritionists have long used very high calcium intakes (up to several grams per day) to treat patients with short bowel syndromes who develop the syndrome of intestinal hyperoxalosis, the principal manifestation of which is severe renal calcinosis and renolithiasis. There have, to date, been no clinical trials of calcium supplementation in stone formers, but two prospective studies have reported an inverse relationship between stone incidence and calcium intake *(36,37)*.

5.3. Hypersensitivity to the Adaptive Response
to Low Calcium Intake

As already noted, cytosolic $[Ca^{2+}]$ functions as a ubiquitous second messenger-mediating cell response to a wide variety of specific control signals. High basal levels presumably trigger inappropriate (i.e., unsignaled) cell responses or, equivalently, lower the response threshold for appropriate stimuli. This effect of PTH is found, for example, in arteriolar smooth muscle, in platelets, and in fat tissue. The first is associated with increased vascular tone, and the last with enhanced lipogenesis. Presumably, the pathogenesis of the premenstrual and polycystic ovary syndromes have an analogous basis.

5.3.1. HYPERTENSIVE DISORDERS

The relationship of the hypertensive disorders to low calcium intake is also discussed in Chapter 4 by Weinberger. Here, we need only mention that, although data from observational studies are mixed, the controlled trials have almost always shown a blood pressure lowering effect of calcium supplementation, and meta-analyses of calcium intervention trials in essential hypertension, preeclampsia, and pregnancy-induced hypertension have unfailingly found a lowering of risk in individuals given augmented calcium intake *(38–41)* even when the data have been assembled so as to minimize the calcium effect size *(41,42)*. At a population level, the effect of high calcium intake is probably small (a blood pressure lowering on the order of 2–5 mm Hg), probably because hypertension is a heterogeneous disorder, with only a fraction of cases exhibiting sensitivity to PTH, and with the calcium effect necessarily confined to only these patients. More recently, the Dietary Approaches to Stop Hypertension (DASH) study exhibited a much larger effect, using food sources of calcium, combined with a high fruit and vegetable diet *(43)*. The full DASH diet effect (which is probably more than the sum of its parts) was estimated to be capable of producing a 27% reduction in stroke and a 15% reduction in coronary artery disease at a population level—the largest effect reported to date. The impressive size of the effect found in this study has been attributed not solely to the calcium content of the diet, but to the higher potassium intake as well, and to the shift to an alkaline ash diet—or both.

It seems likely that the relative resistance of the skeletal remodeling apparatus to PTH in blacks, coupled with their typically low calcium intakes, is a part of the explanation for the high prevalence of hypertensive disease in this racial group. As already noted, blacks exhibit high serum levels of PTH and $1,25(OH)_2D$, both of which, of course, decrease when calcium intake is increased. It may also be that the larger overall response to the high calcium diet in DASH (relative to other calcium supplementation trials) was due precisely to the high proportion of African-Americans in the DASH study cohort (62%).

In addition to the results of calcium intervention trials, there are several corollary lines of evidence implicating dysregulation of the calcium economy in the genesis of the hypertensive disorders. McCarron and associates have shown both a renal calcium leak *(44)* and lower bone mineral density in hypertensives *(45)*, and Brickman and colleagues *(46)* have shown higher circulating PTH and $1,25(OH)_2D$ levels and higher platelet cytosolic $[Ca^{2+}]$ in hypertensives. Such observational studies do not establish the causal direction in the association, but low bone mineral density and high PTH levels are inescapable reflections of negative calcium balance, whether due to inadequate intake or excessive loss. Hence the human data are highly consistent at several levels. Also, it is interesting to note that the salt-sensitive rat models of hypertension require low calcium diets (with consequent elevation of PTH secretion and of $1,25(OH)_2D$ levels) for their expression and, for any given calcium intake level, the spontaneously hypertensive rat (SHR) exhibits lower serum $[Ca^{2+}]$ and higher PTH than normotensive animals *(47,48)*.

Unfortunately, widespread acceptance of the role of calcium in the hypertensive disorders has been impeded by the anti-salt advocates *(49)*, as if sodium sensitivity and calcium dependency could not each be involved in different subsets of the population.

5.3.2. PREMENSTRUAL SYNDROME

Longstanding primary hyperparathyroidism has been classically associated with mood responses, sometimes characterized as "difficult to deal with" and "cussedness." Thys-Jacobs and coworkers, reflecting on the symptom complex known as premenstrual syndrome (PMS), noted a similarity to certain of the symptoms of hyperparathyroidism and hypothesized that there might be a connection between PMS and the PTH-calcium economy. In a small, randomized crossover trial, they showed significant reduction of PMS symptoms on daily supplementation with 1000 mg calcium *(50)*. Because of the inherently subjective character of PMS symptoms, a multicenter trial was organized so as to circumvent potential objections of nonreproducibility *(51)*. This trial, treating 466 women at 12 US medical centers, showed conclusively that supplementation with 30 mmol (1200 mg) calcium reduced PMS symptom severity by as much as 50% or more.

A small number of other studies have yielded concordant collateral data. Thus, Lee and Kanis *(52)* showed that women with established vertebral osteoporosis were more likely to have had severe PMS during their reproductive years than age-matched control subjects. This association between the two conditions is unsurprising, as low calcium intake may be a predisposing factor for each. Similarly, Thys-Jacobs and coworkers *(53)* have shown lower values for bone mass at the spine and hip in menstruating women with PMS than in controls, as well as significantly higher PTH values at the time of the luteinizing hormone peak in women with PMS *(54)*.

As with the hypertensive disorders, there is consistency across all the lines of evidence. Nevertheless, how the pieces of the puzzle fit together remains unclear. Even whether PTH is the trigger is uncertain. However, reduced PTH production is one of the most rapidly occurring changes produced by increasing calcium intake, and elevated PTH can be considered a plausible candidate for the pathogenesis of PMS until proved otherwise. Still, since not every woman with low calcium intake and/or a high PTH gets PMS, and since relief of symptoms with calcium is often not complete, there must be other contributing factors. However, this is true of this entire group of disorders associated with the adaptive response to a low calcium intake.

5.3.3. OBESITY

The linkage of obesity to low calcium intake has only recently become apparent. At least four sets of clinical observations have shown that children and adolescents with high milk intakes weigh less and have less body fat than nonmilk drinkers (e.g., 55,56). Moreover, Zemel and associates (57) have shown, using the NHANES-III database, that risk of obesity exhibits a highly significant stepwise, inverse correlation with dietary calcium intake. In other work, the same authors (57) have demonstrated that low calcium intake increases cytosolic $[Ca^{2+}]$ in the adipocyte (whether through increased PTH or $1,25(OH)_2D$ is unclear). The result of this cell biologic effect is to switch adipose cell metabolism from lipolysis to lipogenesis. This change means a higher average fat content per fat cell in the presence of high PTH levels and provides a plausible mechanism to explain the clinical and epidemiological observations. In transgenic mice expressing the *agouti* gene, low calcium diets provoke obesity, whereas high calcium diets suppress the obesity and elevate core body temperature. Rather than an untoward response (as with blood pressure), this effect may well reflect a primitive adaptation to food shortage. With the primitive diet naturally rich in calcium, low levels of absorbed calcium would signal low food intake and possibly, therefore, impending starvation. Under such circumstances, a shift from fat breakdown to fat synthesis and a reduction in thermogenesis would help conserve critical energy reserves.

It is still unclear how large the effect may be at a population level. Nor are there randomized clinical trial data showing the extent to which high calcium intakes will reduce weight gain or augment weight loss. So the ultimate significance of the observations cited remains uncertain. At very least, this linkage may simply be a fortuitous instance illustrating how PTH can affect the function of cells and tissues not usually considered a part of the calcium homeostatic regulatory system.

5.3.4. POLYCYSTIC OVARY SYNDROME

Also still at an early stage of understanding is the relationship of calcium intake to polycystic ovary syndrome (PCO). PCO is one of the most common causes of infertility today and is generally considered to be a condition of abnormal oocyte differentiation of uncertain etiology. The calcium–PTH–vitamin D axis has not previously been evaluated in PCO. Recently, Thys-Jacobs and colleagues (58) reported a series of 13 patients with PCO who had high serum PTH levels and very low serum 25(OH)D. Although this represented a new finding, interesting in its own right, what is more impressive is the fact that treatment with calcium and vitamin D reversed not only the abnormal indices of the calcium economy, but produced a remission in the syndrome, with two of the patients becoming pregnant.

There are, as yet, no randomized trials of calcium in this disorder, and so the results, however provocative, must be considered tentative. Nor is there yet an experimental basis to explain the effect. The various meiotic and mitotic divisions through which the oocyte goes during its maturation are known to be triggered by rises in cytosolic $[Ca^{2+}]$, so there is at least a plausible area in which to look for an effect of high circulating levels of PTH. But whether such an effect can explain the findings in this syndrome is still only speculative. Nevertheless, the dramatic effect on the disease process produced by lowering serum PTH and raising serum 25(OH)D implicates these substances in the pathogenesis of the disorder (and with them, of course, calcium intake), even if the details of the mechanism must, for now, remain unclear.

6. INTEGRATION

The primitive diet, the one to which human physiology has adapted over the millennia of evolution, was calcium dense, with a calcium content of 70–80 mg/100 kcal (0.42–0.48 mmol/kJ). At energy expenditure levels that prevailed until the very recent advent of private automobiles and other labor-saving devices, such a diet would have provided individuals of contemporary body size with total calcium intakes in the range of 50–75 mmol (2000–3000 mg)/d. Additionally, evolution provided mechanisms to tide us over transient periods of dietary calcium deficiency. Modern diets, based on the calcium-poor foods that served as the basis of the agricultural revolution, provide total calcium intakes far short of those to which our physiologies are adapted. For this reason, the same modern diets cause us to call into constant play the compensatory mechanisms that, under primitive conditions, allowed us to function during what would usually have been transient periods of food shortage. Except for some decline in the size of the calcium reserve, a substantial fraction of contemporary humans appears to be able to do this perfectly well, without sustaining any apparently untoward consequences. But many cannot cope so well. For some, the decreased calcium reserve translates to increased bony fragility. Still others, better able to protect their skeletons, develop hypertension. Others, with a potential for colon carcinogenesis, increase that risk by virtue of absence of a natural protective factor in the food residue from their diets.

For the various reasons reviewed in this chapter, skeletal maintenance must be judged as a necessary, but insufficient, functional endpoint for calcium nutrition. Instead, policymakers need to calculate in terms of *total* health, recognizing that different racial, ethnic, age, and gender groups may have different sensitivities to, or abilities to adjust to, low calcium intakes. As already noted, the skeletal endpoint may not be the right functional indicator of calcium nutritional status in African-Americans, who are manifestly able to amass and maintain strong bones on low calcium intakes. In them, the hypertensive disorders would seem to provide a more relevant indicator, but current data do not allow very precise estimation of the intake needed to minimize the calcium deficiency component of these nonskeletal disorders.

As noted earlier, the rise in the calcium requirement for skeletal health in the elderly reflects mainly a decline in ability to adapt to a low intake. In that sense, the skeletal requirement in the elderly may reflect the true requirement at all ages, i.e., the intakes for which no compensatory adaptive response is required. McKane and associates *(18)* showed substantial involution of the parathyroid glands in healthy elderly women given 60 mmol (2400 mg) calcium for 3 yr. This seemingly high intake did not suppress PTH to subnormal levels; instead, the usually high PTH levels of the elderly were reduced to healthy young adult normal levels. The same study also showed restoration of bone remodeling activity to young adult normal levels. PTH and bone remodeling rise with age, not because these components of the calcium economy fail to adapt, but because the external end organs of the control loop—calcium absorption and renal calcium retention—become less and less responsive with age.

Available data suggest that a calcium intake in the range of 37.5 mmol (1500 mg)/d to 60 mmol (2400 mg)/d may be optimal for all body systems. Lest such an intake be thought "heroic" or "pharmacologic," it is useful to recall that diets with such calcium contents exhibit a calcium nutrient density less than, or in the range of, those of our hominid ancestors, and substantially below those of diets we feed our laboratory animals, including chimpanzees and other primates.

REFERENCES

1. Cosman F, Morgan DC, Nieves JW, Shen V, Luckey MM, Dempster DW, et al. Resistance to bone resorbing effects of PTH in black women. J Bone Miner Res 1997; 12:958–966.
2. Aloia JF, Mikhail M, Pagan CD, Arunacha-Lam A, Yeh JK, Flaster E. Biochemical and hormonal variables in black and white women matched for age and weight. J Lab Clin Med 1998; 132:383–389.
3. Bell NH, Greene A, Epstein S, Oexmann MJ, Shaw S, Shary J. Evidence for alteration of the vitamin D-endocrine system in blacks. J Clin Invest 1985; 76:470–473.
4. Heaney RP. Estrogen-calcium interactions in the postmenopause: a quantitative description. Bone Miner 1990; 11:67–84.
5. Heaney RP, Recker RR, Stegman MR, Moy AJ. Calcium absorption in women: relationships to calcium intake, estrogen status, and age. J Bone Miner Res 1989; 4:469–475.
6. Nordin BEC, Polley KJ, Need AG, Morris HA, Marshall D. The problem of calcium requirement. Am J Clin Nutr 1987; 45:1295–1304.
7. Eaton B and Nelson DA. Calcium in evolutionary perspective. Am J Clin Nutr 1991; 54:281S–287S.
8. Berkelhammer CH, Wood RJ, Sitrin MD. Acetate and hypercalciuria during total parenteral nutrition. Am J Clin Nutr 1988; 48:1482–1489.
9. Sebastian A, Harris ST, Ottaway JH, Todd KM, Morris RC, Jr. Improved mineral balance and skeletal metabolism in postmenopausal women treated with potassium carbonate. N Engl J Med 1994; 330:1776–1781.
10. Schuette SA, Hegsted M, Zemel MB, Linkswiler HM. Renal acid, urinary cyclic AMP and hydroxyproline excretion as affected by level of protein, sulfur amino acid and phosphorus intake. J Nutr 1981; 111:2106–2116.
11. Charles P. Metabolic bone disease evaluated by a combined calcium balance and tracer kinetic study. Danish Med Bull 1989; 36:463–479.
12. Klesges RC, Ward KD, Shelton ML, Applegate WB, Cantler ED, Palmieri GMA, et al. Changes in bone mineral content in male athletes. J Am Med Assoc 1996; 276:226–230.
13. Chapuy MC, Arlot ME, Duboeuf F, Brun J, Crouzet B, Arnaud S, et al. Vitamin D_3 and calcium to prevent hip fractures in elderly women. N Engl J Med 1992; 327:1637–1642.
14. Dawson-Hughes B, Dallal GE, Krall EA, Sadowski L, Sahyoun N, Tannenbaum S. A controlled trial of the effect of calcium supplementation on bone density in postmenopausal women. N Engl J Med 1990; 323:878–883.

15. Dawson-Hughes B, Harris SS, Krall EA, Dallal GE. Effect of calcium and vitamin D supplementation on bone density in men and women 65 years of age or older. N Engl J Med 1997; 337:670–676.

16. NIH Consensus Conference: Optimal Calcium Intake. J Am Med Assoc 1994; 272:1942–1948.

17. Dietary Reference Intakes for Calcium, Magnesium, Phosphorus, Vitamin D, and Fluoride. Food and Nutrition Board, Institute of Medicine, National Academy Press, Washington, DC, 1997.

18. McKane WR, Khosla S, Egan KS, Robins SP, Burritt MF, Riggs BL. Role of calcium intake in modulating age-related increases in parathyroid function and bone resorption. J Clin Endocrinol Metab 1996; 81:1699–1703.

19. Heath H III, Hodgson SF, Kennedy MA. Primary hyperparathyroidism. Incidence, morbidity, and potential economic impact in a community. N Engl J Med 1980; 302:189–193.

20. Heaney RP. Calcium, dairy products, and osteoporosis. J Am Coll Nutr 2000; 19:83S–99S.

21. Orwoll ES, Oviatt SK, McClung MR, Deftos LJ, Sexton G. The rate of bone mineral loss in normal men and the effects of calcium and cholecalciferol supplementation. Ann Int Med 1990; 112:29–34.

22. Nilas L, Christiansen C, Rødbro . Calcium supplementation and postmenopausal bone loss. Br Med J 1984; 289:1103–1106.

23. Heaney RP. Nutrient effects: Discrepancy between data from controlled trials and observational studies. Bone 1997; 21:469–471.

24. Barrett-Connor E. Diet assessment and analysis for epidemiologic studies of osteoporosis. In: Burckhardt P, Heaney RP, eds. Nutritional aspects of osteoporosis. Raven Press, New York, 1991, pp. 91–98.

25. Beaton GH, Milner J, Corey P, McGuire V, Cousins M, Steward E, et al. Sources of variance in 24-hour dietary recall data: Implications for nutrition study design and interpretation. Am J Clin Nutr 1979; 32:2446–2459.

26. Matkovic V and Heaney RP. Calcium balance during human growth. Evidence for threshold behavior. Am J Clin Nutr 1992; 55:992–996

27. Slattery ML, Sorenson AW, Ford MH. Dietary calcium intake as a mitigating factor in colon cancer. Am J Epidemiol 1988; 128:504–514.

28. Garland C, Sliekelle RB, Barrett-Connor E, Criqui MH, Rossof AH, Paul O. Dietary vitamin D and calcium and risk of colorectal cancer. A 19-year prospective study in men. Lancet 1985; 1:307–309.

29. Garland CF, Garland FC. Do sunlight and vitamin D reduce the likelihood of colon cancer. Int J Epidemiol 1980; 9:227–231.

30. Wargovich MJ, Eng VWS, Newmark HL, Bruce WR. Calcium ameliorates the toxic effect of deoxycholic acid on colonic epithelium. Carcinogenesis 1983; 4:1205–1207.

31. Wargovich MJ, Eng VWS, Newmark HL. Calcium inhibits the damaging and compensatory proliferative effects of fatty acids on mouse colon epithelium. Cancer Lett 1984; 23:253–258.

32. Buset M, Lipkin M, Winawer S, Swaroop S, Friedman E. Inhibition of human colonic epithelial cell proliferation in vivo and in vitro by calcium. Cancer Res 1986; 46:5426–5430.

33. Lipkin M, Newmark H. Effect of added dietary calcium on colonic epithelial-cell proliferation in subjects at high risk for familial colon cancer. N Engl J Med 1985; 313:1381–1384.

34. Baron JA, Beach M, Mandel JS, van Stolk RU, Haile RW, Sandler RW, et al., for the Calcium Polyp Prevention Study Group. Calcium supplements for the prevention of colorectal adenomas. N Engl J Med 1999; 340:101–107.

35. Holt PR, Atillasoy EO, Gilman J, Guss J, Moss SF, Newmark H, et al. Modulation of abnormal colonic epithelial cell proliferation and differentiation by low-fat dairy foods. JAMA 1998; 280:1074–1079

36. Curhan GC, Willett WC, Rimm EB, Stampfer MJ. A prospective study of dietary calcium and other nutrients and the risk of symptomatic kidney stones. N Engl J Med 1993; 328: 833–838.

37. Curhan GC, Willett WC, Speizer FE, Spiegelman D, Stampfer MJ. Comparison of dietary calcium with supplemental calcium and other nutrients as factors affecting the risk for kidney stones in women. Ann Intern Med 1997; 126:497–504.

38. Bucher HC, Guyatt GH, Cook RJ, Hatala R, Cook DJ, Lang JD, Hunt D. Effect of calcium supplementation on pregnancy-induced hypertension and preeclampsia. JAMA 1996; 275:1113–1117.

39. Bucher HC, Cook RJ, Guyatt GH, Lang JD, Cook DJ, Hatala D, Hunt D. Effects of dietary calcium supplementation on blood pressure. JAMA 1996; 275:1016–1022.

40. Allender PS, Cutler JA, Follmann D, Cappuccio FP, Pryer J, Elliott P. Dietary calcium and blood pressure: a meta-analysis of randomized clinical trials. Ann Intern Med 1996; 124:825–831.

41. Cappuccio FP, Elliott P, Allender PS, Pryer J, Follman DA, Cutler J. Epidemiologic association between dietary calcium intake and blood pressure: a meta-analysis of published data. Am J Epidemiol 1995; 142:935–945.

42. Birkett NJ. Comments on a meta-analysis of the relation between dietary calcium intake and blood pressure. Am J Epidemiol 1998; 148:223–228.

43. Appel LJ, Moore TJ, Obarzanek E, Vollmer WM, Svetkey LP, Sacks FM, et al., for the DASH Collaborative Research Group.A clinical trial of the effects of dietary patterns on blood pressure. N Engl J Med 1997; 336:1117–1124.

44. McCarron DA, Pingree PA, Rubin RJ, Gaucher SM, Molitch M, Krutzik S. Enhanced parathyroid function in essential hypertension: a homeostatic response to a urinary calcium leak. Hypertension 1980; 2:162–168.

45. Metz, JA Morris CD, Roberts LA, McClung MR, McCarron DA. Blood pressure and calcium intake are related to bone density in adult males. Br J Nutr 1999; 81:383–388.

46. Brickman AS, Nyby MD, von Hungen K, Eggena P, Tuck ML. Calcitropic hormones, platelet calcium, and blood pressure in essential hypertension. Hypertension 1990;16:515–522.

47. McCarron DA, Yung NN, Ugoretz BA, Krutzik S. Disturbances of calcium metabolism in the spontaneously hypertensive rat. Hypertension 1981; 3:1162–1167.

48. Oparil S, Chen Y-F, Jin H, Yang R-H, Wyss JM. Dietary Ca^{2+} prevents NaCl-sensitive hypertension in spontaneously hypertensive rats via sympatholytic and renal effects. Am J Clin Nutr 1991; 54:227S–236S.

49. Taubes G. The (political) science of salt. Science 1998; 281:898–907.

50. Thys-Jacobs S, Ceccarelli S, Bierman A, Weisman H, Cohen M-A, Alvir J. Calcium supplementation in premenstrual syndrome. J Gen Intern Med 1989; 4: 183–189.

51. Thys-Jacobs S, Starkey P, Bernstein D, Tian J, and the Premenstrual Syndrome Study Group. Calcium carbonate and the premenstrual syndrome: effects on premenstrual and menstrual symptoms. Am J Obstet Gynecol 1998; 179:444–452.

52. Lee SJ, Kanis JA. An association between osteoporosis and premenstrual symptoms and postmenopausal symptoms. Bone Miner 1994; 24:127–134.

53. Thys-Jacobs S, Silverton M, Alvir J, Paddison PL, Rico M, Goldsmith SJ. Reduced bone mass in women with premenstrual syndrome. J Women's Health 1995; 4:161–168.

54. Thys-Jacobs S, Alvir MJ. Calcium-regulating hormones across the menstrual cycle: evidence of a secondary hyperparathyroidism in women with PMS.   J Clin Endocrinol Metab 1995; 80:2227–2232.

55. Skinner J, Carruth B, Coletta F. Does dietary calcium have a role in body fat mass accumulation in young children? Scand J Nutr 1999; 43:45S.

56. Teegarden D, Lin Y-C, Weaver CM, Lyle RM, McCabe GP. Calcium intake relates to change in body weight in young women. FASEB J 1999; 13: A873.

57. Zemel MB, Shi H, Greer B, DiRienzo D, Zemel PC. Regulation of adiposity by dietary calcium. FASEB J 2000; 14:1132–1138.

58. Thys-Jacobs S, Donovan D, Papadopoulos A, Sarrel P, Bilezikian JP. Vitamin D and calcium dysregulation in the polycystic ovarian syndrome. Steroids 1999; 64:430–435.

4   Sodium and Other Dietary Factors in Hypertension

Myron H. Weinberger

1. INTRODUCTION

The most recent report of the Sixth Joint National Committee on Prevention, Detection, Evaluation, and Treatment of High Blood Pressure (JNC VI) *(1)* has recommended a trial of lifestyle intervention as initial therapy in individuals with high-normal (130–139 mm Hg systolic/85–89 diastolic) or stage I (140–159/90–99) blood pressure levels without end-organ disease, concomitant cardiovascular disease or diabetes mellitus. This chapter examines the evidence in support of dietary alterations and their effect on blood pressure. The constituents that are considered include calories (body weight), salt (sodium chloride), potassium, calcium, and combinations of these minerals, other dietary components and alcohol. Rather than attempting an encyclopedic review of the studies of all these dietary elements, this chapter succintly summarizes what is currently known about the factors outlined in Table 1.

2. BODY WEIGHT

Body weight has long been linked to blood pressure levels. More recent findings indicate that the distribution of body fat may be a more important determinant of blood pressure elevation and the risk for cardiovascular disease. An increase in visceral abdominal fat (the central or "apple" form) in contrast to the lower body adiposity pattern (the "pear" shape) is linked not only to blood pressure elevation but also to insulin resistance, dyslipidemia and an increased risk for cardiovascular events. These associations have been based largely on epidemiological evidence. However, there are now several intervention trials in which it has been demonstrated that weight loss, often as little as 5 kg rather than a reduction to "ideal" body weight, is associated with a decrease in blood pres-

From: *Frontiers in Nutrition: Strategies for Disease Prevention*
Edited by: T. Wilson and N. J. Temple © Humana Press Inc., Totowa, NJ

Table 1
Review of Nutrition Related Factors that Are Known to Influence Blood Pressure

Factors that increase blood pressure	Factors that decrease blood pressure
Increased sodium intake (Especially for salt-sensitive subjects)	Increased potassium intake
Increased body weight	Increased fruit and vegetable intake
Increased alcohol intake	Increased calcium intake (Especially for salt-sensitive subjects)

sure and an improvement in insulin sensitivity. Studies on both humans and experimental animals suggest that the sympathetic nervous system is involved in the pathophysiology of the weight–blood pressure-insulin resistance relationship, but therapeutic interventions based on these findings are not yet available to confirm this connection.

Another mediator of the body weight-blood pressure relationship appears to be the kidney. In experimental animals, obesity has been associated with alterations in renal blood flow and glomerular filtration rate or intraglomerular pressure. In humans, urinary microalbumin excretion was increased among obese subjects, supporting an abnormality in renal function in humans as well. Moreover, microalbuminuria has been linked to an increased risk of cardiovascular events in hypertensive individuals.

3. SALT (SODIUM CHLORIDE)

The relationship between dietary salt consumption and elevated blood pressure is well known (2). The prevalence of hypertension and its consequences is linearly related to dietary salt intake in societies throughout the world. Hypertension and its sequelae are virtually absent in societies in which habitual salt intake is <50–100 mmol/d. However, there are other differences between these groups and those that habitually consume larger amounts of salt. The "low-salt" societies tend to be isolated, genetically homogeneous, physically fit, and consume increased amounts of potassium and calcium in the form of fresh fruits and vegetables. Increased salt intake is associated with societal "acculturation." This implies a crowded and sedentary lifestyle as well as many other behavioral factors that may affect blood pressure and cardiovascular risk. In addition, the age-related increase in blood pressure is observed only in societies in which salt intake is high. Many of the elderly individuals in low-salt cultures have blood pressure levels that are no higher than those of young adults.

Despite this convincing evidence, controversy still exists concerning the importance of salt in human blood pressure in general, in hypertension, and as a treatment modality. Without considering the various reasons for this controversy, suffice it to say that the magnitude of the effect of salt intake on blood pressure is diluted by the fact that there is substantial heterogeneity in the blood pressure responses of humans to alterations in salt intake (2). Numerous studies have demonstrated that salt-sensitive and salt-resistant individuals can be identified within both the hypertensive and normotensive populations (3). Salt-sensitive subjects will demonstrate a decrease in blood pressure with dietary sodium reduction, usually to the level of 100 mmol/d (2.4 g/d). The human need for sodium is about 10 mmol/d (230 mg/d). Thus, the threshold for blood pressure responsiveness to a reduction in salt intake is many times higher than the physiological requirements. It is often difficult to differentiate between salt-sensitive and salt-resistant subjects without sophisticated research techniques. However, a trial of modest dietary salt restriction or diuretic administration should identify those most likely to benefit from this dietary intervention. Moreover, there have been no adverse reports when a modest reduction in salt intake such as 80–100 mmol/d have been followed.

Certain population groups have been reported to be more likely to be salt sensitive than others (2). Hypertensive individuals are more salt sensitive than those with normal blood pressure. Among hypertensive subjects, salt sensitivity of blood pressure is more frequent among African-Americans (75%) than Caucasians (50%)(3) and increases with increasing age (4). The latter finding is also observed in the normotensive population, with the finding that significant salt sensitivity of blood pressure is not seen until the age decade of 60 yr or more. Individuals with reduced renin responses to sodium and volume depletion, the so-called low-renin subjects, are more likely to be salt sensitive than those with brisk renin responses (5).

In addition to a possible permissive effect of sluggish renin responses to salt sensitivity, a variety of substances have been reported to be involved in the pathophysiology of salt sensitivity of blood pressure. An extensive scientific critique of the many studies that have been conducted in this area is beyond the scope of this chapter; however, note that the sympathetic nervous system, endothelin, insulin sensitivity, atrial natriuretic factor, alterations in renal hemodynamics, and leptin have all been implicated in the pathophysiology of salt, sensitivity. It remains to be determined which of these many factors are primary events and which are simply compensatory responses or epiphenomena.

It has been shown that salt sensitivity requires the administration of sodium as the chloride salt and that other forms of sodium do not have the same pressor effect. However, this is a moot point because over 95% of the sodium found in foods is in the chloride form. Moreover, most of the salt found in food is added in the preparation, processing, and preservation of food and only 15% is added as the discretionary form (as table salt). Thus, it is important for the food preparer as well as the patient to become familiar with identifying the salt content of foods at the grocery store and restaurant as well as in cooking.

Another important recent finding related to salt and blood pressure is the observation that long-term follow-up of salt-sensitive normotensive subjects over a period of 10 yr or more demonstrated an eightfold greater rate of blood pressure increase compared with those who were initially salt-resistant (4). This finding supports the epidemiological observations relating the age-associated rise in blood pressure to increased salt intake.

4. POTASSIUM

As mentioned earlier, in societies in which there is a low prevalence of hypertension and its complications as well as little age-related increase in blood pressure, people tend to consume increased amounts of potassium (and calcium, as discussed in the next section) and follow a reduced salt diet. Fewer studies have examined the relationship between potassium and blood pressure than those involving sodium. However, the findings regarding potassium tend to be consistent. In general, the effect of potassium is smaller than that of sodium based on interventional trials (6). Again, heterogeneity in responsiveness of blood pressure to alterations in potassium intake or balance has been demonstrated. Among potassium-replete normotensive subjects, typically those consuming 60 mmol/d of potassium or more, little effect on blood pressure can be demonstrated with additional potassium administration. However, in hypertensive populations, particularly those comprising substantial numbers of individuals in whom dietary potassium intake is traditionally deficient (the elderly, African-Americans) or those in whom diuretic-induced potassium loss occurs, potassium supplementation has been shown to lower blood pressure. It has also been observed that potassium is more likely to lower blood pressure in hypertensive individuals consuming a high-salt intake, further suggesting a link between sodium and potassium intake in their effects on blood pressure.

The amount of potassium intake required for optimal reduction in blood pressure in those who are sensitive to this mineral is not clear. Most studies indicate that dietary potassium deficiency begins at levels of intake 50 mmol/d and is clearly observed at intakes of 30 mmol/d or less. Dietary sources of potassium are largely fresh fruits and vegetables. In environments where these are scarce, e.g., because of cold climate or high cost, potassium deficiency is more likely. Among a group of normotensive nurses in whom dietary intakes of potassium, calcium, and magnesium were deficient, only potassium supplementation reduced blood pressure (7). Recent studies using diets involving multiple mineral manipulations, such as the Dietary Approaches to Stop Hypertension (DASH) Trial (8) are discussed in the Combination Diets section.

5. CALCIUM

Epidemiological surveys have suggested a relationship between reduced dietary calcium intake and hypertension. Several studies have demonstrated a small and inconsistent effect of calcium supplementation to lower blood pressure. Again, this appears to be largely owing to the heterogeneity in human responses to calcium supplementation. Subgroup analyses of some of the larger studies suggest that those in whom dietary calcium intake is often reduced (African-Americans, the elderly) are more likely to demonstrate a reduction in blood pressure with calcium supplementation than other groups in whom intake is higher. Since both subgroups are traditionally salt sensitive, we conducted a study of calcium supplementation in a group of normal and hypertensive subjects who had been previously categorized with respect to salt sensitivity of blood pressure (9). We found no significant effect of calcium supplementation on blood pressure for the entire group. However, when the subjects were separated on the basis of salt-sensitivity status, we found a significant decrease in blood pressure when the salt-sensitive subjects received calcium supplements and a significant increase in blood pressure when calcium was given to the salt-resistant subjects. These findings suggested a reciprocal relationship between the effects of calcium and sodium on blood pressure that was confirmed by the results of the DASH Trial (*see* Combination Diets Section).

6. OTHER DIETARY CONSTITUENTS

There is, at present, no convincing evidence to link alterations in magnesium intake with blood pressure, and thus the JNC VI report did not advocate an increase in this mineral for the purpose of lowering blood pressure (1). Caffeine may raise blood pressure acutely in caffeine-naïve individuals but does not appear to be a factor in the chronic elevation of blood pressure. Moreover, there is no evidence that withdrawal of caffeine in habitual consumers produces a decrease in blood presssure. While some studies have suggested a beneficial effect of large amounts of omega-3 fatty acids in reducing blood pressure, intolerance of these doses makes this an impractical approach for most individuals.

7. COMBINATION DIETS

A variety of studies have examined the effect of combined dietary approaches on blood pressure as nonpharmacological treatment of hypertension or for the prevention of hypertension in those at increased risk (high-normal blood pressure). These combined studies have been fraught with problems resulting from recidivism, inadequate achievement of dietary goals, or relatively short duration. In general, it can be stated that weight loss appears to be the most effective single intervention as long as the weight loss can be maintained. There does not appear to be an additive benefit when potassium supplementation is combined with modest dietary salt restriction beyond that seen with salt restriction alone. However, in the DASH trial, when a specific diet incorporating modest salt restriction with an increase in fresh fruits and vegetables and low-fat dairy products (presumably increasing potassium, calcium, and magnesium intake) was followed, a significant reduction in blood pressure was observed over the 8-wk study period (8). This benefit appeared to be greatest among African-Americans and those with higher initial blood pressure levels (10). Another study examining multiple dietary changes was a subgroup of the Nurses Health Study II (7), which compared the effects of supplemental potassium, calcium, magnesium, or all three minerals to placebo in normotensive nurses in whom dietary deficiencies of these minerals were documented. As previously mentioned, potassium supplementation alone, but not combination supplementation, lowered blood pressure.

8. ALCOHOL

Alcohol consumption has been shown to have a biphasic effect on blood pressure. Small amounts of alcohol appear to lower blood pressure, presumably secondary to a vasodilator effect, but as alcohol consumption increases, blood pressure rises. The dose-response characteristics vary from individual to individual and may be based on factors such as body surface area, gender, and race. The racial differences may be explicable, in part, by virtue of genetic differences in alcohol metabolism. The mechanism for the alcohol-induced increase in blood pressure appears to be related to activation of, or increased responsiveness to, the sympathetic nervous system. This is manifested by an increase in cardiac output when more than one ounce of alcohol is consumed. Thus, a prudent recommendation to hypertensive subjects is to limit their daily alcohol consumption to no more than 2 oz (60 mL) of 100-proof spirits (or 2.5 oz of 80-proof whiskey), 24 oz (720 mL) of beer or 10 oz (300 mL) of wine. For those hypertensive individuals in whom habitual alcohol consumption exceeds these levels, a reduction in intake may lower blood pressure or make it easier to control.

9. SUMMARY

A variety of dietary and lifestyle factors can influence blood pressure, these factors are reviewed in Table 1. The ideal recommendation for individuals who are hypertensive or are at increased risk for its development are to maintain a body weight as close to ideal as possible; to consume a diet modest in salt content and enriched with fresh fruits, vegetables, and low-fat dairy products, and to consume no more than the recommended optimal amounts of alcohol.

REFERENCES

1. The Joint National Committee on Prevention, Detection, Evaluation, and Treatment of High Blood Pressure: The Sixth Report (JNC VI). Arch Intern Med 1997; 157:2413–2448.
2. Weinberger MH: Salt sensitivity of blood pressure in humans. Hypertension 1996; 27[Part 2]:481–490.
3. Weinberger MH, Miller JZ, Luft FC, et al. Definitions and characteristics of sodium sensitivity and blood pressure resistance. Hypertension 1986; 8 (Suppl 2):127–134.

4. Weinberger MH, Fineberg NS. Sodium and volume sensitivity of blood pressure: Age and blood pressure change over time. Hypertension 1991; 18:67–71.
5. Weinberger MH, Stegner JE, Fineberg NS. A comparison of two tests for the assessment of blood pressure responses to sodium. Am J Hypertens 1993; 6:179–184.
6. Whelton PK, He J, Cutler JA, et al. Effects of oral potassium on blood pressure. JAMA 1997; 277:1624–1632.
7. Sacks FM, Willett WC, Smith A, et al. Effect on blood pressure of potassium, calcium, and magnesium in women with habitual low intake. Hypertension 1998; 31:131–138.
8. Appel LJ, Moore TJ, Obarzanek E, et al. The effect of dietary patterns on blood pressure: results from the Dietary Approaches to Stop Hypertension (DASH) Trial. N Engl J Med 1997; 336:1117–1124.
9. Weinberger MH, Wagner UL, Fineberg NS. The blood pressure effects of calcium supplementation in humans of known sodium responsiveness. Am J Hypertens 1993; 6:799–805.
10. Svetkey LP, Simons-Morton D, Vollmer WM, et al. Effects of dietary patterns on blood pressure: subgroup analysis of the Dietary Approaches to Stop Hypertension (DASH) randomized clinical trial. Arch Intern Med 1999; 159:285–293.

5 Proper Nutritional Habits for Reducing the Risk of Cancer

Carolyn K. Clifford
and Sharon S. McDonald

1. INTRODUCTION

"Cancer" is actually many diseases, with an etiology that comprises genetic and environmental factors, including controllable lifestyle components such as diet. The multistep process of carcinogenesis, the numerous points at which diet-related factors can influence those steps, and the possible interactions among contributing factors, clearly highlight the complexity of cancer etiology, as depicted in Fig. 1 *(1)*. Our current understanding of diet and cancer is based on a large body of solid research evidence from in vitro, animal, epidemiologic, and clinical studies. Overall, this evidence provides strong support for a diet–cancer relationship, suggesting that vegetables and fruits, dietary fiber, certain micronutrients, and physical activity appear to be protective against cancer, whereas fat, excessive calories, and alcohol seem to increase cancer risk *(1–3)*. A recent expert panel suggested that a diet high in vegetables and fruits ranked as the best recommendation for breast cancer prevention, along with avoidance of alcohol *(1)*.

Based on the existence of strong research evidence, dietary guidance that can promote and encourage diet-related behaviors for reducing cancer risk has been formulated by various organizations *(1)*, including the National Cancer Institute (NCI), and is continually being refined as our knowledge of the diet–cancer relationship grows. The NCI dietary guidelines, consistent with those of other organizations, are shown in Table 1. Modification of dietary behaviors and nutritional habits based on current guidelines is a proactive and practical approach to cancer prevention that also is beneficial to overall good health and that can readily be integrated into our daily lives. Evidence supporting the dietary guidelines is reviewed briefly in this chapter.

From: *Nutritional Health: Strategies for Disease Prevention*
Edited by: T. Wilson and N. J. Temple © Humana Press Inc., Totowa, NJ

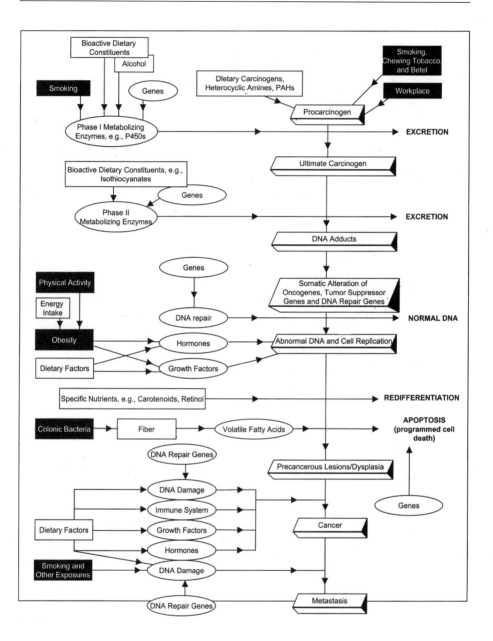

Fig. 1. Diet and the cancer process. Source: ref. *1*.

Table 1
The National Cancer Institute Dietary Guidelines

- Reduce fat intake to less than or equal to 30% of calories.

- Increase fiber intake to 20–30 g/d, with an upper limit of 35 g.

- Include a variety of vegetables and fruits in the daily diet.

- Avoid obesity.

- Consume alcoholic beverages in moderation, if at all.

- Minimize consumption of salt-cured, salt-pickled, or smoked foods.

2. DIETARY FAT

Epidemiologic data, including data from migrant studies, generally suggest a direct relationship between total fat intake or consumption of animal fat or red meat and increased cancer risk at several sites, including the postmenopausal breast, the colon/rectum, and the prostate (1–3). Migrant studies support an increased risk for breast cancer as eating patterns shift from a low-fat, high-fiber diet to a high-fat, low-fiber "Western" diet. In one study, Asian-American women born in the West had a breast cancer risk 1.6 times higher than Asian-American women born in the East (4). Case-control and cohort studies, however, have not found a significant association between fat intake and breast cancer incidence. One meta-analysis of case-control studies found a relative risk (RR) of 1.21 for breast cancer, based on fat intake (5). Two separate meta-analyses of cohort studies reported RRs of 1.01 (5) and 1.05 (6) for the effect of dietary fat on breast cancer risk. Given that dietary fat is closely correlated with other lifestyle factors—including caloric intake, weight gain, obesity, and physical activity—and that dietary assessment methodologies can introduce significant error, inconclusive epidemiologic data for a dietary fat-breast cancer link is not surprising (7).

International correlation studies demonstrate strong, positive associations between colorectal cancer incidence and consumption of red meat and animal fats (2,3,8). Data from case-control and cohort studies generally support the associations with red meat, but data for fat intake are less consistent (9). Cohort data from men in the Health Professionals Follow-Up Study found no significant association of colon cancer with any type of fat, but showed a significantly increased risk associated with red meat intake (10). The Adventist Health Study identified both red meat and white meat as important risk factors for colon cancer (11).

A comprehensive review of dietary fat and prostate cancer concluded that evidence exists for a dietary fat-prostate cancer association, but data are inconclusive and not specific regarding types of fat *(12)*. In the Health Professionals Follow-Up Study, data indicated that prostate cancer risk increased with consumption of red meat (RR = 2.64), but not with fat from poultry, dairy products, or fish *(13)*. One study of the role of diet in the development of prostate cancer in blacks, whites, and Asian-Americans in the United States and Canada reported an overall significant, direct relationship with saturated fat, with the highest risks reported for Asian-Americans *(14)*.

Overall, research findings suggest that the link between fat and cancer risk may be a result of the type of fat consumed rather than or in addition to total fat intake. The cancer-related effects of n-6 polyunsaturated fatty acids (PUFAs) (e.g., linoleic acid) vs those of n-3 PUFAs (e.g., α-linolenic acid, eicosapentanoic acid [EPA], and docosahexanoic acid [DHA]) are of particular interest. Generally, n-6 PUFAs, found in common seed oils, appear to enhance the promotional phase of carcinogenesis in preclinical models for breast, colon, and prostate cancers, whereas n-3 PUFAs—particularly the longer chain n-3 PUFAs such as EPA and DHA, found in fish oil—seem to exert inhibitory effects on cancer *(15–17)*. Overall, data from epidemiologic and clinical studies support a possible protective effect of consumption of fish and n-3 PUFAs on breast and colorectal cancer *(18)*. International comparisons indicate that diets high in n-6 PUFAs are associated with increased breast cancer risk *(8)*, whereas consumption of oleic acid, a monounsaturated fatty acid, and n-3 PUFAs do not increase and may reduce breast cancer risk *(8,19)*. Consumption of olive oil, high in oleic acid, appears to reduce risk of breast cancer in some studies, but not in others *(19)*. In a European multicenter breast cancer study, the ratio of long-chain, n-3 PUFAs in adipose tissue to total n-6 PUFAs showed an inverse relationship with breast cancer risk, indicating that the balance between n-3 PUFAs and n-6 PUFAs may be important *(20)*. These findings are in agreement with ecological mortality data for breast cancer for 24 European countries that show an inverse correlation with fish and fish oil consumption, when expressed as a proportion of animal fat *(15)*. For colorectal cancer, evidence from international correlation and case-control studies do not support an association with vegetable fat *(1–3,10)*. As for breast cancer, epidemiologic data do suggest a protective effect of the consumption of fish or fish oil, expressed as a proportion of animal fat, on colorectal cancer risk *(15)*. For prostate cancer, one review of epidemiologic and experimental evidence suggested that n-3 PUFAs may retard prostate cancer progression *(17)*. Findings from a large cohort study, however, suggested that α-linolenic acid, an n-3 PUFA, increased cancer risk (RR = 3.43), in contrast with saturated fat (RR = 0.95), monounsaturated fat (RR = 1.58), and linoleic acid, an n-6 PUFA (RR = 0.64) *(13)*. It should be noted that although α-linolenic acid is a metabolic precursor of EPA, which has been associated with reduced prostate cancer risk, its conversion to EPA in humans is limited *(17)*. The importance of PUFAs with respect to cancer risk also is discussed in Chapter 13 by de Deckere.

3. PHYSICAL ACTIVITY AND BODY SIZE

Epidemiologic studies have investigated the roles of physical activity (energy expenditure), weight, body size (i.e., body mass index [BMI]), and weight gain in relation to cancer risk. The strongest associations have been found with breast and colon cancer *(1,21)*. Evidence that rapid growth during adolescence and greater adult height increase the risk of breast cancer is convincing *(1)*. Paradoxically, obesity after menopause is associated with increased risk of postmenopausal breast cancer, whereas obesity prior to menopause appears to protect against premenopausal breast cancer *(22)*. Gaining weight after age 18 and being overweight during the premenopausal years, however, appear to increase a woman's risk for breast cancer after the onset of menopause *(22,23)*. Weight loss both prior to and after menopause is associated with reduced risk *(22)*. Studies suggest that moderate physical activity can markedly reduce breast cancer risk *(21,24)*. Sustained physical activity leading to loss of weight and body fat helps reduce circulating levels of estrogen and progesterone, and possibly breast cancer risk. All women should be encouraged to exercise regularly and avoid weight gain. For colorectal cancer, leanness and regular physical activity have been consistently associated with reduced risk in both men and women *(21,24–26)*. Data from the Nurses' Health Study indicated that a BMI greater than 29 kg/m^2 increased risk for colon cancer (RR = 1.45), compared with women with a BMI less than 21 kg/m^2 *(25)*. Current data do not support a relationship between high BMI in adult men and prostate cancer *(1,24)*. However, data from nearly 48,000 men (ages 40–75 yr) in the Health Professionals Follow-Up Study reported that obesity during childhood had a strong inverse association with prostate cancer in adulthood *(27)*. Some data indicate that lean body mass and high percent muscle mass in adult men may increase the risk of prostate cancer, possibly as a result of elevated levels of circulating androgens *(28)*.

4. VEGETABLES, FRUITS, AND WHOLE GRAINS

Epidemiologic data are overwhelmingly supportive of the protective effects of vegetables, fruits, and whole grains on cancer risk. A comprehensive review summarizing the results from 217 case-control and cohort studies found convincing evidence for inverse associations with cancers of the lung, stomach, colon/rectum, esophagus, mouth, and pharynx; a probable protective effect for cancers of the breast, larynx, pancreas, and bladder; and a possible protective effect for cancers of the cervix, ovary, endometrium, prostate, thyroid, liver, and kidney *(1)*. Raw vegetables were protective in 87% of the studies. Vegetables from the *Allium* family (e.g., onion, garlic), carrots, green vegetables, cruciferous vegetables (e.g., broccoli, cauliflower), and tomatoes were protective in approx 70–80% of the studies. Total fruits and citrus fruits were protective in about 65% of the studies. The majority of case-control studies indicate that high vs low consumption of vegetables and fruits reduces cancer risk by approximately half *(29)*. For instance, the relative risk of stomach cancer decreases by about 60% as vegetable intake increases from 100 g/d to 350 g/d and by about 50% as fruit intake increases from 50 g/d to 300 g/d *(1)*. A meta-analysis of 40 case-control studies on whole-grain intake and cancer indicated that increased consumption is associated with decreased risk for various cancers, particularly those of the colon/rectum (pooled OR = 0.79) and stomach (pooled OR = 0.57) *(30)*. Numerous constituents found in vegetables, fruits, and whole-grains—including dietary fiber, micronutrients, and nonnutritive phytochemicals—might contribute to these cancer-protective effects.

4.1. Dietary Fiber

Epidemiologic evidence suggests that colorectal and breast cancer risk, and possibly risk of cancers of the esophagus, mouth, pharynx, stomach, prostate, endometrium, and ovary, may be decreased by increasing intakes of dietary fiber and fiber-rich foods *(1,3,31)*. Based on 25 yr of follow-up data from men in the Seven Countries Study, an increase in fiber intake of 10 g/d was associated with a 33% lower colorectal cancer mortality risk *(32)*. In contrast with the majority of earlier literature, however, 16 yr of follow-up data from the Nurses' Health Study showed no association between dietary fiber intake and colorectal cancer risk in women *(33)*. Overall, study results linking total dietary fiber and cancer are somewhat inconsistent. Dietary fiber from different sources vary in composition, and it is unlikely that all will be equally protective against cancer *(1,3)*. Wheat bran, a rich source of dietary fiber, appears to have protective effects against a range of cancers, especially those of the colon and breast *(34)*, and cereal fiber is consistently protective against colorectal cancer *(35)*. A major confounding factor in examining the association between cancer risk and high-fiber diets is the possible effect on risk caused by micronutrients and phytochemicals in high-fiber foods. The assessment of a cancer-protective effect for dietary fiber can be further complicated by correlations among dietary fiber, dietary fat, and caloric intakes (i.e., high-fiber diets may be relatively low in fat and calories).

4.2. Micronutrients

Reviews of epidemiologic studies that correlated either high intakes of β-carotene-rich vegetables and fruits or high blood concentrations of β-carotene with cancer risk have consistently reported strong support for a significant protective effect of dietary β-carotene on lung cancer *(1,36–39)*. One review noted that associations of β-carotene with reduced cancer risk were most consistent for lung and stomach cancers and that esophageal cancer showed limited but promising risk reduction with respect to dietary β-carotene *(38)*. Reported results for the effects of β-carotene were equivocal for prostate cancer *(40)* and indicated a possible protective effect of β-carotene for breast cancer *(41)*. For colon cancer, data suggested only a modest risk reduction overall *(38)*. Some studies reported significantly reduced risk of colorectal adenomas at high β-carotene intakes *(42)*.

The epidemiologic data that linked high intakes of foods containing β-carotene and high blood levels of β-carotene to reduced risk of lung cancer provided strong support for testing the effect of β-carotene supplements on lung cancer risk in clinical interventions, as was done in high-risk populations in the Alpha-Toco-pherol, Beta-Carotene Cancer Prevention (ATBC) Study *(43)* and the Beta-Caro-tene and Retinol Efficacy Trial (CARET) *(44)*. Unexpectedly, results from these large-scale trials showed adverse treatment effects in terms of increased lung cancer incidence. In the Physicians' Health Study (PHS), however, a general population trial in US physicians that evaluated the effect of aspirin and β-carotene supplementation on the primary prevention of cardiovascular disease and cancer, data showed no significant evidence of either benefit or harm from β-carotene *(45)*. It should be noted that, in addition to β-carotene, vegetables and fruits contain numerous other naturally occurring potential anticarcinogens that may exert their cancer-inhibitory effects through diverse mechanisms. In fact, β-carotene may simply be a marker for the actual protective substances in vegetables and fruits. Results from trials such as the ATBC Study, CARET, and PHS illustrate that definitive clinical evidence of both safety and efficacy is required for individual vegetable and fruit constituents before dietary guidelines more specific than those promoting greater consumption of vegetables and fruits can be formulated.

Few epidemiologic studies have investigated the association of cancer risk with diets high in vitamin E (α-tocopherol). One review concluded that vitamin E possibly decreases risk for lung and cervical cancers, that evidence is insufficient for colon/rectum cancers, and that no relationship exists between vitamin E and breast or stomach cancers *(1)*. In the ATBC Study, 34% fewer cases of prostate cancer and 16% fewer cases of colorectal cancer were diagnosed among male cigarette smokers who received daily vitamin E supplements *(43)*. Although these results suggest a protective effect of vitamin E, prostate and colon cancers were not primary study endpoints; studies targeted at these cancers are needed before conclusions can be reached.

Epidemiologic evidence for a protective effect of diets high in vitamin C-con-taining vegetables and fruits indicates that vitamin C probably decreases risk for stomach cancer, and possibly decreases risk for cancers of the mouth, pharynx, esophagus, lung, pancreas, and cervix *(1)*. One review of more than 50 case-control and cohort studies that investigated intakes of vegetables and fruits, vitamin C, and vitamin E reported that indices of vitamin C computed from vegetable and fruit intakes were associated with lower risk of gastrointestinal and respiratory tract cancers *(46)*.

International correlation studies suggest an inverse association between selenium status and cancer mortality *(47)*. Data from most case-control and cohort studies show a possible protective relationship for lung cancer *(1,37)* but have not been convincing for other cancer sites, including breast, colon/rectum, and stomach *(9,41,48)*. One study reported a reduced risk of advanced prostate cancer (OR = 0.35) at the highest quintile of selenium levels in toenails *(49)*. A clinical intervention trial to determine whether selenium supplementation protects against development of basal or squamous carcinomas of the skin in patients with a history of such carcinomas showed no beneficial effect of selenium *(50)*. Secondary end-point analyses, however, showed significant reductions in total cancer mortality (RR = 0.5), total cancer incidence (RR = 0.63), and incidences of lung (RR = 0.54), colorectal (RR = 0.42), and prostate (RR = 0.37) cancers for patients who received selenium supplements. These clinical findings support the cancer-protective effect of selenium, but must be confirmed in independent intervention trials.

Other micronutrients found in vegetables, fruits, and whole grains—including calcium (green leafy vegetables) and folate (green vegetables, cruciferous vegetables, oranges, whole grains, wheat bran, legumes, and seeds)—have been associated with cancer-protective effects for colorectal cancer. Numerous epidemiologic studies have suggested a weak association between calcium intake and decreased risk of colorectal cancer, but results are inconsistent overall *(1,9,51)*. Folate and methionine, an essential amino acid, also have been linked to reduced risk of colorectal cancers and colorectal adenomas in some, but not all, epidemiologic studies *(1,51,52)*. More evidence is needed before conclusions can be drawn regarding the influence of dietary calcium and folate on cancer risk.

4.3. Phytochemicals

Vegetables, fruits, and whole grains contain various phytochemicals that have been studied for their association with cancer risk *(53,54)*. A short list of phytochemicals and some of their sources include thioethers (garlic, onions, leeks), terpenes (citrus fruits), plant phenols (grapes, strawberries, apples), polyphenols (green tea), indoles and isothiocyanates (cruciferous vegetables), and phytoestrogens (soy, soy products) *(53,54)*. A comprehensive review of the phytochemical-cancer relationship is beyond the scope of this discussion; thus, only selected examples are presented.

Common green, yellow/red, and yellow/orange vegetables and fruits contain more than 40 carotenoids, in addition to β-carotene, that can be absorbed and metabolized by humans, including lutein, zeaxanthin, cryptoxanthin, lycopene, α-carotene, astaxanthin, and canthaxanthin *(55)*. A comprehensive monograph summarizing the current state-of-knowledge on the cancer-preventive effects of carotenoids—a class of compounds that exhibits strong antioxidant activity in vitro—concluded that clear evidence of cancer-protective effects is not available for any of the carotenoids *(56)*. In one population-based study, white male cigarette smokers in the lowest quartile of α-carotene intake had more than twice the risk of lung cancer as those in the highest quartile *(57)*. The corresponding risks associated with intakes of β-carotene and lutein/zeaxanthin increased only about 60%, suggesting that β-carotene is not the dominant protective factor in vegetables and fruits for lung cancer. Findings from an investigation of serum carotenoid levels in Japanese-American men indicated that α-carotene (RR = 0.19), β-carotene (RR = 0.10), β-cryptoxanthin (RR = 0.25), and total carotenoids (RR = 0.22) all significantly reduce the risk of aerodigestive tract cancers (58). A review of 72 studies of tomatoes, tomato-based products, lycopene, and cancer found that evidence of a protective effect was strongest for cancers of the prostate, lung, and stomach; data also suggested reduced risk for cancers of the pancreas, colon and rectum, esophagus, oral cavity, breast, and cervix (59). One recent study reported that the risk for total prostate cancers decreased with increasing quintile of plasma lycopene (OR = 0.75); a stronger inverse association was found for aggressive cancers (OR = 0.56) (60).

Epidemiologic data from studies that investigated the effects of black (oxidized) or green (unoxidized) tea consumption on cancer risk suggest that green tea consumption may reduce overall cancer mortality (61). Data appear to be most consistent for a protective effect of green tea on stomach cancer and do not clearly support a cancer-protective effect of black tea (1). One case-control study in Shanghai reported an inverse association for green tea consumption (highest tertile vs lowest tertile) and cancer risk for colon (men, RR = 0.82; women, RR = 0.67), rectum (men, RR = 0.72; women, RR = 0.57), and pancreas (men, RR = 0.63; women, RR = 0.53) (62). Most animal studies examining the possible effect of tea on cancer incidence have focused on extracts of either black or green tea and on green tea polyphenols (GTP), particularly the catechins—the major catechin in green tea is (–)-epigallocatechin-3-gallate (EGCG) (61,63). Catechins also are present in black tea, but in lesser amounts; black tea contains high amounts of theaflavins, not present in green tea (61). A recent study demonstrated that drinking green tea is an effective way to increase human salivary tea catechin levels; holding the tea in the mouth for a few minutes before swallowing resulted in even higher salivary tea catechin levels (64). The authors suggested that the benefits of drinking tea slowly or using a tea mouthwash or lozenge might be tested in clinical trials for the prevention of oral and esophageal cancer.

5. ALCOHOL

Epidemiologic data support a direct association of alcohol intake with cancers of the oral cavity, pharynx, esophagus, and larynx, where alcohol acts synergistically with smoking to increase risk. Increased risks for liver, breast, colon/rectum, and lung cancers also have been linked to alcohol intake (1,65). A dose-response relationship is observed in most studies (1). For example, in lifelong nonsmokers, risk for esophageal cancer increased with daily consumption of four to eight drinks (RR = 2.7) and eight or more drinks (RR = 5.4), compared with consumption of fewer than four drinks (RR = 1.0) *(66)*. Reports indicate that alcohol consumption and tobacco use have a multiplicative effect on aerodigestive cancers *(1)*. Smoking combined with alcohol consumption increased the risk of oral cancer in Japanese men to three times that of smoking only (OR = 6.2 vs OR = 2.2) *(67)*. A meta-analysis of six prospective studies that included a total of more than 322,000 women evaluated for up to 11 yr indicated that breast cancer risk increases linearly with total alcohol intake, regardless of whether the beverage is beer, wine, or liquor, and that daily alcohol intake equivalent to about 0.75–1 drink is associated with a 9% increase in breast cancer risk *(68)*. Findings from 16 yr of followup in the Nurses' Health Study suggest that the risk of breast cancer associated with alcohol consumption may be reduced by adequate folate intake *(69)*. Epidemiologic data linking alcohol and colorectal cancer have not been consistent *(1,9)*. One review found that 12 of 20 studies reported positive associations between alcohol consumption and colon cancer, and 12 of 19 studies reported positive associations for rectal cancer *(9)*. In a more recent assessment of case-control and cohort studies, data suggested as much as a 1.5–2-fold increase in risk in colorectal cancer for those consuming 30–50 g of alcohol per day, compared with nondrinkers *(1)*. The effects of alcohol on colorectal cancer risk may depend, in part, on methionine and folate intake. In a large cohort study, men in the highest quintiles of methionine and folate intakes who consumed more than 20 g alcohol daily were not at increased risk for colon cancer (RR = 0.79, RR = 1.03, respectively) *(70)*.

6. PRODUCTS OF FOOD PREPARATION AND PRESERVATION

Certain food preparation and preservation methods have been linked to increased risk for some cancers. Epidemiologic data suggest that frequent consumption of grilled and barbecued meat and/or fish may increase risk for both colorectal and stomach cancers; diets high in cured meats may increase colorectal cancer risk; and regular intake of meat and/or fish preserved by smoking may increase stomach cancer risk *(1)*. Dietary carcinogens introduced through food preparation and preservation include heterocyclic aromatic amines (HAAs) and polycyclic aromatic hydrocarbons (PAHs), formed during high-temperature cooking of meats, poultry, and fish; and *N*-nitroso compounds (NOCs), formed in salted and pickled foods cured with nitrate or nitrite *(71–74)*.

A number of HAAs have been determined to be possible carcinogens in humans *(71,72)*. Cooking methods such as panfrying, broiling, grilling, and barbequing, which result in high food surface temperatures, are most likely to produce HAAs, in contrast with stewing, steaming, poaching, and microwaving *(71,75)*. The estimated carcinogenic risk to humans from dietary HAAs is difficult to calculate because of uncertainties in the relative carcinogenicity of specific HAAs, exposures, and interindividual differences in susceptibility *(71)*. In view of the possible role of HAAs in human carcinogenesis, minimizing exposures to HAAs by prudent selection of lower-temperature cooking techniques for meat and by avoiding overcooking may be advisable.

PAHs, formed when fat drips onto hot coals as meats are cooked over an open flame, rise with the smoke and are deposited onto the meat. Benzo(a)pyrene, the most carcinogenic PAH, has been reported at levels up to 50 µg/kg in charcoal-broiled steaks and ground beef, five times greater than levels in some less fatty pork cuts and chicken *(74)*. As with HAAs, it is difficult to arrive at a reliable estimate of the contribution of dietary PAHs to cancer risk *(74,76)*. However, it is prudent to reduce exposures to PAHs by modifying food preparation techniques. Oven cooking, cooking with a heat source above the meat, separation of meat from smoke during cooking, and microwaving all result in food containing minimal amounts of PAHs *(74)*.

Smoked, salted, and pickled meats and fish, as well as salted or pickled vegetables, are dietary sources of NOCs. NOCs also can be formed endogenously at various sites, such as the oral cavity and the stomach, from nitrites and amines present in the diet *(73)*. Epidemiologic studies have demonstrated a direct correlation between exposure to nitrosamines and cancers of the stomach, esophagus, nasopharynx, urinary bladder, liver, and brain *(72,73,77)*. Formation of endogenous NOCs may be inhibited by naturally occurring food constituents and foods—for example, ascorbic acid, tocopherols, phenolic compounds, tea, orange peel, and certain fruit and vegetable juices *(78,79)*. This inhibition may contribute to the generally protective effect of vegetables and fruits on cancer risk that is consistently observed in epidemiologic studies *(1,29,31)*.

7. FUTURE DIRECTIONS

Clearly, impressive progress has been made by the scientific and healthcare communities in establishing the existence of a diet–cancer relationship. This very complex area of research, however, is just beginning to identify and develop approaches to address the broad scope of questions that need to be answered if further significant advances important to cancer prevention are to be achieved. Many gaps in knowledge exist about the fundamental mechanisms of action for dietary patterns and dietary constituents in cancer development, particularly in the context of gene/nutrient interactions. For example, we need a greater understanding of the variations in genetic susceptibility among individuals resulting from polymorphisms in specific genes (e.g., *CYP1A1*, *CPY1A2*, *CYP2D6*, *GSTM1*, and *NAT2*) that cause differences in metabolic or detoxification activities *(80)*. The presence of such polymorphisms in populations targeted in epidemiologic studies may affect certain individuals' responses to dietary constituents and confound study results to some degree, depending on the polymorphisms' prevalence and distribution.

More complete clinical-metabolic information is needed about the pharma-cokinetics of dietary constituents. Information about their absorption, retention, and excretion could facilitate the development of validated biomarkers of dietary intake, which would help to provide more objective measures of intake than the dietary assessment tools currently used in most epidemiologic studies and thus improve measurement accuracy. Developing approaches to separate the interactive effects of diet-related factors—such as those resulting from the complex composition of vegetables and fruits, as well as the close relationship of fat, caloric intake, physical activity, and BMI—is critically important to diet and cancer research, to minimize confounding and aid in interpretation of study results. Also, carefully designed clinical trials to test diet and cancer hypotheses based on epidemiologic and laboratory evidence are essential. For example, the Polyp Prevention Trial tested the effectiveness of a low-fat, high-fiber, high-vegetable and -fruit dietary pattern to prevent recurrence of colorectal adenomatous polyps; no effect on polyp incidence was observed *(81)*. The research areas highlighted here are only a few of the numerous issues that need to be addressed to help ensure the continuation of significant progress that may ultimately make it possible to provide clear, specific dietary guidance for cancer prevention for all individuals.

REFERENCES

1. World Cancer Research Fund/American Institute for Cancer Research. Food, Nutrition and the Prevention of Cancer: A Global Perspective. American Institute for Cancer Research, Washington, DC, 1997.
2. US Department of Health and Human Services. The Surgeon General's Report on Nutrition and Health, DHHS (PHS) Publication No. 88-50210. US Government Printing Office, Washington, DC, 1988.
3. National Academy of Sciences, National Research Council, Commission on Life Sciences, Food and Nutrition Board. Diet and Health: Implications for Reducing Chronic Disease Risk. National Academy Press, Washington, DC, 1989.
4. Ziegler RG, Hoover RN, Hildesheim A, Nomura, AM, Pike MC, West D, et al. Migration patterns and breast cancer risk in Asian-American women. J Natl Cancer Inst 1993; 85:1819–1827.
5. Boyd NF, Martin LJ, Noffel M, Lockwood GA, Tritchler DL. A meta-analysis of studies of dietary fat and breast cancer risk. Br J Cancer 1993; 68:627–636.
6. Hunter DJ, Spiegelman D, Adami H-O, Beeson L, Van den Brandt PA, Folsom AR, et al. Cohort studies of fat intake and the risk of breast cancer - a pooled analysis. N Engl J Med 1996; 334:356–361.
7. Greenwald P. Role of dietary fat in the causation of breast cancer: point. Cancer Epidemiol Biomark Prev 1999; 8:3–7.
8. Hursting SD, Thornquist M, Henderson MM. Types of dietary fat and the incidence of cancer at five sites. Prev Med 1990; 19:242–253.
9. Potter JD. Nutrition and colorectal cancer. Cancer Causes Control 1996; 7:127–146.
10. Giovannucci E, Rimm EB, Stampfer MJ, Colditz GA, Ascherio A, Willett WC. Intake of fat, meat, and fiber in relation to risk of colon cancer in men. Cancer Res 1994; 54:2390–2397.
11. Singh PN, Fraser GE. Dietary risk factors for colon cancer in a low-risk population. Am J Epidemiol 1998; 148:761–774.

12. Kolonel LN, Nomura AMY, Cooney RV. Dietary fat and prostate cancer: current status (review). J Natl Cancer Inst 1999; 91:414–428.
13. Giovannucci E, Rimm EB, Colditz GA, Stampfer MJ, Ascherio A, Chute,CG, Willett WC. A prospective study of dietary fat and risk of prostate cancer. J Natl Cancer Inst 1993; 85:1571–1579.
14. Whittemore AS, Kolonel LN, Wu AH, John EM, Gallagher RP, Howe GR, et al. Prostate cancer in relation to diet, physical activity, and body size in blacks, whites, and Asians in the United States and Canada. J Natl Cancer Inst 1995; 87:652–661.
15. Caygill CPJ, Charlett A, Hill MJ. Fat, fish, fish oil and cancer. Br J Cancer 1996; 74:159–164.
16. Dwyer JT. Human studies on the effects of fatty acids on cancer: summary, gaps, and future research. Am J Clin Nutr 1997; 66:1581S–1586S.
17. Rose DP. Dietary fatty acids and cancer. Am J Clin Nutr 1997; 66:998–1003.
18. De Deckere EAM. Possible beneficial effect of fish and fish n-3 polyunsaturated fatty acids in breast and colorectal cancer. Eur J Cancer Prev 1999; 8:213–221.
19. Lipworth L, Martinez ME, Angell J, Hsieh C-C, Trichopoulos D. Olive oil and human cancer: an assessment of the evidence. Prev Med 1997; 26:181–190.
20. Simonsen N, van't Veer P, Strain JJ, Martin-Moreno JM, Huttunen JK, Navajas JF-C, Martin BC, Thamm M, Kardinaal AFM, Kok FJ, Kohlmeier L. Adipose tissue omega-3 and omega-6 fatty acid content and breast cancer in the EURAMIC Study. Am J Epidemiol 1998; 147:342–352.
21. U.S. Department of Health and Human Services, Centers for Disease Control and Prevention, National Centers for Chronic Disease Prevention and Health Promotion. Physical Activity and Health: A Report of the Surgeon General. U.S. Department of Health and Human Services, Atlanta, 1996.
22. Trentham-Dietz A, Newcomb PA, Storer BE, Longnecker MP, Baron J, Greenberg ER, Willet WC. Body size and risk of breast cancer. Am J Epidemiol 1997; 145:1011–1019.
23. Brinton LA, Swanson CA. Height and weight at various ages and risk of breast cancer. Ann Epidemiol 1992; 2:597–609.
24. McTiernan A, Ulrich C, Slate S, Potter J. Physical activity and cancer etiology: associations and mechanisms. Cancer Causes Control 1998; 9:487–509.
25. Martinez ME, Giovannucci E, Spiegelman D, Hunter DJ, Willett WC, Colditz GA. Leisure-time physical activity, body size, and colon cancer in women. J Natl Cancer Inst 1997; 89:948–955.
26. Colditz GA, Cannuscio CC, Frazier AL. Physical activity and reduced risk of colon cancer: implications for prevention. Cancer Causes Control 1997; 8:649–667.
27. Giovannucci E, Rimm EB, Stampfer MJ, Colditz GA, Willett WC. Height, body weight, and risk of prostate cancer. Cancer Epidemiol Biomark Prev 1997; 6:557–563.
28. Andersson S-O, Wolk A, Bergstrom R, Adami H-O, Engholm G, Englund A, Nyren O. Body size and prostate cancer: a 20-year follow-up study among 135,006 Swedish construction workers. J Natl Cancer Inst 1997; 89:385–389.
29. Steinmetz KA, Potter JD. Vegetables, fruit, and cancer. I. Epidemiology. Cancer Causes Control 1991; 2:325–357.
30. Jacobs DR, Jr, Marquart L, Slavin J, Kushi LH. Whole-grain intake and cancer: an expanded review and meta-analysis. Nutr Cancer 1998; 30:85–96.
31. Steinmetz KA, Potter J D. Vegetables, fruit, and cancer prevention: a review. J Am Diet Assoc 1996; 96:1027–1039.
32. Jansen MCJF, Bueno-de-Mesquita HB, Buzina R, Fidanza F, Menotti A, Blackburn H,et al. for the Seven Countries Study Group. Dietary fiber and plant foods in relation to colorectal cancer mortality: the Seven Countries Study. Int J Cancer 1999; 81:174–179.
33. Fuchs CS, Giovannucci EL, Colditz GA, Hunter DJ, Stampfer MJ, Rosner B, et al. Dietary fiber and the risk of colorectal cancer and adenoma in women. N Engl J Med 1999; 340:169–176.
34. Ferguson LR, Harris PJ. Protection against cancer by wheat bran: role of dietary fibre and phytochemicals. Eur J Cancer Prev 1999; 8:17–25.
35. Hill MJ. Cereals, cereal fibre and colorectal cancer risk: a review of the epidemiological literature. Eur J Cancer Prev 1998; 7:S5–S10.

36. Peto R, Doll R, Buckley JD, Sporn MB. Can dietary beta-carotene materially reduce human cancer rates? Nature 1981; 290:201–208.
37. Ziegler RG, Mayne ST, Swanson CA. Nutrition and lung cancer. Cancer Causes Control 1996; 7:157–177.
38. van Poppel G, Goldbohm RA. Epidemiologic evidence for β-carotene and cancer prevention. Am J Clin Nutr 1995; 62:1393S–1402S.
39. Cooper DA, Eldridge AL, Peters JC. Dietary carotenoids and lung cancer: a review of recent research. Nutr Rev 1999; 57:133–145.
40. Kolonel LN. Nutrition and prostate cancer. Cancer Causes Control 1996; 7:83–94.
41. Hunter DJ, Willett WC. Nutrition and breast cancer. Cancer Causes Control 1996; 7:56–68.
42. Enger SM, Longnecker MP, Chen M-J, Harper JM, Lee ER, Frankl HD, Haile RW. Dietary intake of specific carotenoids and vitamins A, C, and E, and prevalence of colorectal adenomas. Cancer Epidemiol Biomark Prev 1996; 5:147–153.
43. Heinonen OP, Huttunen JK, Albanes D. for the Alpha-Tocopherol Beta-Carotene Cancer Prevention Study Group. The effect of vitamin E and beta carotene on the incidence of lung cancer and other cancers in male smokers. N Engl J Med 1994; 330:1029–1035.
44. Omenn GS, Goodman GE, Thornquist MD, Balmes J, Cullen MR, Glass A, et al. Effects of a combination of beta carotene and vitamin A on lung cancer and cardiovascular disease. N Eng J Med 1996; 334:1150–1155.
45. Hennekens CH, Buring JE, Manson JE, Stampfer M, Rosner B, Cook NR, et al. Lack of effect of long-term supplementation with beta carotene on the incidence of malignant neoplasms and cardiovascular disease. N Eng J Med 1996; 334:1145–1149.
46. Byers T, Guerrero N. Epidemiologic evidence for vitamin C and vitamin E in cancer prevention. Am J Clin Nutr 1995; 62:1385S–1392S.
47. Schrauzer GN, White DA, Schneider CJ. Cancer mortality correlations studies III: statistical associations with dietary selenium intakes. Bioinorg Chem 1997; 7:23–34.
48. Kono S. Hirohata T. Nutrition and stomach cancer. Cancer Causes Control 1996; 7:41–55.
49. Yoshizawa K, Willett WC, Morris SJ, Stampfer MJ, Spiegelman D, Rimm EB, Giovannucci E. Study of prediagnostic selenium level in toenails and the risk of advanced prostate cancer. J Natl Cancer Inst 1998; 90:1219–1224.
50. Clark LC, Combs GF, Jr, Turnbull BW, Slate EH, Chalker DK, Chow J, et al. Effects of selenium supplementation for cancer prevention in patients with carcinoma of the skin. J AMA 1996; 276:1957–1963.
51. Potter JD. Colorectal cancer: molecules and populations. J Natl Cancer Inst 1999; 91:916–932.
52. Kune GA. Diet, In: Causes and Control of Colorectal Cancer: A Model for Cancer Prevention. Kluwer Academic Publishers, Boston, 1996, pp. 69–115.
53. Wattenberg LW. Inhibition of carcinogenesis by minor dietary constituents. Cancer Res 1992; 52:2085s–2091s.
54. Huang M-T, Ferarro T, Ho C-T. Cancer chemoprevention by phytochemicals in fruits and vegetables. An overview, In: Huang M-T, Osawa T, Ho C-T, Rosen RT, eds. Food Phytochemicals for Cancer Prevention I. Fruits and Vegetables. American Chemical Society, Washington, DC,1994, pp. 2–16.
55. Khachik F, Nir Z, Ausich RL, Steck A, Pfander H. Distribution of carotenoids in fruits and vegetables as a criterion for the selection of appropriate chemopreventive agents, In: Ohigashi H, Osawa T, Terao J, Watanabe S, Yoshikawa T, eds. Food Factors for Cancer Prevention. Springer-Verlag, New York, 1997, pp. 204–208.
56. IARC Working Group. IARC Handbooks of Cancer Prevention: Carotenoids (vol. 2). International Agency for Research on Cancer, Lyon, France,1998.
57. Ziegler RG, Colavito EA, Hartge P, McAdams MJ, Schoenberg JB, Mason TJ, Fraumeni JF, Jr. Importance of α-carotene, β-carotene, and other phytochemicals in the etiology of lung cancer. J Natl Cancer Inst 1996; 88:612–615.

58. Nomura AMY, Ziegler RG, Stemmermann GN, Chyou P-H, Craft NE. Serum micronutrients and upper aerodigestive tract cancer. Cancer Epidemiol Biomark Prev1997; 6:407–412.

59. Giovannucci E. Tomatoes, tomato-based products, lycopene, and cancer: review of the epidemiologic literature. J Natl Cancer Inst 1999; 91:317–331.

60. Gann PH, Ma J, Giovannucci E, Willett W, Sacks FM, Hennekens CH, Stampfer MJ. Lower prostate cancer risk in men with elevated plasma lycopene levels: results of a prospective analysis. Cancer Res 1999; 59:1225–1230.

61. Kuroda Y, Hara Y. Antimutagenic and anticarcinogenic activity of tea polyphenols. Mutation Res 1999; 436:69–97.

62. Ji B-T, Chow W-H, Hsing AW, McLaughlin JK, Dai Q, Gao Y-T, et al. Green tea consumption and the risk of pancreatic and colorectal cancers. Int J Cancer 1997; 70:255–258.

63. Ahmad N, Mukhtar H. Green tea polyphenols and cancer: biologic mechanisms and practical implications. Nutr Rev 1999; 57:78–83.

64. Yang CS, Lee M-J, Chen L. Human salivary tea catechin levels and catechin esterase activities: implication in human cancer prevention studies. Cancer Epidemiol Biomark Prev 1999; 8:83–89.

65. Longnecker MP. Alcohol consumption and risk of cancer in humans: an overview. Alcohol 1995; 12:87–96.

66. Tavani A, Negri E, Franceschi S, La Vecchia C. Risk factors for esophageal cancer in lifelong nonsmokers. Cancer Epidemiol Biomark Prev 1994; 3:387–392.

67. Takezaki T, Hirose K, Inoue M, Hamajima N, Kuroishi T, Nakamura SK, et al. Tobacco, alcohol and dietary factors associated with the risk of oral cancer among Japanese. Jpn J Cancer Res 1996; 87:555–562.

68. Smith-Warner SA, Spiegelman D, Yuan S-S, van den Brandt PA, Folsom AR, Goldbohm RA, et al. Alcohol and breast cancer in women: a pooled analysis of cohort studies. J Am Med Assoc1998; 279:535–540.

69. Zhang S, Hunter DJ, Hankinson SE, Giovannucci EL, Rosner BA, Colditz GA, et al. A prospective study of folate intake and the risk of breast cancer. J Am Med Assoc 1999; 281:1632–1637.

70. Giovannucci E, Rimm EB, Ascherio A, Stampfer MJ, Colditz GA, Willett WC. Alcohol, low-methionine-low-folate diets, and risk of colon cancer in men. J Natl Cancer Inst 1995; 87:265–273.

71. Skog KI, Johansson MAE, Jagerstad MI. Carcinogenic heterocyclic amines in model systems and cooked foods: a review on formation, occurrence and intake. Food Chem Toxicol 1998; 36:879–896.

72. IARC Working Group. IARC Monographs on the Evaluation of Carcinogenic Risks to Humans (vol. 56). International Agency for Research on Cancer, Lyon, France, 1993.

73. Eichholzer M, Gutzwiller F. Dietary nitrates, nitrites, and *N*-nitroso compounds and cancer risk: a review of the epidemiologic evidence. Nutr Rev 1998; 56:95–105.

74. Lijinsky, W. The formation and occurrence of polynuclear aromatic hydrocarbons associated with food. Mutat Res 1991; 259:251–261.

75. Layton DW, Bogen KT, Knize MG, Hatch FT, Johnson VM, Felton JS. Cancer risk of heterocyclic amines in cooked foods: an analysis and implications for research. Carcinogenesis 1995; 16:39–52.

76. Schoket B. DNA damage in humans exposed to environmental and dietary polycyclic aromatic hydrocarbons. Mutation Res 1999; 424:143–153.

77. Tricker AR, Preussmann R. Carcinogenic *N*-nitrosamines in the diet: occurrence, formation, mechanisms and carcinogenic potential. Mutation Res 1991; 259:277–289.

78. Helser MA, Hotchkiss JH, Roe DA. Influence of fruit and vegetable juices on the endogenous formation of *N*-nitrosoproline and *N*-nitrosothiazolidine-4-carboxylic acid in humans on controlled diets. Carcinogenesis 1992; 13:2277–2280.

79. Xu GP, Song PJ, Reed PI. Effects of fruit juices, processed vegetable juice, orange peel and green tea on endogenous formation of N-nitrosoproline in subjects from a high-risk area for gastric cancer in Moping County, China. Eur J Cancer Prev 1993; 2:327–335.
80. Perera FP. Molecular epidemiology: insights into cancer susceptibility, risk assessment, and prevention. J Natl Cancer Inst 1996; 88:496–509.
81. Schatzkin A, Lanza E, Corle D, Lance P, Iber F, Caan B, et al. Polyp Prevention Trial Study Group. Lack of effect of a low-fat, high-fiber diet on the recurrence of colorectal adenomas. N Engl J Med 2000; 342:1149–1155.

6 Health Benefits of Soy Isoflavones

Ted Wilson and Patricia A. Murphy

1. INTRODUCTION

Asian populations have a relatively low rate of breast cancer and heart disease when compared to persons in the United States and Europe consuming a Western diet *(1)*. These populations tend to differ with respect to lifestyle and genetic makeup, but most importantly, they differ with respect to dietary composition. The traditional Western diet tends to differ from its Asian counterpart that contains reduced amounts of red meat and saturated fats, but higher quantities of soy. When the diet of Japanese persons is converted to a Western diet, the low breast cancer and cardiovascular disease (CVD) rates climb to those of Western countries. Furthermore, the observation of worsening cardiovascular health in the Japanese population has been suggested to be a result of a slow conversion to a Western diet *(2)*.

Soy foods are a rich source of dietary protein. Soy consumption in Western countries is increasing due to the relatively high quality of its protein content and the low cost. As a result, soy–protein isolates have become major components of foods such as infant formula and other second-generation foods *(3)*. Soy-based foods are rich in a class of compounds called isoflavones (*see* Fig. 1). Isoflavones have chemical structures that are similar to the hormone estrogen, hence they are commonly called phytoestrogens. Phytoestrogens can bind to estrogen receptors in the body, although with low affinity, and have biological activities in the body that often times mimic that of estrogen *(4)*. Paradoxically, phytoestrogens can also exert a weak antiestrogenic effect as well *(5)*. The three most common phytoestrogens in soy products are daidzein, genistein, and glycitein. In addition to their phytoesterogenic activities, daidzein and genistein are also known to have powerful in vivo antioxidant effects that may be physiologically important *(6)*. Ultimately, the content of daidzein, genistein, and glycitein present in a food appears to determine the extent of health protection received by consumers of a traditional Asian diet.

From: *Nutritional Health: Strategies for Disease Prevention*
Edited by: T. Wilson and N. J. Temple © Humana Press Inc., Totowa, NJ

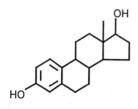

estrogen

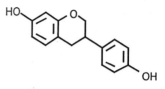

equol

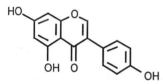

genistein

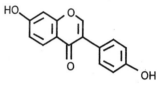

daidzein

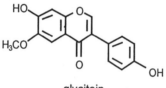

glycitein

Fig. 1. Polyphenolic structures of estradiol, genistein, daidzein, glycitein, and equol.

This chapter discusses how the consumption of soy isoflavones appears to result in health benefits for cancer, heart disease, menopausal hot flushes, and osteoporosis. The physiological mechanisms for these soy biological activities is briefly addressed, although the mechanisms are not definitively understood. This chapter also reviews how differences in mechanistic effects can be a result of differences in the nutritional content of isoflavones in food products. Finally, the chapter suggests a conservative estimate of the amount of soy needed in the diet and a description of when soy is most useful for providing these health promotional activities.

2. WHAT ARE THE BIOLOGICALLY ACTIVE CONTENTS OF SOY?

Only soybeans, alfalfa sprouts, clover sprouts, and garbanzo beans (or chickpeas) of leguminous plant foods contain large amounts of a class of compounds called isoflavones. The three most important soy isoflavones, with respect to content and biological activity, are genistein, daidzein, and glycitein (*see* Fig. 1). Isoflavones have a phenyl-ring structure with a series of attached hydroxyl groups that give them their unique biological activities *(8)*. A close structural similarity exists between the structure of the isoflavones and estradiol (Fig. 1). A potentially important isoflavone metabolite is equol (Fig. 1). Equol is unique because it has a higher estrogenic activity than its precursor, daidzein. It is also unique because only 35% of individuals in the United States have the intestinal flora responsible for its production *(9)*. The nutritional importance of equol formation and excretion remains to be more completely understood. The genistein metabolite, *p*-ethylphenol, appears to have no activity. Metabolites of glycitein have not as yet been identified. All three soy isoflavones are glucoronidated in the intestinal cells prior to entering the bloodstream *(10)*.

Isoflavones in raw soy-food products are typically found conjugated to a glycosidic group. The glucose can be as a 6"-*O*-acetylglucose or a 6"-*O*-malonylglucose with the malonyl form the predominant one in raw soybeans. This structural property is called a β-glycosidic linkage or more commonly a glycone structure. When consumed by humans, glycones are not absorbed from the intestinal tract *(11)*. Cleavage of the sugar moiety by the gut flora creates a compound referred to as an aglycone, resulting in a substantial increase in absorption from the gastrointestinal tract and improved bioavailabilty of consumed soy isoflavones *(11)*.

When isoflavone glycosides are converted to their aglycone forms, the isoflavones are known to be readily absorbed from the intestinal tract; however, until recently, little was known about their bioavailability and pharmacokinetics. King and Bursill *(11)* studied the plasma and urinary kinetics of isoflavones following consumption of a single soy-flour meal. They determined that peak urinary isoflavones were achieved 6–12 h following meal consumption, with peak plasma concentrations of 3.1 μ*M* and 4.1 μ*M* for daidzein and genistein, respectively. Mean urinary recovery was 62 and 22% for daidzein and genistein, respectively. The halftime of elimination for daidzein and genistein was 4.7 and 5.7 h, respectively. Xu and colleagues reported a similar halftime for daidzein and genestein *(12)* Zhang and colleagues *(10)* recently reported that glycitein was more bioavailable than daidzein. Isoflavones undergo degradation by gut microflora, as considerable intersubject variations in fecal isoflavone excretion have been observed *(13,14)*.

The magnitude of the microfloral degradation of the gut isoflavones directly impacts the plasma and urinary level of isoflavones. Human subjects with high rates of isoflavone degradation have low levels in plasma and in fecal and urinary isoflavone excretion. In contrast, subjects with low rates of isoflavone degradation have high levels in plasma and in fecal and urinary isoflavone excretion *(13)*.

3. EFFECTS OF SOY ON CARDIOVASCULAR DISEASE

Asian populations with high soy intakes have CVD rates that are characteristically lower than their counterparts consuming a Western diet *(15)*. When compared to Americans, 40–69-yr-old Japanese have CVD death rates that are six- and eightfold lower for males and females, respectively. It has been suggested that the difference is due to the presence of soy products in the Japanese diet. Soy isoflavones have been proposed to affect several CVD risk factors, exerting their primary effect by improving the plasma lipid profile and the antioxidant capacity of low-density lipoprotein (LDL) particles.

3.1. Effects of Soy on the Lipid Profile

Soy protein and soy isoflavones appear to exert powerful effects on the plasma lipid profile. Soy products are naturally cholesterol free, and their consumption appears to result in a lowering of plasma triglyceride, total- and LDL cholesterol concentrations. A meta-analysis *(16)* on data from 38 studies of human soy–protein consumption where the average intake was 47 g/d soy–protein determined that, when compared to animal protein consumption, soy protein consumption caused (on average) decreases of 10.5% for triglycerides, 9.3% for total cholesterol, and 12.9% for LDL cholesterol. These reductions were observed to be more pronounced in consumers with preexisting hypercholesterolemia.

Raw soy and soy–protein fractions both appear to exert a lipid lowering effect. However, soy products that have been stripped of their isoflavone content tend to be less effective in lowering plasma lipids *(17)*. Furthermore, it has been suggested that the effects associated with soy protein are due to isoflavones that remain associated with soy–protein fractions *(18)*. It has been estimated that soy–protein diets must contain 1.5 mg isoflavone/g soy protein to provide the cholesterol-lowering effects in humans *(19)*.

A theory to explain the lipid-lowering properties of soy was put forward by Forsythe and colleagues *(20)*, who postulated that it occurs because soy consumption increases thyroxine levels. It is known that hypothyroidemia is associated with a reduction in hepatic LDL receptors and hypercholesterolemia from poor removal of circulating LDL cholesterol. Clinically, the condition is reversible when thyroxine is administered. It is possible that soy isoflavones stimulate the production of thyroid-stimulating hormone, resulting in increased thyroxine levels and increased hepatic LDL receptors. Because apolipoprotein B-100 (apo B-100) has a thyroxine-binding site, it is also possible that thyroxine may affect the affinity of LDL for receptor-mediated uptake *(21)*. Although direct thyroxine/soy interactions have not been investigated in humans, pigs maintained on a high-soy diet for 14 wk showed a marked hypocholesterolemia that was associated with significant elevations of plasma thyroxine and thyroid-stimulating hormone *(20)*.

3.2. Effects of Soy on LDL Oxidation

Oxidative damage to LDL particles leads to lipid peroxidation and damage to the apolipoprotein B-100 protein of LDL. This event causes oxidized LDL to be recognized by the scavenger receptors localized within the arterial wall (22). LDL uptake via scavenger receptors is unregulated and is known to cause rapid accumulation of LDL cholesterol, promoting plaque formation. Animal and human studies have determined that dietary antioxidants, such as α-tocopherol, can prevent plaque formation and possibly lead to plaque regression. Soy isoflavones have a hydroxylated diphenolic structure that confers an antioxidant activity relative to the prevention of LDL oxidation (6).

The ability of soy isoflavonoids to improve the antioxidant capacity of apo B-100–containing particles has been recently confirmed by two studies. Rats consuming soy protein isolates for 3 wk develop a VLDL (very-low-density lipoprotein)/LDL fraction that becomes significantly more resistant to oxidative damage, although the antioxidant improvement in the low-genistein group was only slightly less than that observed in the high-genistein group (23). A more recent study of humans consuming soy diets confirmed these observations. Human volunteers were fed soy bars enriched with genistein (12 mg) and diadzein (7 mg) three times daily (6). LDL from soy consumers showed a dramatic increase in resistance to cupric ion-mediated oxidation following 2 wk of soy consumption. This oxidative resistance was not associated with isoflavonoids bound to the LDL particles themselves. The observed protective effect was transient, however, and 12 d following discontinuation of the soy diet, LDL oxidative susceptibility had returned to baseline.

4. SOY EFFECTS ON CANCER

4.1. Breast Cancer

The incidence of breast cancer in Western countries is much greater than in Asian populations where soy intake is relatively high. When Asians convert their diet to that of Western countries, the cancer risk returns to near that of Western countries, although it remains slightly lower (24). Phytoestrogen consumption has been suggested to be the agent responsible for providing soy-linked breast cancer protection. Genistein and daidzein, and possibly their metabolites, have been suggested to affect breast cancer by suppressing tumor initiation and proliferation (4). Furthermore, recent studies indicate that genistein may also inhibit angiogenesis, thus preventing vascularization in cancerous tissues and thereby limiting tumor growth (25). Large-scale randomized clinical trials to determine if soy consumption reduces the risk of breast cancer development have not been performed.

The exact mechanism for the soy-dependent anti-breast cancer effect observed in the epidemiological studies remains to be conclusively determined. Isoflavones, such as genistein, can bind to the estrogen receptor, but binding affinity is only 0.001 that of estrogen *(4)*. However, given that plasma isoflavones reach levels that are in the micromolar range, whereas plasma estrogens are typically in the nanomolar range, these weak estrogenic effects may still be important. Additionally, the plasma isoflavones are present as glucoronides, which appear to have one-tenth the esterogenic receptor binding affinity of isoflavone aglycones *(10)*. Paradoxically, isoflavones are also known to inhibit estrogen from binding to its true receptors; this has been termed an antiestrogenic effect *(5)*. Determination of a chronic effect is also confusing because soy isoflavones have not been found to exert significant effects on circulating hormone levels *(26)*.

Breast cancer risk tends to be higher in women with shorter menstrual cycles *(27)*; significantly, women consuming soy (60 g/d; 45 mg isoflavones/d) have follicular phases that are 2.5 d longer *(28)*. During the follicular cycle, the mitotic index is about four times greater than during the rest of the cycle. This high rate of cell division occurs when tumor initiation is thought to be most likely to occur. By reducing the number of days spent in the high-risk phase, and maximizing the number of days spent in the low-risk portion of the cycle, soy is thought to lower breast cancer risk. However, most studies in this area have been conducted for less than two menstrual cycles, and therefore, the long-term effect is difficult to predict.

4.2. Other Types of Cancer

In addition to its primary effects on breast cancer, soy-containing diets may also have a protective role with respect to other types of cancer. In a case-control study in Hawaii, consumers of a diet rich in soy had significantly fewer cases of endometrial cancer *(29)*. In the rat model, consumption of soybeans and soy flour has been found to reduce the early stages of colon cancer, an effect that may be similar to that observed with respect to human colorectal cancer *(30)*.

Soy diets also appear to beneficially affect prostate cancer development. The disease is far less common in Japan than in the United States *(31)*. When soy-consuming mice are injected with prostate cancer cells, the degree of apoptosis stimulation and inhibition of tumor angiogensis is positively correlated to the level of soy in the diet *(30)*. However, because dietary fat is a known cancer risk factor, and because soy diets are lower in fat content, it has also been suggested that the protective effect may simply be due to a reduction in the fat content of soy consumers *(33)*.

5. EFFECT OF SOY CONSUMPTION ON OSTEOPOROSIS

Osteoporosis is a disease of the elderly where bone density and calcium content is progressively decreased due to osteoclast overactivity, leading to an increase in the pelvic fracture rate especially in postmenopausal women. Epidemiological studies have observed that, when compared with Western populations, bone density is greater and hip fractures less frequent in Asian populations consuming large amounts of soy in the form of tofu, miso, and tempeh. This is despite the generally low levels of milk consumption in Asian populations. Promotion of increased bone density can be achieved with hormone replacement therapy, but increased risks of breast cancer has been an important factor leading investigators to pursue alternatives to estradiol. Raloxifene is a pharmacoligical alternative that shares significant structural similarities to soy isoflavones (34); it inhibits osteoclast activity and bone resorption, promoting increased bone density.

Randomized human trials of soy effects on osteoporosis have also been performed, although outcomes are less definitive. A recent study fed postmenopausal women low and high isoflavone soy protein diets and looked at changes in bone density (35). After 6 mo, the bone density of the lumbar spine was significantly increased in women consuming the high isoflavone diet. However, a recent Dutch study found no correlation between urinary isoflavone consumption and the rate of bone resorption (36). This negative result may also simply reflect a lack of isoflavone consumption in the entire participant population. Given the ease of soy administration and its low cost, if a given amount of soy in the diet could be found to consistently provide protection from osteoporosis in the elderly, health and quality of life could be significantly improved.

Human studies of soy effects on osteoporosis are complicated due to the slow nature of changes in bone density. Rats make useful models for evaluating lifetime effects of soy consumption on osteoporosis. Ovarectomized (lacking endogenous esterogen production) rats fed a 22% soy protein diet were found to have a level of bone loss suppression equivalent to that of estrogen supplemented rats (37). Furthermore, in ovarectomized rats fed a regular isoflavone-rich soy or an isoflavone-depleted soy diet, antiosteoporotic effects were only associated with consumption of the isoflavone-rich diet. These observed effects are possibly due to soy-dependent suppression of osteoclasts (38).

6. MENOPAUSE AND HOT FLUSH SYMPTOMS

Approximately 85% of North American women will experience symptoms of postmenopausal hot flushes. Hot flushes among climacteric women are debilitating symptoms that are typically treated with hormone replacement therapies. Approximately 85% of women with hot flushes experience some relief with estrogen replacement therapy (39); however, this comes at the cost of increased risk for uterine and breast cancer. In contrast to women in the United States, hot flush symptoms are observed only in 25% of climacteric women in Japan (40). It has been suggested that soy protein consumption by Japanese women is responsible for this protective effect.

The effect of soy supplementation on hot flushes in menopausal women was recently evaluated (41). Participants received 60 g/d soy. After 12 wk, soy recipients had significantly fewer hot flushes (reduced by 43%) than did the control group where a 31% reduction was observed. This modest improvement was not associated with changes in plasma hormone levels. In contrast, Murkies and colleagues (42) administered 45 g/d of soy. After 12 wk, significant increases in urinary isoflavone excretion were observed in the soy-supplemented group; significant differences in hot flush symptoms were not observed, however.

Clinical trials examining the efficacy of soy as a treatment for hot flushes have not been conclusive. Given the strength of the existing epidemiological data, future studies will certainly want to clarify the relationship between soy intake and hot flush symptoms. Perhaps the protective effect of soy requires a longer duration to be observed, or perhaps the processing techniques used in the production of the soy protein products used in these studies modified their content of protective compounds.

7. FOOD PROCESSING AND SOY CONTENT

The isoflavone content of foods is largely derived from soybeans although alfalfa and clover sprouts, chickpeas (garbanzo beans) can also provide a source of isoflavones. Recently, an electronic database became available for isoflavone contents of soy foods and soy ingredients and can be accessed at http://www.nal.usda.gov/fnic. Table 1 presents ranges of isoflavone content reported in the database.

Soy oil removed during the defatting process is popular for cooking. It is a common misconception that soy oil is also isoflavone rich. The isoflavone content of most oils is zero because the hydroxyl groups of genistein and diadzein give these isoflavonoids very low lipid solubilities (43). In spite of their lack of isoflavone contents, soy oils may still be beneficial for health because of their cholesterol-free status and their relatively high content of mono- and polyunsaturated fats. A more detailed description of how polyunsaturated fats affect plasma lipid profiles and coronary heart disease risk is found in Chapter 9 by Clarke and Frost, and Chapter 13 by de Deckere.

The isoflavone content of soybeans is quite variable and is a complicating factor with regards to study replication and dietary recommendations (43,44). The isoflavone content of a single Clark cultivar grown in the same location in Illinois on two consecutive years varied by 30%. The isoflavone content of a single cultivar grown in different regions of Illinois during the same year can vary by as much as threefold. Similar variations are also known to occur with respect to cultivars grown in Iowa (45).

Soy-containing foods can be divided into the following categories: ingredients, second-generation food products, and beverages/supplements/flours 1. Each soy product type is associated with a unique processing history isoflavone content. The isoflavone content of foods available in Hawaii

Table 1
Range of Isoflavone Content of Representative Soy Foods (mg/100 g wet weight)

			Total		
	% M[a]	Dein[b]	Gein	Glein	Total
Soybeans	8	9.88–91.30	20.67–134.10	4.80–16.70	36.20–220.90
Soy isolate	5	7.70–68.89	27.17–105.10	5.40–26.40	46.50–199.25
Soy concentrate					
Ethanol washed					
	6	0.79–21.09	1.29–10.73	1.57	2.08–31.82
Water washed					
	3	16.68–91.05	40.29–75.95	4.27–6.05	61.23–167.00
Texturized soy protein					
	5	1.65–123.25	2.75–144.02	15.60–28.28	4.40–295.55
Soy germ	8	855.2	288.3	769.60	1913.10
Kinako (toasted soy flour)					
	5	87.65–119.20	70.74–126.90	14.40–18.40	131.70–260.50
Soymilk	89	1.14–9.84	1.12–11.28	0.36–0.86	1.26–21.13
Tofu A[c]	83	7.35–9.10	11.10–13.80	1.70–2.20	20.15–25.10
Tofu L[d]	86	8.55–13.71	12.85–18.31	2.40–2.40	23.80–32.02
Miso[d]	53	7.10–36.64	11.70–52.39	2.30–3.80	22.70–89.20
Tempeh[e]	61	4.67–27.30	1.11–39.77	0.90–3.20	6.88–62.50
Natto[f]	59	16.02–31.46	21.52–45.53	6.89–13.01	46.40–86.99
Edamame	68	6.62–12.20	5.94–14.40	1.29–4.29	16.49–26.60
Chicken analog[g]					
Raw	74	3.45	7.90	0.85	12.20
Soy hot dog					
Raw	59	1.00–3.40	2.05–8.20	0.30–3.40	3.35–15.00
Soy burger[h]					
Raw	63	2.95	5.28	1.07	9.30
Soy/beef burger[i]					
Raw	63	0.20–0.55	0.35–1.10	0.00–0.10	0.55–1.75

[a]Moisture.

[b]Dein = daidzein; Gein = genistein; Glein = glycitein; Total = moles of isoflavone × molecular weight of isoflavone.

[c]Tofu A = Azumaya, extrafirm, composite; L = Mori-Nu, firm, silken, 6-city composite.

[d]Miso = shiro (white), 6 bag composite from supplier.

[e]Tempeh, raw, 5-city composite, White Wave.

[f]Sumibi natto.

[g]Chicken = Worthington Foods FriChik, 5-city, 2-can/city composite.

[h]Harvest burger.

[i]School lunch USDA commodity patty, 6-patty composite.

Taken from the USDA–Iowa State University Isoflavone Database.

and Singapore was recently evaluated by Franke and colleagues *(47)*. Murphy and colleagues *(48)* reported the isoflavone levels in retail and institutional soy-food samples nationally based on retail sales volume. Soy ingredients, such as soy flour, isolate, and textured vegetable (or soy) protein (TVP) typically have the highest protein content. Soy flour is probably the richest source of isoflavones, with an average dry weight value of 2570 mg/kg. In contrast, soy concentrate, used in many soy analog products, may have no isoflavones because of the ethanol-washing step in its production that removes isoflavones. Soy nuts, produced by roasting or frying soybeans typically have the highest isoflavone content, as the water has been removed from the intact soybean. Traditional soy food products include foods like tofu, tempeh, and miso.

Traditional soy foods tend to have the highest total isoflavone concentrations of all soy food products, with firm unfermented tofu isoflavone content ranging from 297–355 mg/kg. Second-generation tofu products include soy burgers and cheeses; these products have an extremely variable isoflavone content, with soy burgers at 51 mg/kg and from 9–301 mg/kg for cheeses. The isoflavone content of soy protein-enriched drink products have the greatest degree of variability. Soy milk had 35 mg/kg and a soy chocolate shake (Light and Fit) had over 1000 mg/kg. Low- and no-fat soymilks and tofus are produced by adding additional soy protein to dilute out the fat content or by skimming the soymilk, in a process similar to that used for cow's milk processing. When soy protein is added during production, the type of soy added greatly alters the isoflavone content of the product. The isoflavone content of the soy protein can vary from almost zero to reasonable amounts, if soy isolate is used. The consumer has no way to estimate isoflavones in the low- and no-fat products unless the manufacturer makes a claim on the package. Direct food comparisons for these products are further complicated because of their variable water content.

8. CONCLUSIONS

Asian populations have for generations consumed soy as the primary dietary source of protein. Epidemiological studies have determined that, relative to consumers of the traditional Western diet, soy consumers in Asia are well protected from coronary heart disease (CHD), breast cancer, prostate cancer, osteoporosis, and hot flush symptoms. As the dietary habits of Asians change to favor the Western diet, the disease protection that these people once enjoyed is beginning to erode. The traditional Asian diet is lower in cholesterol, saturated fat, and total fat, all of which are associated with promotion of CHD and cancer (for further reviews, *see* Chapter 9 by Clarke and Frost, and Chapter 5 by Clifford and McDonald). However, there is increasing evidence that only part of the health benefit of soy is because of reductions in fat and cholesterol intake.

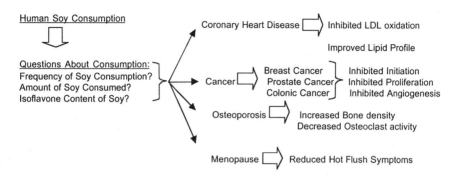

Fig. 2. Review of diseases affected by soy consumption and potential mechanisms.

Soy contains a group of compounds called isoflavones. Epidemiological, animal, and human studies are confirming that isoflavones in soy are responsible for a large part of the protective effects observed in Asian populations. Figure 2 reviews the proposed diseases affected by soy consumption and potential mechanisms. When soy products are depleted of their isoflavone content, they tend to become less effctive or ineffective with respect to cancer and CHD risk factor reduction. When soy isoflavones are studied in animals or humans under in vitro or controlled dietary conditions, protective effects are generally observed with respect to CHD, cancer, osteoporotic, and menopausal symptoms.

Determination of the amount of consumed dietary soy needed to provide these benefits is clouded by the fact that the content of isoflavones in soybeans is highly variable, as is the total content of soy in the foods that are typically eaten in Western countries. The estimate of 48 g soy protein/d of Anderson and associates *(16)* provides a good starting point with respect to the prevention of cardiovascular disease, assuming that the isoflavone content of the soy protein remains intact. This represents a quantity of soy isoflavones that could be obtained in one 100 g serving of tofu or 25 mg of isoflavones. Recently, the FDA has approved a health claim for soy protein and cardiovascular disease prevention at 25 g soy protein per day in 6 g per serving. The isoflavones associated with this level of human consumption would come close to the range of values associated with protection with respect to cancer, osteoporosis, and hot flush symptoms. As we learn more about the relative individual contributions of isoflavones for protection from these diseases, we will undoubtedly be able to fine tune these dietary recommendations.

REFERENCES

1. Alderceutz H, Mazur W. Phyto-oesterogens and western diseases. Ann Med 1997; 29:95–120.
2. Weisburger JH. Dietary fat and risk of chronic disease: mechanistic insights from experimental studies. J Am Diet Assoc 1997; 97(7 Suppl): S16–S23.

3. Klein KO. Isoflavones, soy-based infant formulas and relevance to endocrine function. Nutr Rev 1998; 56:193–204.

4. Zava DT, Duwe G. Estrogenic and antiproliferative properties of genistein and other flavonoids in human breast cancer cells in vitro. Nutr Cancer 1997; 27:31–40.

5. Martinez-Campos A, Amara JF, Dannies P. Antiesterogens are partial esterogen agonists for prolactin production in priomary pituitary cultures. Mol Cell Endocrinol 1986; 48:127–133.

6. Tikkanen MJ, Wahala K, Ojala S, Vihma V, Aldercreutz H. Effect of soybean phytoestrogen intake on low density lipoprotein oxidation resistance. Proc Natl Acad Sci USA 1998; 95:3106–3110.

7. Song T, Hendrich S, Murphy PA. Esterogenic activity of glycitein, a soy isoflavone. J Agric Food Chem 1999; 147:1607–1610.

8. Ruiz-Larrea MB, Mohan AR, Paganga G, Miller NJ, Bolwell GP, Rice-Evans CA. Antioxidant activity of phytoestrogenic isoflavones. Free Rad Res 1997; 26:63–70.

9. Slavin JL, Karr SC, Hutchins AM, Lampe JW. Influence of soybean processing, habitual diet, and soy dose on urinary isoflavonoid excretion. Am J Clin Nutr 1998; 68:1492S–1495S.

10. Zhang Y, Wang G-J, Song TT, Murphy PA, Hendrich S. Differences in disposition of the soybean isoflavones glycitein, diadzein and genestein in humans with moderate fecal isoflavone degradation activity. J Nutr 1999; 129:957–962.

11. King RA, Bursill DB. Plasma and urinary kinetics of the isoflavones daidzein and genistein after a single soy meal in humans. Am J Clin Nutr 1998; 67:867–872.

12. Xu, X, Wang H-J, Cook LR, Murphy PA, Hendrich S. Daidzein is a more bioavailable soymilk isoflavone to young adult women than is genistein. J Nutr 1994; 124:825–832.

13. Hendrich S, Wang G-J, Lin H-K, Xu X, Tew B-Y, Wang H-J, Murphy PA. Isoflavone metabolism and bioavailability. In: Papas AM, ed. Antioxidant Status, Diet, Nutrition, and Health. CRC Press LLC, Boca Raton, FL; 1998, pp. 211–230.

14. Karr SC, Lampe JW, Hutchins AM, Slavin JL. Urinary isoflavonoid excretion in humans is dose dependent at low to moderate levels of soy–protein consumption. Am J Clin Nutr 1997; 66:46–51.

15. Beaglehole R. International trends in heart disease mortality, morbidity, and risk factors. Epidemiol Rev 1990; 12:1–15.

16. Anderson JW, Johnstone BM, Cook-Newell ME. Meta-analysis of the effects of soy protein intake on serum lipids. New Engl J Med 1995; 322:276–282.

17. Anthony MS, Clarckson TB, Bullock BC, Wagner JD. Soy protein versus soy phytoesterogens in prevention on diet-induced coronary artery atherosclerosis of male cynomolgus monkeys. Arterioscler Thromb Vasc Biol 1997; 17:2524–2531.

18. Greaves KA, Parks JS, Williams JK, Wagner JD. Intact dietary soy protein, but not adding an isoflavone-rich extract to casein, improves plasma lipid in ovarectomized cynomolgus monkeys. J Nutr 1999; 129:1585–1592.

19. Crouse JR, Morgan T, Terry JF, Ellis J, Vitolins M, Burke GL. A randomized trial comparing the effect of casein with that of soy protein containing varying amouns of isoflavones on plasma concentrations of lipids and lipoproteins. Arch Intern Med 1999; 159:2070–2076.

20. Forsythe III WA. Soy protein, thyroid regulation and cholesterol metabolism. J Nutr 1995; 125:619S–623S.

21. Benvenga S, Cahnmann HJ, Robbins J. Localization of the thyroxine binding sites in apolipoprotein B-100 of human low density lipoproteins. Endocrinology 1990; 127:2241–2246.

22. Steinberg D. Oxidative modification of low density lipoprotein and atherosclerosis. Circulation. 1997; 95:1062–1071.

23. Anderson JW, Diwadkar VA, Bridges SR. Selective effects of different antioxidants on oxidation of lipoproteins from rats. Proc Soc Exp Biol Med 1998; 218:376–381.

24. Wu AH, Zeigler RG, Nomura AM, West DE, Kolonel LN, Horn-Ross PL, et al. Soy intake and risk of breast cancer in Asians and Asian Americans. Am J Clin Nutr 1998; 68:1437S–1443S.

25. Fotis T, Pepper M, Aldercreutz H, Fleischemann G, Hase T, Montesano R, Scheiger L. Genistein, a dietary-derived inhibitor of in vitro angiogenesis. Proc Natl Acad Sci USA 1993; 90:2690–2694.

26. Duncan AM, Merz BE, Xu X, Nagel TC, Phipps WR, Kurzer MS. Soy isoflavones exert modest hormonal effects in premenopausal women. J Clin Endo Metab 1999; 84:192–197.

27. Olsson H, Landin-Olsson M, Gullberg B. Retrospective assessment of menstrual cycle length in patients with breast cancer, in patients with benign breast disease, and in women without breast disease. J N C I 1983; 70:17–20.

28. Cassidy A, Bingham S, Setchell KDR. Biological effects of a diet of soy protein rich in isoflavones on the menstrual cycle of premenopausal women. Am J Clin Nutr 1994; 60:333–340.

29. Goodman MT, Wilkens LR, Hankin JH, Lyu L-C, Wu AH, Kolonel LN. Association of soy and fiber consumption with the risk of endometrial cancer. Am J Epid 1997; 146:294–306.

30. La Marchand L, Hankin JH, Wilkens LR, Kolonel LN, Englyst HN. Dietary fiber and colorectal cancer risk. Epidemiology 1997; 7:658–665.

31. Messina MJ, Persky V, Stetchell KD, Barnes S. Soy intake and cancer risk: a review of the in vitro and in vivo data. Nurt Cancer 1994; 21:113–131.

32. Zhou JR, Gugger ET, Tanaka T, Guo Y, Blackburn GL, Clinton SK. Soybean phytochemicals inhibit the growth of transplantable human prostate carcinoma and tumor angiogenesis in mice. J Nutr 1999; 129:1628–1635.

33. Fair WR, Fleshner NE, Heston W. Cancer of the prostate: a nutritional disease? Urology 1997; 50:840–848.

34. Balfour, JA, Goa KL. Raloxifene. Drugs Aging 1998; 12:335–341.

35. Potter SM, Baum JA, Teng H, Stillman RJ, Shay NF, Erdman JW. Soy protein and isoflavones: their effects on blood lipids and bone density in postmenopausal women. Am J Clin Nutr 1998; 68:1375S–1379S.

36. Kardinaal AF, Morton MS, Bruggeman-Rogans IE, van Beresteijn EC. Phyto-oestrogen excretion and rate of bone loss in postmenopausal women. Eur J Clin Nutr 1998; 52:850–855.

37. Harrison E, Adjei AA, Ameho C, Yamamoto S, Kono S. The effect of soybean protein on bone loss in a rate model of postmenopausal osteoporosis. J Nutr Sci Vitaminol (Tokyo) 1998; 44:257–268.

38. Gao YH, Yamaguchi M. Suppressive effect of genistein on rat bone osteoclasts: apoptosis is induced through Ca^{2+} signaling. Biol Pharm Bull 1999; 22:805–809.

39. Haas S, Walsh B, Evans S, Krache M, Ravnikar V, Schiff I. The effect of transdermal estradiol on hormone and metabolic dynamics over a 6-week period. Obstet Gynecol 1988; 71:671–676.

40. Notelovitz M. Esterogen replacement therapy indications, contraindications, and agent selection. Am J Obstet Gynecol 1989; 161:8–17.

41. Albertazzi P, Pansini F, Bonaccorsi G, Zanotti L, Forini E, De Alyosio D. The effect of dietary soy supplementation on hot flushes. Obstet Gynecol 1998; 91:6–11.

42. Murkies AL, Wilcox G, Davis SR. Clincal review 92: phytoestrogens. J Clin Endocrinol Metab 1992; 83:297–303.

43. Eldridge, AC, Kwolek WF. Soybean isoflavones: Effect of environment and variety on composition. J Agric Food Chem 1983; 31:394–396.

44. Farmakalidis E, Murphy PA. Isolation of 6"-O-acetygenistein and 6"-O-acetydaidzin from toasted defatted soyflakes. J Agric Food Chem 1985; 33:385–389.

45. Wang H, Murphy PA. Isoflavone composition of American and Japanese soybeans in Iowa: Effects of variety, crop year and location. J Agric Food Chem 1994a; 42:1674–1680.

46. Wang H, Murphy PA. Isoflavone content in commercial soybean foods. J Agric Food Chem 1994b; 42:1666–1673.

47. Franke AA, Hankin JH, Mimi CY, Mastarinec G, Low SH, Custer LJ. Isoflavone levels in soy foods consumed by multiethnic populations in Singapore and Hawaii. J Agric Food Chem 1999; 47:977–986.
48. Murphy PA, Song T, Buseman G, Barua K, Beecher GR, Trainer D, Holden J. Isoflavones in retail and institutional foods. J Agric Food Chem 1999; 47:2697–2704.

7

Antioxidants in Health and Disease

Norman J. Temple and Artur Machner

1. INTRODUCTION

In recent years, two lines of investigation have converged to some extent. A large body of convincing evidence demonstrates that fruits and vegetables are strongly protective against various types of cancer. At the same time, growing evidence reveals an association between the intake of antioxidants, oxidative stress, and various disease states.

There has been a tendency to see antioxidants and fruits and vegetables as merely two sides of the same coin. Although antioxidants undoubtedly provide a partial explanation for the health-giving properties of fruits and vegetables, they are far from the whole story. It is crucially important to bear in mind one of the fundamental rules of epidemiology: association does not mean causation. This was well expressed by Sies *(1)*, who noted that the decline in the stork population of Germany parallels the declining birth rate.

2. BIOCHEMISTRY OF OXIDATIVE STRESS

Sleep, slimness, and sunshine are all fine in the right amount, but they illustrate that you can have too much of a good thing. The same may be said of oxygen: some is good but too much is bad.

Oxidative stress is a condition in which either reactive oxygen species (ROS) or reactive nitrogen species (RNS), or both, overwhelm the body's antioxidant defense mechanisms and start damaging vital cellular components *(2,3)*. This state is reached either by excessive exposure to ROS or RNS, or by inadequate antioxidant defenses.

ROS include free radicals such as superoxide, hydroxyl, peroxyl, alkoxyl, hydroperoxyl, as well as certain highly reactive nonradicals such as hydrogen peroxide, hypochlorous acid, ozone, and singlet oxygen. RNS include some

From: *Nutritional Health: Strategies for Disease Prevention*
Edited by: T. Wilson and N. J. Temple © Humana Press Inc., Totowa, NJ

radicals such as nitric oxide and nitrogen dioxide, in addition to such nonradicals as nitrous acid, dinitrogen tetroxide, peroxynitrite, and the nitronium cation.

As noted, several of the most prominent ROS and RNS are free radicals. They are highly reactive and unstable species that contain one or more unpaired electrons in their atomic orbits. Free radicals can be generated in the body by numerous mechanisms including leakage of electrons from biological membranes; by activated phagocytes such as neutrophils, macrophages, and monocytes; by reactions with polyunsaturated fats; and by reduction of tissue oxygen by transition metals such as copper and iron. In addition, there are various exogenous sources of free radicals including radiation, air pollution, and smoking.

ROS and RNS cause damage to proteins, lipids, and DNA. Antioxidants protect against this damage using four main mechanisms: the sequestration of transition metal ions into complexes, scavenging or quenching free radicals and other ROS and RNS, breaking chain reactions by free radicals, and repairing molecules damaged by free radicals.

Several proteins are known to bind and potentially stabilize transition metals, thereby protecting against oxidative damage. Albumin is the major protein in plasma where it chelates copper and iron. It may also possess some direct free radical scavenging ability. Transferrin is the main iron transport protein in the blood but also carries zinc. Ceruloplasmin chelates copper for transport in the blood. Ferritin and hemoseridin, present in bone marrow, liver, and other organs, are intracellular storage proteins for iron, making it unavailable for catalyzing free radical reactions.

Uric acid is a nitrogenous waste product as an end product of purine metabolism and is ubiquitous in body fluids. It is also very important as a free radical scavenger. According to one estimate, uric acid and albumin are the two major antioxidants in human plasma, contributing 24 and 33%, respectively, of the total antioxidant activity *(4)*.

Reduced glutathione (GSH) is a water-soluble tripeptide that is mainly present inside cells. High levels are found in the lower respiratory tract. This is of particular importance, as air may contain ROS and RNS such as ozone and nitrogen dioxide. GSH is also responsible for providing antioxidant protection to red blood cells.

GSH has numerous other antioxidant properties. It can react directly with ROS and RNS by virtue of its thiol group (–SH). GSH can break the disulfide bridges formed inside and between proteins by the action of oxidants. In its antioxidant action GSH forms an intermolecular disulfide nonradical end product, glutathione disulfide (GSSG). This can either be exported from the cell or transformed back to GSH by the combined action of GSH reducatase and NADPH. GSH also acts as an antioxidant indirectly by regenerating ascorbate (vitamin C) from dehydroascorbate, and α-tocopherol (vitamin E) from a tocopheroxyl radical. This property is very important in maintaining tissue levels of these antioxidant vitamins.

Several enzymes have an important antioxidant function. Glutathione peroxidase breaks down hydrogen peroxide, using GSH and selenium as cofactors. Catalase also breaks down hydrogen peroxide, producing water and oxygen. Superoxide dismutase (SOD) converts superoxide into hydrogen peroxide and oxygen. Equally important to the presence of these antioxidant enzymes are the minerals that serve as cofactors, e.g., zinc, copper, and selenium.

Ascorbate has numerous antioxidant properties. It is able to directly scavenge several free radicals. It acts as a chain-breaking antioxidant in lipid peroxidation. Ascorbate is believed to regenerate vitamin E from its tocopheroxyl radical form, but this requires confirmation. It inhibits nitrosamine carcinogenesis by the direct reduction of that compound, an action that may be important in protection against gastric cancer.

Vitamin E is, in actuality, a group of eight related substances that exhibit the activity of α-tocopherol. Their richest dietary source is seed oils. The vitamin is fat soluble and is located in lipids, the lipid portion of membranes, and lipoproteins. It is highly efficient at protecting polyunsaturated fats in these cellular components from lipid peroxidation by terminating chain reactions and by scavenging ROS. In the process, vitamin E is converted to a tocopheroxyl radical, but can be regenerated by ascorbic acid, by GSH, and by coenzyme Q. Coenzyme Q (ubiquinone) can be obtained from food but can also be synthesized by humans.

Twenty years ago, β-carotene was seen merely as a precursor of retinol (vitamin A). Over 600 related compounds (carotenoids) have been identified, although only 10% can be converted to retinol. It is now known that carotenoids have the capacity to efficiently quench several free radicals, singlet oxygen in particular. They are obtained from a wide range of fruits and vegetables and their antioxidant capacity varies with their structure.

Many phenolic compounds from vegetables and fruits have been suggested to act as antioxidants. One important group is the flavonoids, which are widely distributed in many foods; rich sources are black tea, red wine, cranberry juice, broccoli, onions, and apples. Flavonoids are often associated with pigmentation in plants, although in the case of quercetin in the onion no pigmentation occurs. Two synthetic phenols, BHA (butylated hydroxyanisole) and BHT (butylated hydroxyphenol), have been widely used as food preservatives. They act by preventing lipid peroxidation.

3. OXIDATIVE STRESS AND DISEASE

Many studies have been carried out in which the degree of oxidative stress was determined in different states of body dysfunction. The degree of oxidative stress has been reported based on a variety of measures: low levels of enzymes, which have an antioxidant function; low levels of antioxidant substances (e.g., vitamin E, urate), and raised levels of substances produced as a result of oxidative stress (e.g., damaged DNA, malondialdehyde, F_2-isoprostanes).

DNA is susceptible to damage by ROS and RNS. This produces various chemical modifications of its bases; examples of this are methylation, deamination, and oxidation. However, cells also possess DNA repair systems. Perhaps the most well-known example of an oxidation product apparently leading to disease is that of oxidized low-density lipoprotein (LDL). This oxidative change to LDL is seen as a step on the road to atherosclerosis (*see* Chapter 8 by Woodside and Young) *(5)*.

There are many other pathological conditions associated with oxidative stress, including an impaired immune system and increased risk of infectious disease *(6)*; cancer *(7)*; diabetes (both non-insulin-dependent and insulin-dependent diabetes) *(8,9)*; autoimmune conditions including rheumatoid arthritis *(10)* and ankylosing spondylitis *(8)*; various respiratory diseases *(11)*; eye disease, including cataracts *(12)* and retinal damage leading to age-related macular degeneration *(13)*; Alzheimer's disease *(14)*; and schizophrenia *(15)*.

Hollywood likes to present a black and white view of the world. "Terrorists" fit neatly into that ludicrously simple world view as the epitome of evil, to be destroyed by the superhero. Free radicals seem to have a similar image at the cellular level: disease is reduced to a conflict between free radicals and antioxidants. What we consider now is the extent to which this viewpoint accords with the evidence.

4. FRUIT, VEGETABLES, ANTIOXIDANTS, AND DISEASE

4.1. Cancer

Impressive evidence has emerged in recent years demonstrating the potent protective action of fruit and vegetable consumption against a host of diseases. The most convincing evidence concerns cancer. Well over 200 studies have shown an inverse relationship between the intake of these foods and the risk of most types of cancer *(16)*. The overall risk reduction for cancer is about 40–50% (i.e., based on comparison between those with the highest and lowest intakes) *(17)*.

Another line of investigation has been to assess the relationship between consumption of micronutrients and cancer risk (*see* Chapter 5 by Clifford and McDonald). Numerous studies have shown an inverse relationship between intake of vitamin C and risk of several cancers, especially oral cavity, esophagus, and stomach and, to a lesser extent, colon and lung *(18,19)*. The most well-known association is that for β-carotene. There is a strong inverse association between both dietary intake and blood level on one hand, and the risk of several cancers, especially lung and stomach, on the other *(20)*. Further support for the preventive action of β-carotene has come from intervention studies, which have demonstrated that supplemental doses of the nutrient prevent precancerous changes of the oral cavity *(21,22)* and cause partial regression of precancerous changes of the stomach *(23)*.

The close association between β-carotene intake and cancer risk was the inspiration for three intervention studies, which aimed to prevent cancer by giving supplements. The results from these trials, however, produced not an iota of evidence that β-carotene supplements prevent cancer *(24–28)*. These negative results led to a great deal of debate that is far from over. As a result, attention has shifted to other substances in fruits and vegetables that may account for the cancer-preventive properties of these foods. Carotenoids are still considered prime candidates. In particular, lycopene, the red substance in tomatoes, is attracting much interest because of its pronounced negative association with various cancers, particularly those of the prostate, lung, and stomach *(29)*.

We must not lose sight of the fact that as yet there is no hard evidence that antioxidants are truly involved in the fruit, vegetable, and cancer story. We must again remind ourselves that "association does not prove causation." There are many other substances beside antioxidants that may be the common denominator between fruits, vegetables, and the prevention of cancer. Here are some examples.

The cruciferous vegetables—broccoli, cabbage, cauliflower, and brussels sprouts—contain a group of phytochemicals whose sex appeal has been eclipsed by β-carotene *(30)*. These substances induce the synthesis of detoxifying enzymes, which may help eliminate carcinogens.

A vitamin that has recently emerged as a possible anticarcinogen is folate *(31)*. Fruits and vegetables are an important source. Recently, Zhang and colleagues *(32)* published results from the Nurses' Health Study that showed a strong inverse association between folate intake and risk of breast cancer. However, this was only seen among nurses consuming alcohol. In another report from the Nurses' Health Study Giovannucci and colleagues *(33)* reported that long-term use of folate-containing supplements was associated with a reduced risk of colon cancer. They referred to other correlation studies that have also highlighted the possible protective action of folate against cancer and adenomas of the colon.

Which of the substances discussed here is the most plausible candidate that explains why fruits and vegetables prevent cancer? If this was a multiple-choice exam, the smart answer would be "all the above."

The epidemiological evidence is mostly inconclusive for a protective role for vitamin E in cancer, though it does appear to be negatively associated with colorectal adenomas *(24)*. In one intervention study, 50 mg/d of vitamin E apparently reduced the incidence of prostate and colorectal cancer by 36 and 16%, respectively *(34)*. In another study, 400 mg/d caused partial regression of precancerous changes of the stomach *(23)*. (Note: These doses are far above the usual daily intake; the US RDA is 8–10 mg/d.)

Selenium is another nutrient that functions as a cofactor in several antioxidant systems and merits discussion. Evidence from international correlation studies and from animal experiments strongly supports the view that this mineral has an anticancer action *(24)*. Data from the Health Professionals Follow-Up Study indicate that selenium is protective against prostate cancer *(35)*. One controlled intervention study has been carried out and reported that when a supplement of 200 µg/d was given, total cancer mortality fell by half *(36)*. Clearly, this exciting finding requires confirmation. As noted earlier selenium is a cofactor for the enzyme GSH peroxidase, thereby giving it an antioxidant action. However, it is not known if this is relevant to its anticancer properties.

4.2. Coronary Heart Disease

It has been estimated that increased consumption of fruits and vegetables could potentially reduce levels of coronary heart disease (CHD) by 15% *(37)*. The presumption is that much of this benefit is because antioxidants provided by fruits and vegetables enhance the resistance of LDL to oxidative change (*see* Chapter 8 by Woodside and Young). However, as with cancer, we must be very cautious before concluding that the credit does indeed belong to antioxidants. Certainly, a negative association has been reported between intake of both vitamin C and carotenoids and the risk of CHD *(5)*. A negative association has also been described between intake of carotenoids with vitamin A activity and carotid artery plaques *(38)*. But, as with cancer, these associations might easily reflect confounding by associated substances present in fruits and vegetables. Indeed, the intervention trials that aimed—and failed—to prevent cancer using supplements of β-carotene also showed no beneficial effect with regard to CHD *(26–28)*.

The credit for the relatively low level of CHD in France has often been bestowed on red wine. However, there is a hole in this assumption: evidence from case-control and prospective studies indicates that red wine has no greater protective association with CHD than any other type of alcoholic beverage *(39)*.

Other nutrients contained in fruits and vegetables might play a more important role in explaining why fruits and vegetables help prevent CHD. Evidence, which was reviewed in Chapter 8 by Woodside and Young, suggests that folate may protect against CHD by lowering the blood level of homocysteine. Similarly, Chapter 4 by Weinberger discussed the blood pressure lowering effect of both potassium and of fruits and vegetables. Law and Morris *(37)* recently argued that folate and potassium fully explain the relationship between fruit, vegetables, and CHD.

Results from various epidemiological investigations suggest that vitamin E may be protective against CHD (*see* Chapter 8 by Woodside and Young). In particular, in two prospective studies, total vitamin E intake (diet plus supplements) was inversely associated with risk of CHD *(40,41)*. Moreover, vitamin E is protective against atherosclerosis in experimental animals *(5)*. On the other hand, intervention trials using supplements of vitamin E have failed to provide clear evidence of protection *(37; see* Chapter 8 by Woodside and Young).

4.3. Antioxidants and Other Diseases

Evidence from case-control and prospective studies suggests that vitamin C protects against cataracts *(12)*, asthma *(11)*, and loss of pulmonary function *(42)*. But we cannot conclude from such evidence that we are looking at cause-and-effect relationships. It is at least as likely that these are merely more examples of confounding, and that the true protective factors are substances closely associated in the diet with vitamin C. In the case of vitamin C and asthma, however, there is some evidence from intervention studies that vitamin C itself is protective *(11)*.

Studies in diabetics have indicated a beneficial action of supplemental vitamin E based on lowered levels of triglyceride and glycosylated hemoglobin (an index of blood glucose) *(43)*. In addition, supplemental vitamin E reportedly improves immune function *(6)*.

4.4. How Important Are Antioxidants?

Everyone knows that if we stop breathing, the effects are seriously unpleasant. But it would be wrong to conclude that we should therefore breathe deeply. So it is with oxidative stress. Because oxidative stress is associated with various disease states, we cannot necessarily conclude that consuming more antioxidants will make us healthier. Indeed, ascorbate and various other flavonoids also have prooxidant activity, especially at high concentrations and in the presence of iron or copper. This emphasizes that it is simplistic to say that antioxidants always act for the good.

Everything is a matter of balance. Over millions of years of evolution, animals have developed systems that maintain a delicate balance between the need for oxygen and the harm done by oxidative stress. When we shift the balance in favor of oxidative stress by breathing polluted air, smoking, taking excess iron, or being deficient in antioxidant nutrients, we certainly do harm. But it does not automatically follow that more antioxidants mean less oxidative stress and better health. As a rule, when we shift the balance in a natural system by meddling, the result is usually both unpredictable and unwelcome. This probably explains why large supplements of β-carotene appear to do more harm than good: they somehow upset the natural balance. If the health of nonsmoking individuals who eat a well-balanced diet could be improved simply by quenching oxidative stress with antioxidants, this would beg the following question: Why did evolution not do a better job of protecting humans by increasing the tissue concentration of antioxidants?

If oxidative stress played a major role in disease, then we should expect clear evidence that supplements of antioxidants prevent disease. But this is simply not the case. The failure of supplements of β-carotene to prevent cancer and CHD was discussed earlier. Three randomized trials have been conducted in which elderly subjects received vitamin C (50–200 mg/d) or placebo for periods of 6 mo–2 yr *(44)*. The overall relative risk showed an increase in mortality of 8%

(not significant). On the positive side, supplemental doses of β-carotene and vitamin C each reportedly improve immune functioning *(6)* and help prevent oxidative damage of DNA *(45,46)*.

Evidence that was discussed previously suggests that relatively high doses of vitamin E, in the range 50–500 mg/d (i.e., many times more than can be obtained from the diet), may reduce the risk of cancer, CHD, and other diseases. However, we must stress the lack of clear evidence that vitamin E will prevent any disease.

Combining the evidence from studies of β-carotene and vitamins C and E, these antioxidants have very limited potency in disease prevention. The obvious inference from this is that if augmenting the body's antioxidant defenses does little to prevent disease, then conversely, oxidative stress plays only a minor role in disease causation. Halliwell *(2,3)* also cautioned against jumping to the conclusion that oxidative stress has a causal role in disease. He pointed out that oxidative stress might often be a consequence of tissue injury rather than a cause of it. However, as discussed earlier, we have convincing evidence that oxidative stress is associated with various diseases. It seems unlikely that we can have so much smoke without at least a small fire. The interrelationships between nutrients, oxidative stress, and disease described in this chapter can probably best be explained as the sum of the following:

1. First, oxidative stress does have a certain role in disease. Our environment contributes an excessive burden of oxidative stress (e.g., cigarette smoke and pollution). Simultaneously, large numbers of people have a suboptimal intake of antioxidants. As a result of the combined effect of these two problems, there is very commonly an imbalance between oxidative stress and tissue level of antioxidants. This may be part of the reason why fruits and vegetables help prevent cancer and other diseases.

2. A diet rich in fruits and vegetables provides an increased intake of particular nutrients that are often consumed in suboptimal amounts and that help prevent disease by mechanisms unrelated to oxidative stress. For instance, folate and potassium are especially important in connection with CHD and hypertension.

3. Phytochemicals, obtained from a wide variety of foods, play an important, though poorly understood, role in health protection. They have diverse properties, including acting as antioxidants. For instance, in Chapter 6, Wilson and Murphy described soy isoflavones and how their estrogenic action may help prevent cancer and CHD. Flavonoids are a related family of phytochemicals that have been credited with disease-preventing properties. It has been speculated that flavonoids may protect against CHD, but the supporting evidence is far from clear *(47)*. As discussed earlier, cruciferous vegetables (broccoli, cabbage, cauliflower, and brussels sprouts) contain phytochemicals that have been credited with anticarcinogenic properties. The phytochemicals are almost certainly an important reason why fruits and vegetables (and the antioxidants they contain) manifest such a strong protective association with disease, especially with cancer.

In 1927, Heisenberg, a great physicist, formulated his uncertainty principle as follows: "The more precisely we determine the position, the more imprecise is the determination of velocity in this instant." Perhaps we should formulate an analogous uncertainty principle with regard to the problem of how fruits and vegetables prevent disease: "The more precisely we study specific nutrients and phytochemicals, the more imprecisely can we determine their role in disease."

5. FUTURE INTERVENTION TRIALS

Much medical research can be characterized as "reductionism," the strategy of attempting to explain the whole in terms of the sum of the parts. In some cases, as with the relationship between folate and neural tube defects, this approach has been successful. In the great majority of cases, however, the complete picture remains elusive. So it is likely to prove with the relationship between fruit, vegetables, and health: there are simply too many factors that may plausibly be involved. Epidemiological studies can only take us so far because a diet rich in fruits and vegetables is also rich in hundreds of substances that these foods contain, therefore making it extremely difficult to identify the protective substances. Intervention trials that test individual substances are also limited in their usefulness, as it is not feasible to separately test all promising substances.

The foregoing arguments dictate that the most appropriate strategy for future intervention trials is supplementation with mixtures of fruits and vegetables (MFV) *(48)*. Let us start with cancer. A person planning an intervention trial using just one or two substances has the daunting task of selecting the most promising agents. But, as stressed above, we really do not know what substances deserve the credit for the anticarcinogenic potency of fruits and vegetables. Indeed, the true protective agent might not yet have been discovered. Even if we were to carry out dozens of long-term intervention trials using pure substances, we may still miss the real answer, as protection may very well come not from a "magic bullet," but from a "team" of substances, each of which is needed for optimal effectiveness. Such trials could therefore end up being no more successful than those using β-carotene. However, using MFV ensures that all active ingredients are present, whether they are merely one or two substances or a hundred.

There are additional reasons why it makes sense to use MFV. As discussed earlier fruits and vegetables also help prevent CHD and remedy hypertension. The most likely substances responsible for this, folate and potassium, are almost certainly different than those responsible for the anticarcinogenic effect. Therefore, the use of MFV is the one sure way to prevent both cancer and CHD while also treating hypertension. The case becomes even stronger when we consider other conditions related to oxidative stress. Cataracts have a negative association with vitamin C intake but, in reality, we have little hard evidence as to the true protective substances. MFV should also prove an effective prophylactic agent for this condition.

6. WHERE ARE WE AT?

A person navigating through the world of antioxidants might feel somewhat like Christopher Columbus: when he left, he did not know where he was going, when he got there, he did not know where he was, and when he got back he did not know where he had been.

Ideally, we would like to formulate a supplement that provides a safe, cheap, and effective means to prevent degenerative diseases and to help preserve bodily functions into old age. Clearly, we are still a long way from that goal. What we do have is an excellent substitute: fruits and vegetables. Although we have overwhelming evidence for advising a generous intake of these foods, the evidence is scanty and contentious that supplements of the antioxidant nutrients and phytochemicals provided by these foods (such as vitamin C and the carotenoids) will prevent disease.

The same may be said of whole grains. Evidence from may case-control studies on cancer *(49,50)* and a prospective study on CHD *(51)* indicates that a generous intake of whole grains reduces the risk of both diseases by about one-third. However, we are still far from being able to formulate a supplement that will duplicate these benefits.

This is not to deny that there are some promising leads. As discussed earlier, we have suggestive evidence that lycopene, selenium, and (in high doses) vitamin E may all have a protective action against disease, especially cancer. It would be premature, however, to conclude that supplements of these should be recommended. One obvious danger is that supplements may give a false sense of security and detract from a healthy diet.

REFERENCES

1. Sies H. A new parameter for sex education. Nature 1988; 332:337.
2. Halliwell B. Free radicals, antioxidants and human disease: curiosity, cause or consequence? Lancet 1994; 344:721–724.
3. Halliwell B. Antioxidants in human health and disease. Ann Rev Nutr 1996; 16:33–50.
4. Miller NJ, Rice-Evans CA. Spectrophotometric determination of antioxidant activity. Redox Report 1996; 2:161–171.
5. Kritchevsky D, Kritchevsky SB. Antioxidants and their role in coronary heart disease prevention. In: Basu TK, Temple NJ, Garg ML, eds. Antioxidants in Human Health and Disease. CAB International, Wallingford, Oxon, UK, 1999, pp. 151–164.
6. Bendich A. Immunological role of antioxidant vitamins. In: Basu TK, Temple NJ, Garg ML, eds. Antioxidants in Human Health and Disease. CAB International, Wallingford, Oxon, UK, 1999, pp. 27–41.
7. Ames BN, Shigenaga MK, Hagen TM. Oxidants, antioxidants and the degenerative diseases of aging. Proc Natl Acad Sci, USA 1993; 90:7915–7922.
8. Dusinska M, Lietava J, Olmedilla B, Raslova K, Southon S, Collins AR. Indicators of oxidative stress, antioxidants and human health. In: Basu TK, Temple NJ, Garg ML, eds. Antioxidants in Human Health and Disease. CAB International, Wallingford, Oxon, UK, 1999, pp. 411–422.
9. Hannon-Fletcher M, Hughes C, O'Kane MJ, Moles KW, Barnett CR, Barnett YA. An investigation of in vivo antioxidant status and DNA damage in patients with IDDM. In: Basu TK, Temple NJ, Garg ML, eds. Antioxidants in Human Health and Disease. CAB International, Wallingford, Oxon, UK, 1999, pp. 259–269.

10. Halliwell B. Oxygen radicals, nitric oxide and human inflammatory joint disease. Ann Rheum Dis 1995; 54:505–510.
11. Young IS, Roxborough HE, Woodside JV. Antioxidants and respiratory disease. In: Basu TK, Temple NJ, Garg ML, eds. Antioxidants in Human Health and Disease. CAB International, Wallingford, Oxon, UK, 1999, pp. 293–311.
12. Taylor A, Jacques P, Epstein E. Nutrition and the risk of cataract. In: Basu TK, Temple NJ, Garg ML, eds. Antioxidants in Human Health and Disease. CAB International, Wallingford, Oxon, UK, 1999, pp. 271–284.
13. Nath R, Gupta A, Prasad R, Pandav SS, Thakur R. Reactive oxygen species and age-related macular degeneration. In: Basu TK, Temple NJ, Garg ML, eds. Antioxidants in Human Health and Disease. CAB International, Wallingford, Oxon, UK, 1999, pp. 285–292.
14. Martins RN, Chan CW, Waddington E, Veurink G, Laws S, Croft K, Dharmarajan AM, Beta-amyloid and oxidative stress in the pathogenesis of Alzheimer's disease. In: Basu TK, Temple NJ, Garg ML, eds. Antioxidants in Human Health and Disease. CAB International, Wallingford, Oxon, UK, 1999, pp. 367–391.
15. Reddy R, Yao JK. Schizophrenia: role of oxidative stress and essential fatty acids. In: Basu TK, Temple NJ, Garg ML, eds. Antioxidants in Human Health and Disease. CAB International, Wallingford, Oxon, UK, 1999, pp. 351–366.
16. Steinmetz KA, Potter JD. Vegetables, fruit, and cancer prevention: a review. J Am Diet Assoc 1996; 96:1027–1039.
17. Block G, Patterson BH, Subar AF. Fruit, vegetables, and cancer prevention: a review of the epidemiological evidence. Nutr Cancer 1992; 18:1–29.
18. Block G. Vitamin C and cancer prevention: the epidemiological evidence. Am J Clin Nutr 1991; 53:270S–282S.
19. Byers T, Guerrero N. Epidemiologic evidence for vitamin C and vitamin E in cancer prevention. Am J Clin Nutr 1995; 62:1385S–1392S.
20. Van Poppel G, Goldbohm RA. Epidemiologic evidence for β-carotene and cancer prevention. Am J Clin Nutr 1995; 62:1393S–1402S.
21. Garewal HS, Meyskens FL, Killen D, Reeves D, Kiersch TA, Elletson H, et al. Response of oral leukoplakia to β-carotene. J Clin Oncol 1990; 8:1715–1720.
22. Stitch HF, Stitch W, Rosin MP, Vallejera MO. Use of the micronucleus test to monitor the effect of vitamin A, beta-carotene and canthaxanthin on the buccal mucosa of betel nut/tobacco chewers. Int J Cancer 1984; 34:745–750.
23. Bukin YV, Draudin-Krylenko VA. The role of carotene and vitamin E in the treatment of early gastric premalignant lesions: biochemical and clinical aspects. In: Basu TK, Temple NJ, Garg ML, eds. Antioxidants in Human Health and Disease. CAB International, Wallingford, Oxon, UK, 1999, pp. 235–248.
24. Greenwald P, McDonald SS. Antioxidants and the prevention of cancer. In: Basu TK, Temple NJ, Garg ML, eds. Antioxidants in Human Health and Disease. CAB International, Wallingford, Oxon, UK, 1999, pp. 217–234.
25. Omenn GS, Goodman GE, Thornquist MD, Balmes J, Cullen MR, Glass A, et al. Risk factors for lung cancer and for intervention effects in CARET, the β-Carotene and Retinol Efficacy Trial. J Natl Cancer Inst 1996; 88:1550–1559.
26. Hennekens CH, Buring JE, Manson JE, Stampfer M, Rosner B, Cook NR, et al. Lack of effect of long-term supplementation with carotene on the incidence of malignant neoplasms and cardiovascular disease. N Engl J Med 1996; 334:1145–1149.
27. Omenn GS, Goodman GE, Thornquist MD, Balmes J, Cullen MR, Glass A, et al. Effects of a combination of carotene and vitamin A on lung cancer and cardiovascular disease. N Engl J Med 1996; 334:1150–1155.
28. Alpha-Tocopherol Beta-Carotene Cancer Prevention Study Group. The effect of vitamin E and carotene on the incidence of lung cancer and other cancers in male smokers. N Engl J Med 1994; 330:1029–1035.

29. Giovannucci E. Tomatoes, tomato-based products, lycopene, and cancer: review of the epidemiological literature. J Natl Cancer Inst 1999; 91:317–332.

30. Nestle M. Broccoli sprouts in cancer prevention. Nutr Rev 1998; 56:127–130.

31. Mason JB, Levesque T. Folate: effects on carcinogenesis and the potential for cancer chemoprevention. Oncology 1996; 10:1727–1743.

32. Zhang S, Hunter DJ, Hankinson SE, Giovannucci EL, Rosner BA, Colditz GA, et al. A prospective study of folate intake and the risk of breast cancer. JAMA 1999; 281:1632–1637.

33. Giovannucci E, Stampfer MJ, Colditz GA, Hunter DJ, Fuchs C, Rosner BA, et al. Multivitamin use, folate, and colon cancer in women in the Nurses' Health Study. Ann Intern Med 1998; 129:517–524.

34. Heinonen OP, Albanes D, Virtamo J, Taylor PR, Huttenen JK, Hartman AM, et al. Prostate cancer and supplementation with α-tocopherol and β-carotene: incidence and mortality in a controlled trial. J Natl Cancer Inst 1998; 90:440–446.

35. Yoshizawa K, Willett WC, Morris SJ, Stampfer MJ, Spiegelman D, Rimm EB, Giovannucci E. Study of prediagnostic selenium level in toenails and the risk of advanced prostate cancer. J Natl Cancer Inst 1998; 90:1219–1224.

36. Clark LC, Combs GF, Turnbull BW, Slate EH, Chalker DK, Chow J, et al. Effects of selenium supplementation for cancer prevention in patients with carcinoma of the skin. JAMA 1996; 276:1957–1963.

37. Law MR, Morris JK. By how much does fruit and vegetable consumption lower the risk of ischaemic heart disease? Eur J Clin Nutr 1998; 52:549–556.

38. Kritchevsky SB, Tell GS, Shimakawa T, Dennis B, Li R, Kohlmeier L, Steere E, Heiss G. Provitamin A carotenoid intake and carotid artery plaques: the Atherosclerosis Risk in the Communities Study. Am J Clin Nutr 1998; 68:726–733.

39. Rimm EB, Klatsky A, Grobbee D, Stampfer MJ. Review of moderate alcohol consumption and reduced risk of coronary heart disease: is the effect due to beer, wine, or spirits? BMJ 1996; 312:731–736.

40. Rimm EB, Stampfer MJ, Ascherio A, Giovannucci E, Colditz GA, Willett WC. Vitamin E consumption and the risk of coronary heart disease in men. N Engl Med 1993; 328:1450–1456.

41. Stampfer MJ, Hennekens CH, Manson JE, Colditz GA, Rosner GA, Willett WC. Vitamin E consumption and the risk of coronary disease in women. N Engl J Med 1993; 328:1444–1449.

42. Hu G, Zhang X, Chen J, Peto R, Campbell TC, Cassano PA. Dietary vitamin C intake and lung function in rural China. Am J Epidemiol 1998; 148:594–599.

43. Jain SK. Oxidative stress, vitamin E and diabetes. In: Basu TK, Temple NJ, Garg ML, eds. Antioxidants in Human Health and Disease. CAB International, Wallingford, Oxon, UK, 1999, pp. 249–257.

44. Ness A, Egger M, Davey Smith G. Role of antioxidant vitamins in prevention of cardiovascular diseases. BMJ 1999; 319:577.

45. Duthie SJ, Ma A, Ross MA, Collins AR. Antioxidant supplementation decreases oxidative DNA damage in human lymphocytes. Cancer Res 1996; 56:1291–1295.

46. Panayiotidis M, Collins AR. Ex vivo assessment of lymphocyte antioxidant status using the comet assay. Free Radic Res 1997; 27:533–537.

47. Temple NJ. Dietary flavonoid intake and risk of cardiovascular disease in postmenopausal women. Am J Epidemiol 2000;151:634.

48. Temple NJ. Fruit, vegetables, and cancer prevention trials. J Natl Cancer Inst 1999; 91:1164.

49. Jacobs DR, Marquart L, Slavin J, Kushi LH. Whole-grain intake and cancer: an expanded review and meta-analysis. Nutr Cancer 1998; 30:85–96.

50. Chatenoud L, Tavani A, La Vecchia C, Jacobs DR, Negri E, Levi F, Franceschi S. Whole grain food intake and cancer risk. Int J Cancer 1998; 77:24–28.

51. Jacobs DR, Meyer KA, Kushi LH, Folsom AR. Whole-grain intake may reduce the risk of ischemic heart disease death in postmenopausal women: the Iowa Women's Health Study. Am J Clin Nutr 1998; 68:248–257.

8 Dietary Antioxidants and Protection from Coronary Heart Disease

Jayne V. Woodside and Ian S. Young

1. INTRODUCTION

This chapter discusses evidence linking antioxidant nutrients with the inhibition of low-density lipoprotein (LDL) oxidation. The possibility that increasing antioxidant intake could protect against coronary heart disease (CHD) is reviewed. The chapter also provides information regarding what ideal antioxidant intakes should be.

Hypercholesterolemia is universally accepted as a major risk factor for atherosclerosis. However, at any given concentration of plasma cholesterol, there is still great variability in the occurrence of cardiovascular events. One of the major breakthroughs in atherogenesis research has been the realization that oxidative modification of LDL may be a critically important step in the development of the atherosclerotic plaque. The formation of foam cells from monocyte-derived macrophages in early atherosclerotic lesions is not caused by native LDL but only following modification of LDL by various chemical reactions such as oxidation *(1; see* Fig. 1).

The cholesterol-laden foam cell is a characteristic feature of the atherosclerotic lesion. The rapid uptake of oxidatively modified LDL occurs through scavenger receptors, which are not down regulated by cholesterol accumulation *(2)*. Recognition of LDL by the scavenger receptor depends on alteration of key lysine residues of apolipoprotein B, which can be brought about by aldehydes produced during the spontaneous decomposition of lipid hydroperoxides *(3)*.

Some reports have suggested the presence of oxidatively modified LDL in plasma *(4)*, but most oxidation is believed to occur in the arterial wall. There, LDL may be in a microenvironment where the antioxidants, which normally prevent lipid peroxidation, can become depleted. All the cells of the vessel wall—endothelial cells, smooth muscle cells, macrophages, and lymphocytes—can modify LDL in vitro *(5–7)*. LDL oxidation is believed to be caused by highly

From: *Nutritional Health: Strategies for Disease Prevention*
Edited by: T. Wilson and N. J. Temple © Humana Press Inc., Totowa, NJ

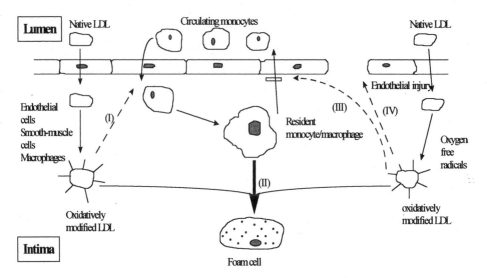

Fig. 1. Mechanisms by which oxidation of LDL may contribute to atherogenesis. Oxidized LDL is chemotactic for circulating monocytes (I), which are phenotypically modified and become macrophages. Oxidized LDL is recognized by the scavenger receptor on the macrophage and becomes internalized rapidly. As more lipid is ingested by the macrophage, a foam cell is formed (II). This eventually bursts and a fatty streak, the first phase of an atherosclerotic lesion, results. Oxidized LDL inhibits the motility of resident macrophages and therefore their ability to leave the intima (III). Oxidized LDL is cytotoxic to endothelial cells, leading directly to endothelial cell damage (IV). Oxidation can occur via the effects of reactive oxygen species or due to the oxidation of the cell's own lipids. Adapted from Steinberg et al. (1989). *(123)*

reactive free radicals but the nature and source of these have yet to be fully defined. Several mechanisms are likely to be involved, including transition metal ion-mediated generation of hydroxyl radicals *(8)*, production of reactive oxygen species by enzymes such as myeloperoxidase and lipoxygenase, and direct modification by reactive nitrogen species *(9)*.

Oxidized LDL may also be atherogenic by mechanisms other than its rapid uptake into macrophages via the scavenger receptor. Oxidized forms of LDL are chemotactic for circulating macrophages and smooth muscle cells and facilitate monocyte adhesion to the endothelium and entry into the subendothelial space *(11)*. Oxidized LDL is also cytotoxic toward arterial endothelial cells and inhibits the release of nitric oxide and the resulting endothelium-dependent vasodilation *(13)*. There is therefore a potential role for oxidized LDL in altering vasomotor responses, perhaps contributing to vasospasm in diseased vessels. In addition, oxidized LDL is immunogenic; autoantibodies against various epitopes of oxidized LDL have been found in human serum, and immunoglobulin (IgG) specific for epitopes of oxidized LDL can be found in lesions *(14,15)*. Oxidized LDL may be able to induce arterial wall cells to produce chemotactic factors, adhesion molecules, cytokine, and growth factors that have an important role in the development of the plaque *(16)*.

Evidence for LDL oxidation in vivo is now well established. In immunocytochemical studies, antibodies against oxidized LDL stain atherosclerotic lesions but not normal arterial tissue *(17)*. LDL extracted from animal and human lesions has been shown to be oxidized and is rapidly taken up by macrophage scavenger receptors *(18)*. In young myocardial infarction (MI) survivors, an association has been demonstrated between increased susceptibility of LDL to oxidation and the degree of coronary atherosclerosis *(19)*, while the presence of ceroid, a product of lipid peroxidation, has been shown in advanced atherosclerotic plaques *(20)*. A recent study, however, has suggested that atherosclerotic plaques contain very little oxidized LDL compared to the amounts of activated complement and enzymatically altered LDL *(21,22)*, an observation that requires further study.

2. DIETARY ANTIOXIDANTS AND LDL OXIDATION

The role of dietary factors in protecting against the change from native to oxidized LDL has received considerable attention. The antioxidant vitamins are derived from fresh fruits and vegetables, and from vegetable oil and polyunsaturated margarine to which vitamin E is usually added as an antioxidant; they cannot be synthesized from simple precursors. Thus, dietary intake, absorption, metabolism, and storage determine concentrations of vitamins in plasma and body tissues. An overview of epidemiological research suggests that individuals with the highest intake of antioxidant vitamins, whether through diet or supplements, tend to experience 20–40% lower risks of CHD than those with the lowest intake or blood levels *(23)*. Vitamin E is the major lipid-soluble antioxidant present in LDL, preventing the formation of lipid hydroperoxides from polyunsaturated fatty acids. Vitamin C can scavenge free radicals in the aqueous phase and may also regenerate vitamin E *(24)*. β-Carotene, a vitamin A precursor, does not have a confirmed antioxidant mechanism *(25)*, although it and other carotenoids are contained within LDL *(26)*. There is some evidence that carotenoids may protect LDL against oxidation more efficiently at low pO_2 levels, which could have relevance to the levels of protection provided in the arterial wall in vivo.

When LDL is exposed to oxidative stress in vitro, lipid peroxidation can only proceed after the sequential loss of its antioxidants in the order ubiquinol-10, α-tocopherol, γ-tocopherol, lycopene, and β-carotene *(27–29)*. Accordingly, LDL supplemented with vitamin E in vitro *(27,30)* or in vivo *(31)* is much harder to oxidize in vitro. Similarly, the α-tocopherol content of the LDL has been shown to be the most important determinant of susceptibility to oxidation in an in vitro model *(32)*.

In addition to antioxidant content of LDL, several other factors can influence the susceptibility to oxidation. Polyunsaturated fatty acids appear to be the most vulnerable moiety following the application of oxidative stress. The fatty acid composition of the diet is, therefore, an important factor determining the susceptibility of LDL to oxidation, with monounsaturated fatty acids protecting LDL against oxidation (33). Small dense LDL particles are also easier to oxidize than more buoyant particles (34). The binding of LDL particles to proteoglycans, glycation, and the presence of preformed lipid peroxides are also important factors (35).

3. INTERVENTION STUDIES IN ANIMALS

Studies of antioxidant supplementation in laboratory animals have provided evidence of the importance of oxidized LDL in vivo. Many such studies have been performed, and they generally provide support for the antioxidant hypothesis. For example, in a study in atherosclerotic rabbits, uptake of LDL into foam cells was approx 4 times greater for oxidized LDL than for native LDL. Adding of vitamin E to the system resulted in a 30–55% decrease in accumulated radiolabeled LDL in plaques and foam cells (36,37). The effects of a diet high in saturated fat with and without fruits and vegetables and antioxidant vitamins (C, E, and β-carotene) on oxidative stress and development of atherosclerosis has also been evaluated in rabbits. Blood lipid peroxide levels decreased significantly in rabbits supplemented with fruits and vegetables or antioxidant vitamins. In contrast, blood lipid peroxide levels increased significantly in the unsupplemented groups and precipitated coronary thrombosis (38).

4. INTERVENTION STUDIES IN HUMANS
WITH BIOCHEMICAL ENDPOINTS

A number of studies have evaluated the effects of vitamin E on copper-catalyzed LDL oxidation in healthy volunteers. In one study, men supplemented with 268, 537, or 805 mg vitamin E per day for 8 wk showed a decreased susceptibility of LDL to oxidation. There was no significant effect of daily supplementation with 40 or 134 mg (39). In a study of the effects of low-dose vitamin E supplementation (100 mg/d for 1 wk, then 200 mg/d for 3 wk), there was a significant increase in lag time before the onset of LDL oxidation and a significant decrease in the propagation rate (40). Princen and associates (41) have evaluated the minimal supplementary dose of vitamin E necessary to protect LDL against oxidation in vitro in healthy young adults. Resistance of LDL to oxidation increased in a dose-dependent manner with resistance time differing significantly from baseline even after ingestion of only 17 mg/d of vitamin E. However, the progression of lipid peroxidation in LDL was only reduced after intake of 268 and 536 mg/d. In a study of 200 mg α-tocopherol supplementation over a 2-mo period in smoking men, lag time was increased in LDL + VLDL after both copper induction and hemin/hydrogen peroxide induction. Plasma α-tocopherol, VLDL + LDL α-tocopherol, and LDL total antioxidant capacity were all increased in the intervention group *(42)*. Vitamin E supplementation appears to promote a clear reduction in the susceptibility of LDL to oxidation. The case for β-carotene and vitamin C, however, is less clear cut.

The effect of high-dose vitamin C supplementation (1000 mg/d) on LDL oxidation was evaluated in a study of 19 smokers. The vitamin C-supplemented group had a significant reduction in the susceptibility of LDL to oxidation after 4 wk *(43)*. Two months of vitamin C supplementation with freshly squeezed orange juice (estimated 500 mg/d) also produced a significant increase in lag time in 36 healthy males consuming a diet high in saturated fatty acids *(44)*. Jialal and associates *(45)* found that supplementation with β-carotene (1–2 μmol) inhibited the oxidative modification of LDL in healthy subjects. By contrast, Lin and colleagues *(46)* reported that a natural-food diet containing 0.93 μmol β-carotene per day was insufficient to alter either plasma or LDL β-carotene or carbonyl groups in LDL. A higher dose of 6.2 μmol β-carotene per day did increase both plasma and LDL β-carotene and reduce LDL carbonyl production.

When the effectiveness of β-carotene, vitamin C, and vitamin E supplements were compared by Reaven and associates *(31)*, susceptibility of LDL to oxidation did not change during β-carotene supplementation (60 mg/d) but decreased 30–40% with the addition of a vitamin E supplement (1600 mg/d). Addition of vitamin C supplementation (2 g/d) did not further reduce the susceptibility to oxidation. In another study, a combined supplement—β-carotene (30 mg/d), vitamin C (1 g/d), and vitamin E (530 mg/d)—was given to men for 3 mo. It produced a twofold prolongation of the lag phase of LDL oxidation and a 40% reduction in the oxidation rate *(47)*. The effects of combined antioxidant supplementation were not significantly different from the effects of vitamin E supplementation alone. Finally, we have recently shown that a combination of low-dose antioxidant vitamins (150 mg ascorbic acid, 67 mg α-tocopherol, 9 mg β-carotene daily) over a period of 8 wk significantly prolonged the lag time to oxidation *(48)*.

The effects of antioxidant supplementation on LDL oxidation may depend on smoking status. In a group of smokers and nonsmokers, resistance of LDL to oxidation increased significantly and the rate of LDL oxidation decreased significantly after vitamin E supplementation (671 mg/d for 7 d). There was some indication of a small increase in the resistance of LDL to oxidation in smokers after supplementation with β-carotene (20 mg/d for 2 wk, then 40 mg/d for 12 wk) *(49)*.

In summary, therefore, experimental evidence suggests that antioxidant vitamins can reduce the susceptibility of LDL to oxidation in vitro. Vitamin E would appear to be the most effective antioxidant; both β-carotene and vitamin C have produced extensions in lag time to oxidation only in a minority of studies, although it remains possible that they may have a beneficial effect in individuals with poor baseline status.

5. EPIDEMIOLOGICAL STUDIES LINKING ANTIOXIDANTS AND LDL OXIDATION

5.1. Vitamin E

Two large longitudinal studies in the United States examined the association between vitamin E intake and risk of CHD (50,51). In a group of 39,910 male health professionals, those who took vitamin E supplements in doses of at least 100 IU per day for over 2 yr had a 37% lower relative risk of CHD compared to men who did not take vitamin E supplements, after adjustment for age, coronary risk factors, and intake of vitamin C and β-carotene. In the Nurses' Health Study of 87,245 female nurses, women who took vitamin E supplements for more than 2 yr had a 41% lower relative risk of major coronary disease. This effect persisted after adjustment for age, smoking, obesity, exercise, blood pressure, plasma cholesterol, and use of postmenopausal estrogen replacement, aspirin, vitamin C, and β-carotene (51).

It must be noted that this effect was limited to vitamin E supplement use. High vitamin E intakes from dietary sources were not associated with a significant decrease in risk, although even the highest dietary vitamin E intakes were far lower than intakes among supplement users (51).

Support from case-control studies based on biological samples is sparse, although Gey and coworkers (52) found that plasma levels of vitamin E in men aged 40–49 yr correlated strongly and inversely with the age-specific mortality from CHD in 16 European regions. A population case-control study also evaluated the relation between undiagnosed angina pectoris and plasma antioxidant levels in men aged 35–54 yr. Plasma levels of vitamin C, vitamin E, and carotene manifested a significant inverse correlation with undiagnosed angina. The inverse association between vitamin E levels and angina remained significant after adjustment for smoking habits, age, blood pressure, relative weight, and blood lipid levels (53). However, these results have been offset by several negative studies. There was no association between plasma vitamin E and prevalence of CHD in a cross-sectional survey of 1132 Finnish men (54). Similarly, most nested case-control studies found no relationship between plasma vitamin E levels and subsequent coronary mortality (55,56) or risk of MI (57,58). The reason for these disparate results is unknown, but may include changes in diet following disease diagnosis, poor classification of controls, and lack of variation in plasma levels within populations not using supplements.

5.2. Vitamin C

The evidence linking the water-soluble vitamin C with cardiovascular disease is less strong than that for vitamin E. In the Physicians' Follow-Up Study, a high intake of vitamin C was not associated with a lower risk of CHD in men (50), whereas in women from the Nurses Health Survey, an initial effect was attenuated after adjustment for multivitamin use *(59)*. Only one prospective study, which involved 11,348 adults, demonstrated an inverse relationship between vitamin C intake and cardiovascular mortality *(60)*. This effect was due largely to the use of vitamin C in supplements and may have been a reflection of other antioxidant vitamins in multivitamin preparations. A link between intake and carotid artery wall thickness has also been suggested *(61)*. Plasma levels were not correlated with coronary mortality rates among four European populations *(62)*, or with prevalent coronary disease in Finland *(54)*. In the Basle Prospective Study, low levels of vitamin C alone did not increase the risk of CHD, although the risk of disease at low levels of both vitamin C and β-carotene was greater than that for β-carotene alone *(63)*. However, a prospective population study of 1605 healthy men aged 42–60 in Finland has recently shown that men who had vitamin C deficiency had a relative risk of MI of 2.5 after adjusting for the main risk factors for MI *(64)*.

5.3. β-Carotene

There is some indication that increased dietary intake of β-carotene is associated with reduced risk of CHD although again the evidence is less convincing than that for vitamin E. In the prospective Nurses Health Survey, consumption of vitamin A and β-carotene in food and supplements weakly predicted the incidence of CHD *(65)*; Gaziano and Hennekens reported a 22% risk reduction for women in the highest quintile of β-carotene compared with those in the lowest *(66)*. No adjustment was made for the potentially confounding effect of other antioxidant vitamins in multivitamin preparations. However, a small prospective study on 1271 elderly people also demonstrated an inverse relationship between β-carotene intake in fruit, and vegetables and subsequent cardiovascular death *(67)*. Similar findings have been shown for serum carotenoid level and CHD risk *(68)*, and carotenoid intake and carotid artery plaque thickness *(61)*. Several studies indicate that dietary and circulating levels of β-carotene affect smokers more than nonsmokers *(50,58,69)*. In the Health Professionals Follow-Up Study, high β-carotene intake was associated with reduced CHD risk in current smokers and exsmokers (70% risk reduction) but not never-smokers, after adjustment for cardiovascular risk factors and vitamin C and E intake *(50)*. It was suggested that a high dietary intake of β-carotene is especially important in smokers who have both an increased demand for antioxidants (to combat smoking-induced free radicals) and a correspondingly lower circulating level for a given dietary intake *(70)*. However, β-carotene supplements in smokers may have harmful effects as discussed in the next section.

5.4. Intervention Studies in Humans with Clinical Endpoints

Observational studies, of course, only infer a cause-and-effect relationship. Even in the most well-designed observational studies, the amount of uncontrolled and uncontrollable confounding could easily be as large as the small to moderate reductions in risk that are most plausible *(71)*. Individuals who select higher intakes of antioxidants may also adopt other dietary or nondietary lifestyle characteristics that account for the apparent benefits of antioxidants seen in observational studies. Prospective studies with a clinical endpoint are required, and only randomized trials of sufficient sample size, dose, and duration of treatment and follow-up can provide reliable data. The limitations of intervention trials are that they can often only be interpreted for the particular study population, and for the antioxidant dose provided during the trial. Numerous intervention studies designed to test the hypothesis that increased antioxidant intake will protect against atherosclerosis are currently in progress. In general, these studies are using supplements of antioxidant vitamins or other antioxidants, and results so far have not been encouraging.

The Alpha-Tocopherol, Beta-Carotene Cancer Prevention Trial (ATBC), conducted among 29,133 male heavy smokers in Finland, found no reduction in CHD morbidity or mortality during 5–8 yr of treatment with vitamin E (50 mg/d) or β-carotene (20 mg/d). Those assigned vitamin E had no significant decrease in CHD deaths, but a 50% excess of deaths from cerebral hemorrhage, whereas those assigned to β-carotene experienced an 11% increase in CHD deaths *(72)*. In a further analysis, a subgroup of the original subjects with a previous MI were considered *(73)*. The endpoint of this substudy was the first major coronary event after randomization. The proportion of major coronary events was not decreased with either α-tocopherol or β-carotene supplements. In fact, β-carotene conferred an excess of fatal CHD (75% increase in risk). There was a beneficial effect of vitamin E on nonfatal MI with a risk reduction of 38%.

The CARET (Beta-Carotene and Retinol Efficacy Trial), designed to test the effects of a combined supplement of 30 mg β-carotene and 25,000 IU retinol daily among 18,314 cigarette smokers and individuals with occupational asbestos exposure, was ended early when researchers detected an elevated risk of death from lung cancer in those receiving β-carotene *(74)* and, again, no beneficial effect on cardiovascular disease (CVD) was found. For CVD mortality, there was a nonsignificant 26% increase in the treated group ($p = 0.06$).

The Physicians Health Study followed more than 22,000 US male doctors treated with 50 mg β-carotene or placebo every other day for an average of 12 yr *(75)*. The trial appears to have been conducted meticulously and its results would seem to seriously question any beneficial effect with such supplementation on CVD in well-nourished populations. There were no significant effects on individual outcomes, or on a combined endpoint of nonfatal MI, nonfatal stroke, and cardiovascular death, for which the relative risk was 1.0. There was also no evidence of harm (or benefit) among the 11% of participants who were current smokers at baseline.

Greenberg and associates *(76)* studied the effect of β-carotene supplementation (50 mg/d) in 1720 male and female subjects for a median period of 4.3 yr with a median follow-up of 8.2 yr. Subjects whose plasma levels of β-carotene were in the highest quartile at the beginning of the study had the lowest risk of death from all causes compared with those in the lowest quartile. Supplementation, however, had no effect on either all-cause or cardiovascular mortality.

Thus for β-carotene supplementation, it would appear that there are no overall benefits among individuals with a good nutritional status who are at low or average risk of developing CHD. The situation may be different, however, for those with a previous history of such disease.

5.5. Intervention Studies in Humans—Secondary Prevention

Hodis and coworkers *(77)* have shown a reduction in CHD progression (as measured angiographically) in men given 100 IU vitamin E daily, although no benefit was found for vitamin C. Singh and colleagues *(78)* found that a combination of vitamins A, C, E, and β-carotene administered within a few hours after acute MI and continued for 28 d led to significantly fewer cardiac events and a lower prevalence of angina pectoris in the supplemented group. The Cambridge Heart Antioxidant Study (CHAOS), a trial of vitamin E supplementation on 2002 patients with angiographic evidence of coronary disease, was carried out with a mean treatment duration of 1.4 yr. This short-term supplementation with α-tocopherol (268 or 537 mg/d) reduced CHD morbidity in patients (77% decreased risk of subsequent nonfatal MI). No benefit was found, however, in terms of cardiovascular mortality, with a nonsignificant excess among vitamin E-allocated participants *(79)*. The recently published GISSI-P trial investigated the independent and combined effects of n-3 PUFA and vitamin E on morbidity and mortality after MI *(80)*. Although n-3 PUFA reduced the primary combined endpoint of death, nonfatal MI, and stroke, vitamin E had no benefit. When each supplement was compared with no treatment in a four-way analysis, however, there was a nonsignificant reduction of 11% in events by vitamin E (the study was designed so that only a reduction of 20% in events would be statistically significant).

5.6. Summary and Evaluation of Human Intervention Studies

Thus, for vitamin E in Western populations, the only available trial data in primary prevention are from the ATBC trial *(72)*, which shows a negative effect. In secondary prevention, the accumulating trial data for vitamin E are more encouraging, particularly in terms of nonfatal endpoints *(73,79,80)*, but far from conclusive in demonstrating net benefits. Each of these studies is open to specific criticism—the CHAOS study was too small to measure mortality, hemodynamic data were limited to only 706 of the 2002 patients, the amount of vitamin E was changed during the trial, and the patients were only followed up for 17 mo on average. Subjects in the ATBC study received a relatively low dose (50 mg) of vitamin E; there are doubts about the length of treatment; and it is uncertain whether the potential vitamin E-mediated protective effect could have any impact in such high-risk subjects (middle-aged heavy smokers). This last uncertainty also applies to the CARET study where those treated were already at elevated risk for lung cancer due to exposure to asbestos or cigarette smoking *(81–84)*; therefore, preclinical cancerous change may already have been present.

How should we interpret the discordance between data from cohort studies and the results so far available from clinical trials? In general, it may be that the duration of clinical trials is too short to show a benefit, and that antioxidant intake over many years is required to prevent atherosclerosis. Thought needs to be given to trial design; with dose, duration of treatment and follow-up period, initial antioxidant levels and dietary intake, and extent and distribution of existing atherosclerosis being taken into consideration. Animal models have nearly always tested the effects of antioxidants on the early atherosclerotic lesions. Whether or not antioxidants have inhibitory effects on the later stages remains to be seen. In addition, the complex mixture of antioxidant micronutrients found in a diet high in fruit and vegetables may be more effective than large doses of one or a small number of antioxidant vitamins. It could be that several of these compounds work together but have no effect individually, or that other dietary components (e.g., trace elements) may be effectors of carotenoid action.

The significant results linking antioxidant intake with CHD risk observed in cohort studies may be due to confounding by other lifestyle behaviors. Slattery and associates *(85)* examined dietary antioxidants and plasma lipids in the Coronary Artery Risk Development in Young Adults (CARDIA) study and found that a higher intake of antioxidants was associated with other lifestyle factors such as physical activity and not smoking. Plasma concentrations of antioxidants are linked with social class, being higher in more affluent groups *(86)*. Although these variables can be individually controlled for in analyses, it may be that a complex lifelong behavior pattern needs to be studied before conclusions regarding antioxidants and CHD can be made. For example, passive smoking has recently been shown to have an atherogenic effect on LDL *(87)*, yet exposure to smoke is a difficult lifestyle variable to control for in cohort analyses and is rarely measured.

5.7. Further Clinical Trials of Antioxidant Supplementation

There are several clinical trials of antioxidant supplementation underway at present that are designed to clarify the effects of antioxidant supplementation on CVD. In each of these trials, doses of vitamin E greater than 200 mg/d are being used, which should be sufficient to increase serum levels at least two- to three-fold. The Women's Health Study is a primary prevention trial investigating the effects of vitamin E, β-carotene, and aspirin on CVD and cancer in 40,000 women aged 50 yr and over *(88)*. In France, the Supplementation Vitamins,

Minerals and Antioxidant (SU.VI.MAX) Trial is testing a combination of anti-oxidant vitamins including vitamin E, vitamin C, and β-carotene in 15,000 healthy men and women (89). The Heart Protection Study in Oxford is investi-gating the effects of vitamin E, vitamin C, and β-carotene in 18,000 subjects with above average risk of MI (90), and a secondary prevention trial using the same three vitamins in 8000 women has been established in the United States (Women's Antioxidant Cardiovascular Disease Trial, WACDR) (91). The Heart Outcomes Protection Study is also assessing vitamin E in 9000 persons with previous MI, stroke, or peripheral vascular disease and diabetic patients (92).

6. WHOLE FOODS AND LDL OXIDATION

Although intervention trials are important in evaluating possible beneficial effects of antioxidants against development or progression of CHD, they have limitations and should be considered as only one component in the totality of available research evidence. It may be that a lifetime of intake is required to show a protective effect, or that a mixture of natural antioxidants found in fruits and vegetables provide the necessary protective mixture. A number of studies of people who eat a diet rich in fruit and vegetables, and therefore rich in antioxidant nutrients, have tried to test the hypothesis that fruits and vegetables lower the risk of CHD (93–96). In general, observational studies of vegetarians and those with diets rich in fruits and vegetables support the hypothesis that such a diet might lower the risk of CHD. Vegetarians generally have high intakes of cereals, nuts, vegetable oils, vegetables, and fruit. However, vegetarians differ from the rest of the population in a number of important ways: they tend to smoke less, have a lower BMI and alcohol intake, and come predominantly from higher social classes, all of which are known to confer a health advantage.

Few studies have looked at the effects of whole foods on biochemical end-points. A recent study asked subjects with normal lipid concentrations who ate three or fewer servings of fruit and vegetables daily to consume eight servings per day (97). Plasma concentrations of vitamin C, retinol, α-tocopherol, α- and β-carotene, lipids, and lipoproteins were assessed before and after an 8-wk inter-vention period. The plasma vitamin C, α-carotene, and β-carotene concentra-tions increased, whereas concentrations of retinol, α-tocopherol, lipids and lipoproteins remained unchanged, despite some increase in dietary vitamin E and a small reduction in saturated fat intake. An interesting addition to the results would have been the inclusion of data on the susceptibility of LDL to oxidation. The authors concluded that more specific dietary advice to modify fat intake may be necessary to reduce the risk of CVD.

By contrast, Singh and colleagues (98) found over a 12-wk period that fruit and vegetable administration to subjects at high risk of CHD lowered total and LDL cholesterol and triglyceride levels, and increased HDL-cholesterol. Another study by Wise and coworkers *(99)* using dehydrated fruit and vegetable extracts over a period of 28 d in 15 healthy adults aged 18–53 yr produced increases of 50–2000-fold in plasma carotenoid and tocopherol levels. During the same intervention period, plasma lipid peroxides decreased fourfold, with much of this lowering taking place during the first week *(99)*.

Other antioxidant micronutrients may be important in increasing the resistance of LDL to oxidation. Flavonoids are plant-derived compounds that inhibit in vitro copper-catalyzed LDL oxidation *(100–103)*. The inhibition of oxidation of human LDL by consumption of red wine or tea has been attributed to the presence of antioxidants such as flavonoids and other polyphenols in red wine and catechin in tea *(104)*. Isoflavonoids such as genistein also reportedly increase LDL resistance to oxidation *(105,106)*, although this has not been confirmed *(107)*, whereas aged garlic extract has recently been shown to have antioxidant properties *(108)*. Ubiquinol-10 is another effective lipid-soluble antioxidant that inhibits LDL oxidation due to aqueous or lipid-phase peroxyl radicals *(109)*. The effect of antioxidant supplementation may be sex-specific with 17 β-estradiol at physiological levels increasing the resistance of LDL to oxidation in some studies *(110)*. Further studies, especially in humans, are required to validate the role of these antioxidants in inhibiting LDL oxidation.

7. OTHER ANTI-ATHEROGENIC EFFECTS OF ANTIOXIDANTS

The difficulty in linking inhibition of LDL oxidation with inhibition of atherosclerosis may stem from the dynamic nature of CHD *(111)*. CHD involves not only the development of an atherosclerotic plaque, but also plaque rupture, vasoconstriction, and local thrombosis, resulting in partial or total arterial obstruction. Some antioxidants may limit the clinical expression of atherosclerosis by stabilizing the plaque rather than by affecting its size *(111)*. Scavenger receptor activity has been shown to be downregulated in macrophages after incubation with α-tocopherol *(112)*. Several other mechanisms can contribute to the vascular effects of α-tocopherol: it has been shown to reduce monocyte adhesion and transmigration into the intima *(11)*, it can inhibit the proliferation of smooth muscle cells *(113)*, and it prevents the cytotoxic effects of oxidized LDL by reducing endothelial cell damage *(114, 115)*.

Oxidized LDL also impairs the release of nitric oxide from normal arteries, which usually prevents inappropriate adhesion of leukocytes and platelets, and vasospasm *(116)*. Thus, the presence of oxidized LDL might contribute to the platelet adhesion and vasospasm that are involved in the pathogenesis of acute coronary syndromes. LDL derived from patients treated with Probucol (a synthetic antioxidant) and oxidized in vitro does not impair the action of nitric oxide to the same degree as LDL derived from normal subjects *(116)*. Antioxidant protection of LDL by Probucol and improved endothelial function has also been found in patients treated for hypercholesterolemia *(117)*.

These alternative vascular effects of antioxidants and decreased LDL oxidation may explain the positive findings for antioxidants in the prevention of secondary CHD or the clinical expression of established CHD, rather than in primary prevention or the initial development of atherosclerotic lesions *(111)*.

8. LEVELS OF ANTIOXIDANT INTAKE FROM FOOD SOURCES

In the absence of conclusive evidence linking antioxidant intake with a reduced risk of CHD, dietary recommendations are difficult. Vitamin C and β-carotene are available from fruits and vegetables, and vitamin E from vegetable oils. Results from southern European countries consuming the classical Mediterranean diet show that high plasma levels of these antioxidants can be achieved. This diet is characterized by a preference for fresh products and frequent consumption of fruits, vegetables, legumes, and oils with a high vitamin E content. In contrast, major parts of populations in the United States or in northern parts of Europe do not consume optimal amounts of antioxidant nutrients. The availability of lower-priced convenience foods in the United States acts against the consumption of freshly prepared foods. Thus, only 40% of Americans consume five servings of fruit and vegetables daily *(118)*, as recommended by the US national food guide, the Food Guide Pyramid. Only a quarter consumed fruits or vegetables rich in vitamin C or the carotenoids, and on any given day 54% ate no fruit at all *(119)*. A recent reanalysis of the Second National Health and Nutrition Examination Survey (NHANES II) data showed that vitamin supplements are the major contributors of the principal antioxidant micronutrients in the US diet (28% of vitamin C and 46% of vitamin E) *(120)*.

Estimates of the requirement for micronutrients are based on the minimum quantity necessary to prevent a deficiency. The translation of minimum requirement to a dietary recommendation for population groups necessitates that allowance be made for a number of variables, including (1) periods of low intake, (2) increased utilization, (3) individual variability, and (4) bioavailability. In the United States, the Recommended Daily Allowances (RDAs) incorporate "margins of safety" intended to be sufficiently generous to encompass the variability in the minimum requirement among people, and bioavailability from different food sources.

To date, recommendations on micronutrient intake have therefore been primarily intended to prevent clinically overt deficiencies such as scurvy. If, however, observational and experimental evidence continues to show that the prevention of slow multistage processes such as CVD and cancer might require a higher intake of some essential antioxidants, then a recommended intake should be devised referring to amounts considered sufficient for the avoidance of these disease states. Gey *(121)* suggests that the present recommendations will require either an upgrading or an additional term, e.g., a recommended optimum intake

(ROI) that will vary with gender and age, with special requirements for smokers, pregnancy, and the elderly. The ROI could be defined as sufficient (culture- and/or region-specific) intake to achieve blood levels associated with the observed minimum relative risk of disease *(121)*. For example, Carr and Frei *(122)* have suggested a doubling of the current RDA for vitamin C for optimum reduction in chronic disease risk. A ROI would simply quantify specific dietary constituents of conceivably crucial importance within the still desirable "five servings of fruit and vegetables daily."

9. CONCLUSION

There is strong evidence to support a link between antioxidant intake and a protective effect on the susceptibility of LDL to oxidation, but the relevance of this to CHD, and the possibility of other important bioactive micronutrients and phytochemicals in vegetables and fruit, require further research.

REFERENCES

1. Witztum JL, Steinberg D. Role of oxidized LDL in atherogenesis. J Clin Invest 1991; 88:1785–1792.
2. Brown MS, Goldstein JL. Lipoprotein metabolism in the macrophage: implications for cholesterol deposition in atherosclerosis. Ann Rev Biochem 1983; 52:223–261.
3. Steinbrecher UP, Lougheed M, Kwan WC, Dirks M. Recognition of oxidized low density lipoprotein by the scavenger receptor of macrophages results from derivatization of apolipoprotein B by products of fatty acid peroxidation. J Biol Chem 1989; 264:15,216–15,223.
4. Itabe H, Yamamoto H, Imanaka T, Shimamura K, Uchiyama H, Kimura J, et al. Sensitive detection of oxidatively modified low-density lipoprotein using a monoclonal antibody. J Lipid Res 1996; 37:45–53.
5. Morel DW, DiCorleto PE, Chisholm GM. Endothelial and smooth muscle cells alter low density lipoprotein in vitro by free radical oxidation. Arteriosclerosis 1984; 4:357–364.
6. Henriksen T, Mahoney EM, Steinberg D. Enhanced macrophage degradation of low density lipoprotein previously incubated with cultured endothelial cells: recognition by the receptor for acetylated low density lipoproteins. Proc Natl Acad Sci USA 1981; 78:6499–6503.
7. Esterbauer H, Gebicki J, Puhl H, Jurgens G. The role of lipid peroxidation and antioxidants in oxidative modification of LDL. Free Rad Biol Med 1992; 13:341–390.
8. Smith C, Mitchinson MJ, Aruoma OI, Halliwell B. Stimulation of lipid peroxidation and hydroxyl radical generation by the contents of human atherosclerotic lesions. Biochem J 1992; 286:901–905.
9. Heinecke JW. Mechanisms of oxidative damage of low density lipoprotein in human atherosclerosis. Curr Opin Lipidol 1997; 8:268–274.
10. Quinn MT, Parthasarathy, S, Fong, LG, Steinberg, D. Oxidatively modified low density lipoproteins: a potential role in recruitment and retention of monocyte/macrophages during atherogenesis. Proc Natl Acad Sci USA 1987; 84:2995–2998.
11. Navab M, Imes S, Hama S, Hough GP, Ross LA, Bork RW, et al. Monocyte transmigration induced by modifications of LDL in cocultures of human aortic wall cells is due to induction of monocyte chemotactic protein I synthesis and is abolished by HDL. J Clin Invest 1991; 88:2039–2046.
12. Hessler JR, Robertson AL, Chisolm GM. LDL cytotoxicity and its inhibition by HDL in human vascular smooth muscle and endothelial cell culture. Atherosclerosis 1979; 32: 213.

13. Kugiyama K, Kerns SA, Morrisett JD, Roberts R, Henry PD. Impairment of endothelial-dependent arterial relaxation by lysolecithin in modified low-density lipoproteins. Nature 1990; 344:160–162.
14. Salonen JT, Yla-Herttuala S, Yamamoto R, Butler R, Korpela H, Salonen R, Nyyssonen K, Palinski W, Witztum JL. Autoantibody against oxidised LDL and progression of carotid atherosclerosis. Lancet 1992; 339:883–887.
15. Libby P, Hansson GK. Involvement of the immune system in human atherogenesis: current knowledge and unanswered questions. Lab Invest 1991; 64:5–15.
16. Witztum JL. Role of oxidized low-density lipoprotein in atherogenesis. Br Heart J 1993; 69: S12–S18.
17. Palinski W, Rosenfeld ME, Yla-Herttuala S, Gurtner GC, Socher SS, Butler SW, et al. Low density lipoprotein undergoes oxidative modification in vivo. Proc Natl Acad Sci USA 1989; 86:1372–1376.
18. Yla-Herttuala S, Palinski W, Rosenfeld ME, Parthasarathy S, Carew TE, Butler S, et al. Evidence for the presence of oxidatively modified low density lipoprotein in atherosclerotic lesions of rabbit and man. J Clin Invest 1989; 84:1086–1095.
19. Regnstrom J, Nilsson J, Tornvall P, Landou C, Hamsten A. Susceptibility to low-density lipoprotein oxidation and coronary atherosclerosis in man. Lancet 1992; 339:1183–1186.
20. Ball, RY, Carpenter, KL, Mitchinson, MJ. What is the significance of ceroid in human atherosclerosis? Arch Pathol Lab Med 1987; 111:1134–1140.
21. Bhakdi S. An alternative hypothesis of the pathogenesis of atherosclerosis. Herz 1998; 23:163–167.
22. Torzewski M, Klouche M, Hock J. Immunohistochemical demonstration of enzymatically modified human LDL and its colocalization with the terminal complement complex in early atherosclerotic lesions. Atheroscler Thromb Vasc Biol 1998; 18:369–378.
23. Gaziano JM, Manson, JE, Hennekens CH. Natural antioxidants and cardiovascular disease: observational epidemiologic studies and randomized trials. In: Frei B, ed. Natural Antioxidants in Human Health. Academic Press, Inc., San Diego, pp. 387–409.
24. Leake DS. Oxidised low density lipoproteins and atherogenesis. Br Heart J 1993; 69:476–478.
25. Frei B. Cardiovascular disease and nutrient antioxidants: role of low-density lipoprotein oxidation. Crit Rev Food Sci Nutr 1995; 35: 83–98.
26. Duthie GG, Wahle KJ. Smoking, antioxidants, essential fatty acids and coronary heart disease. Biochem Soc Trans 1990; 18:1051–1054.
27. Esterbauer H, Striegl G, Puhl H, Rotheneder M. Continuous monitoring of in vitro oxidation of human low density lipoprotein. Free Rad Res Commun 1989; 6:67–75.
28. Jessup, W, Rankin, SM, de Whalley, CV, Hoult, JRS, Scott, J, Leake, DS. Alpha-tocopherol consumption during low-density-lipoprotein oxidation. Biochem J 1990; 265:399–405.
29. Stocker, R, Bowry, VW, Frei, B. Ubiquinol-10 protects human low-density lipoprotein more efficiently against lipid peroxidation than does alpha-tocopherol. Proc Natl Acad Sci USA 1991; 88:1646–1650.
30. Esterbauer, H, Puhl, H, Dieber-Rotheneder, M, Waeg, G, Rabl, H. Effect of antioxidants on oxidative modification of LDL. Ann Med 1991; 23:573–581.
31. Reaven PD, Khouw A, Beltz WF, Parthasarathy S, Witztum JL. (1993) Effect of dietary antioxidant combinations in humans. Protection of LDL by vitamin E but not by beta-carotene. Arterioscler Thromb. 1993; 13:590–600.
32. Leonhardt, W, Hanefeld, M, Schaper, F. Diminished susceptibility to in vitro oxidation of low-density lipoprotein in hypercholesterolemia: key role of alpha-tocopherol content. Atherosclerosis 1999; 144:103–107.
33. Parthasarathy S, Khoo JC, Miller E, Barnett J, Witztum JL Steinberg D. (1990) Low density lipoprotein rich oleic acid is protected against oxidative modification: Implications for dietary prevention of atherosclerosis. Proc Natl Acad Sci USA 1990; 87:3894–3898.

34. Tribble DL, Holl LG, Wood PD, Krauss RM. Variations in oxidative susceptibility among six low density lipoprotein subfractions of differing density and particle size. Atherosclerosis 1992; 93:189–199.

35. Maxwell SRJ, Lip GYH. Free radicals and antioxidants in cardiovascular disease. Br J Clin Pharmacol 1997; 44:307–317.

36. Wiklund O, Mattson L, Bjoernheden T, Camejo G, Bondjiers G. Uptake and degradation of low-density lipoproteins in atherosclerotic rabbit aorta: role of local LDL modification. J Lipid Res 1991; 32:55–62.

37. Kummerow FA, Mahfouz MM Zhou Q. (1999) Effects of antioxidants on atherogenesis. In: Basu TK, Temple NJ, Garg ML, eds. Antioxidants in Human Health and Disease. CABI, Oxon, pp.165–173.

38. Singh RB, Niaz AM, Ghosh S, Agarwal P, Ahmad S, Begum R, et al. Randomized, controlled trial of antioxidant vitamins and cardioprotective diet on hyperlipidemia, oxidative stress and development of experimental atherosclerosis: the Diet and Antioxidant Trial on Atherosclerosis (DATA). Cardiovasc Drugs Ther 1995; 9:763–771.

39. Jialal I, Grundy SM. Effect of dietary supplementation with alpha-tocopherol on the oxidative modification of low-density lipoprotein. J Lipid Res 1992; 33:899–906.

40. Suzukawa M, Ishikawa T, Yoshida H, Makamura H. Effect of in vivo supplementation with low-dose vitamin E on susceptibility of low-density lipoprotein and high density lipoprotein to oxidative modification. J Am Coll Nutr 1995; 14:46–52.

41. Princen HMG, van Duyvenvoorde W, Buytenhek R, van der Laarse A, van Poppel G, Leuven JAG, van Hinsberg VWM. Supplementation with low doses of vitamin E protects LDL from lipid peroxidation in men and women. Arterioscler Thromb Vasc Biol 1995; 15:325–333.

42. Porkkala-Sarataho EK, Nyyssonen MK, Kaikkonen JE, Poulsen HE, Hayn EM, Salonen RM, Salonen JT. A randomized, single-blind, placebo-controlled trial of the effects of 200 mg α-tocopherol on the oxidation resistance of atherogenic lipoproteins. Am J Clin Nutr 1998; 68:1034–1041.

43. Fuller CJ, Grundy SM, Norkus EP, Jialal I. Effect of ascorbate supplementation on low-density lipoprotein oxidation in smokers. Atherosclerosis 1996; 119:139–150.

44. Harats D, Chevion S, Nahir M, Norman Y, Sagee O, Berry EM. Citrus fruit supplementation reduces lipoprotein oxidation in young men ingesting a diet high in saturated fat: presumptive evidence for an interaction between vitamins C and E in vivo. Am J Clin Nutr 1998; 67:240–245.

45. Jialal I, Norkus EP, Cristol L, Grundy SM. Beta-carotene inhibits the oxidative modification of low-density lipoprotein. Biochem Biophys Acta 1991; 1086:134–138.

46. Lin Y, Burri BJ, Neidlinger TR, Muller HG, Dueker SR, Clifford AJ. Estimating the concentration of β-carotene required for maximal protection of low-density lipoproteins in women. Am J Clin Nutr 1998; 67:837–845.

47. Jialal I, Grundy SM. Effect of combined supplementation with α-tocopherol, ascorbate and beta carotene on low-density lipoprotein oxidation. Circulation 1993; 88:2780–2786.

48. Woodside JV, Yarnell JWG, McMaster D, Young IS, Roxborough HE, McCrum EE, et al. Antioxidants, but not B-group vitamins increase the susceptibility of LDL to oxidation: a randomised, factorial design, placebo-controlled trial. Atherosclerosis 1999; 144:419–427.

49. Princen HMG, van Poppel G, Vogelezang C, Buytenhek R, Kok FJ. Supplementation with vitamin E but not beta-carotene in vivo protects low-density lipoprotein from lipid peroxidation in vitro. Effect of cigarette smoking. Arterioscler Thromb 1992; 212:554–562.

50. Rimm EB, Stampfer MJ, Ascherio A, Giovannucci E, Colditz GA, Willett WC. Vitamin E consumption and the risk of coronary heart disease in men. N Engl J Med 1993; 328:1450–1456.

51. Stampfer MJ, Hennekens CH, Manson JE, Colditz GA, Rosner B, Willett WC. Vitamin E consumption and the risk of coronary heart disease in women. N Engl J Med 1993; 328:1444–1449.

52. Gey KG, Puska P, Jordan P, Moser UK. Inverse correlation between vitamin E and mortality from ischaemic heart disease in cross-cultural epidemiology. Am J Clin Nutr 1991; 53:S326–S334.

53. Riemersma RA, Wood DA, MacIntyre CCA, Elton RA, Gey KF, Oliver MF. Risk of angina pectoris and plasma concentrations of vitamins A, C and E and carotene. Lancet 1991; 337:1–5.

54. Salonen JT, Salonen R, Seppanen K, Kantola M, Parviainen M, Alfthan G, et al. Relationship of serum selenium and antioxidants to plasma lipoproteins, platelet aggregability and prevalent ischaemic heart disease in Eastern Finnish men. Atherosclerosis 1988; 70:155–160.

55. Salonen JT, Salonen R, Penttila I, Herranen J, Jauhianen M, Kantola M, et al. Serum fatty acids, apolipoproteins, selenium and vitamin antioxidants and the risk of death from coronary artery disease. Am J Cardiol 1985; 56:226–231.

56. Kok FJ, de Bruijn AM, Vermeeren R, Hofman A, Vanlaar A, Debruin M, et al. Serum selenium, vitamin antioxidants, and cardiovascular disease mortality: a 9-year follow-up study in the Netherlands. Am J Clin Nutr 1987; 45:462–468.

57. Hense HW, Stender M, Bors W, Keil U. Lack of association between serum vitamin E and myocardial infarction in a population with high vitamin E levels. Atherosclerosis 1993; 103:21–28.

58. Street DA, Comstock GW, Salkeld RM, Schuep W, Klag MJ. Serum antioxidants and myocardial infarction. Circulation 1994; 90:1154–1161.

59. Manson JE, Stampfer MJ, Willett WC, Colditz GA, Rosner B, Speizer FE, Hennekens CH. A prospective study of vitamin C and incidence of coronary heart disease in women (Abstract). Circulation 1992; 85:865.

60. Enstrom JE, Kanim LE, Klein MA. Vitamin C intake and mortality among a sample of the United States population. Epidemiology 1992; 3:194–202.

61. Kritchevsky, SB, Shimakawa, T, Tell, GS, Dennis, B, Carpenter, M, Eckfeldt, JH, et al. Dietary antioxidants and carotid artery wall thickness. The ARIC Study. Circulation 1995; 92:2142–2150.

62. Riemersma RA, Oliver M, Elton RA, Alfthan G, Vartiainen E, Salo M, et al. Plasma antioxidants and coronary heart disease: vitamins C, E, and selenium. Eur J Clin Nutr 1990; 44:143–150.

63. Gey KF, Stahelin HB, Eichholzer M. Poor plasma status of carotene and vitamin C is associated with higher mortality from ischaemic heart disease and stroke: the Basle Prospective Study. Clin Invest 1993; 71:3–6.

64. Nyyssonen K, Parviainen MT, Salonen R, Tumilehto J, Salonen JT. Vitamin C deficiency and risk of myocardial infarction: prospective population study of men from eastern Finland. BMJ 1997; 314:634–638.

65. Manson JE, Stampfer MJ, Willett WC, Colditz GA, Rosner B, Speizer FE, Hennekens CH. (1991) A prospective study of antioxidant vitamins and incidence of coronary heart disease in women (abstract). Circulation 84, 546.

66. Gaziano JM, Hennekens CH. (1993) The role of beta-carotene in the prevention of cardiovascular disease. Ann NY Acad Sci 691, 148–155.

67. Gaziano JM, Manson JE, Branch LG, Colditz GA, Buring JE, Hennekens CH. (1992) A prospective study of beta-carotene in fruits and vegetables and decreased cardiovascular mortality in the elderly (Abstract). Am. J. Epidemiol. 136, 985.

68. Morris DL, Kritchevsky SB, Davis CE. Serum carotenoids and coronary heart disease. The Lipid Research Clinics Coronary Primary Prevention Trial and follow-up study. JAMA 1994; 272:1439–1441.

69. Kardinaal AFM, Kok FJ, Ringstad J, Gomez-Aracena J, Mazaev VP, Kohlmeier L, et al. Antioxidants in adipose tissue and risk of myocardial infarction: the EURAMIC study. Lancet 1993; 342:1379–1384.

70. Margetts BM, Jackson AA. Interactions between people's diet and their smoking habits: the dietary and nutritional survey of British adults. BMJ 1993; 307:1381–1384.
71. Hennekens CH, Buring JE. Epidemiology in Medicine. Little, Brown & Co., Boston, 1987.
72. Alpha-Tocopherol, Beta Carotene Cancer Prevention Study Group. The effect of vitamin E and beta carotene on the incidence of lung cancer and other cancers in male smokers. N Engl J Med 1994; 330:1029–1035.
73. Rapola JM, Virtamo J, Ripatti S, Huttunen JK, Albanes D, Taylor PR, Heinonen OP. Randomised trial of α-tocopherol and β-carotene supplements on incidence of major coronary events in men with previous myocardial infarction. Lancet 1997; 349:1715–1720.
74. Omenn GS, Goodman GE, Thornquist MD, Balmes J, Cullen MR, Glass A, et al. Effects of a combination of beta carotene and vitamin A on lung cancer and cardiovascular disease. N Engl J Med 1996; 334:1150–1155.
75. Hennekens CH, Buring JE, Manson JE, Stampfer M, Rosner B, Cook NR, et al. Lack of effect of long-term supplementation with beta carotene on the incidence of malignant neoplasms and cardiovascular disease. N Engl J Med 1996; 334:1145–1149.
76. Greenberg ER, Baron JA, Karagas MR, Stukel TA, Merenberg DW, Stevens MM, et al. Mortality associated with low plasma concentration of beta-carotene and the effect of oral supplementation. JAMA 1996; 275:699–703.
77. Hodis HN, Mack WJ, LaBrec L, Cashin-Hemphill L, Sevanian S, Johnson R, Azen SP. Serial coronary angiographic evidence that antioxidant vitamin intake reduced progression of coronary artery atherosclerosis. JAMA 1995; 273:1849–1854.
78. Singh RB, Niaz MA, Rastogi SS, Rastogi S. Usefulness of antioxidant vitamins in suspected acute myocardial infarction. Am J Cardiol 1996; 77:232–236.
79. Stephens NG, Parsons A, Schofield PM, Kelly F, Cheeseman K, Mitchinson MJ, Brown MJ. Randomised controlled trial of vitamin E in patients with coronary disease: Cambridge Heart Antioxidant Study (CHAOS). Lancet 1996; 347:781–786.
80. GISSI-Prevenzione Investigators. Dietary supplementation with n-3 polyunsaturated fatty acids and vitamin E after myocardial infarction: results of the GISSI-Prevenzione trial. Lancet 1999; 354:447–455.
81. Greenberg ER, Sporn MB. Antioxidant vitamins, cancer, and cardiovascular disease. N Engl J Med 1996; 334:1189–1190.
82. Steinberg D. Clinical trials of antioxidants in atherosclerosis: are we doing the right thing? Lancet 1995; 346:36–38.
83. Riemersma RA. Coronary heart disease and vitamin E. Lancet 1996; 347:776–777.
84. Hennekens CH. Antioxidant vitamins and cardiovascular disease: current perspectives and future directions. Eur Heart J 1997; 18:177–179.
85. Slattery ML, Jacobs DR, Dyer A, Benson J, Hilmer JE, Caan BJ. Dietary antioxidants and plasma lipids: the CARDIA study. J Am Coll Nutr 1995; 14:635–642.
86. Gregory J, Foster K, Tyler H, Wiseman M. The Dietary and Nutritional Survey of British Adults. London: HMSO, 1990.
87. Valkonen M, Kuusi T. Passive smoking induces atherogenic changes in low-density lipoprotein. Circulation 1998; 92:2012–2016.
88. Buring JE, Hennekens CH. The Women's Health Study: Rational and background. J Myocardial Ischemia 1992; 4:30–40.
89. Gaziano JM. Antioxidant vitamins and coronary artery disease risk. Am J Med 1994; 97:3A–18A.
90. Sleight P. Can vitamins and cholesterol-lowering drugs help guard against heart disease? MRC News 1995; 66:35–39.
91. Manson JE, Gaziano JM, Spelsberg A, Ridker PM, Cook NR, Buring JE, et al. A secondary prevention trial of antioxidant vitamins and cardiovascular disease in women: rationale design and methods. Ann Epidemiol 1995; 5:261–269.

92. HOPE Investigators. The HOPE (Heart Outcomes Prevention Evaluation) Study. The design of a large, simple randomised trial of an angiotensin converting enzyme inhibitor (ramipril) and vitamin E in patients at high risk of cardiovascular events. Can J Cardiol 1995; 12:127–137.

93. Thorogood M, Mann J, Appleby P, McPherson K. Risk of death from cancer and ischaemic heart disease in meat and non-meat eaters. BMJ 1994; 308:1667–1671.

94. Chang-Claude J, Frentzel-Beyme R, Eilber U. Mortality pattern of German vegetarians after 11 years of follow-up. Epidemiology 1992; 3:395–401.

95. Key T, Thorogood M, Appleby P, Burr M. Dietary habits and mortality in 11,000 vegetarians and health conscious people: results of a 17 year follow up. BMJ 1996; 313:775–779.

96. Phillips RL, Kuzma JW, Beeson WL, Lotz T. Influence of selection versus lifestyle on risk of fatal cancer and cardiovascular disease among Seventh-Day Adventists. Am. J. Epidemiol 1980; 112:296–314.

97. Zino S, Skeaff M, Williams S, Mann J. Randomised controlled trial of effect of fruit and vegetable consumption on plasma concentrations of lipids and antioxidants. BMJ 1997; 314:1787–1791.

98. Singh RB, Rastogi SS, Niaz MA, Ghosh S, Singh R, Gupta S. Effect of fat-modified and fruit-enriched and vegetable-enriched diets and blood lipids in the Indian Diet Heart Study. Am J Cardiol 1992; 70:869–874.

99. Wise JA, Morin RJ, Sanderson R, Blum K. Changes in plasma carotenoid, alpha-tocopherol, and lipid peroxide levels in response to supplementation with concentrated fruit and vegetable extracts—a pilot study. Curr Ther Res Clin Exp 1996; 57:445–461.

100. Mangiapane H, Thompson J, Salter A, Brown S, Bell DG, White D. The inhibition of oxidation of low-density lipoprotein by catechin: a naturally occurring flavonoid. Biochem Pharmacol 1992; 43:445–450.

101. Hertog MGL, Feskens EJM, Hollman PCH, Katan MB, Kromhout D. Dietary antioxidant flavonoids and risk of coronary heart disease. The Zutphen Elderly Study. Lancet 1993; 342:1007–1011.

102. Hertog MGL, Kromhout D, Aravanis C, Blackburn H, Buzina R, Fidanza F, et al. Flavonoid intake and long-term risk of coronary heart disease and cancer in the Seven Countries Study Arch Int Med 1995; 55:381–386.

103. Aviram M, Fuhrman B. Polyphenolic flavonoids inhibit macrophage-mediated oxidation of LDL and attenuate atherogenesis. Atherosclerosis 1998; 137:S45–S50.

104. Nigdikar SV, Williams NR, Griffin BA Howard AN. Consumption of red wine polyphenols reduces the susceptibility of low-density lipoproteins to oxidation in vivo. Am. J. Clin. Nutr. 1998; 68:258–265.

105. Tikkanen MJ, Wahala K, Ojala S, Vihma V, Adlercreutz H. Effect of soybean phytoestrogen intake on low density lipoprotein oxidation resistance. Proc Natl Acad Sci USA 1998; 95:3106–3110.

106. Kerry N, Abbey M. The isoflavone genistein inhibits copper and peroxyl radical mediated low density lipoprotein oxidation in vitro. Atherosclerosis 1998; 140:341–347.

107. Woodside JV, Denholm EE, Campbell MJ, Young IS, Honour J, Leathem AJC. The effect of phyto-estrogen supplementation on antioxidant status. Proc Nutr Soc 2000; 59:48A.

108. Munday JS, James KA, Fray LM, Kirkwood SW, Thompson KG. Daily supplementation with aged garlic extract, but not raw garlic, protects low density lipoprotein against in vitro oxidation. Atherosclerosis 1999; 143:399–404.

109. Stocker R, Bowry VW, Frei B. Ubiquinol-10 protects human low density lipoprotein more efficiently against lipid peroxidation than does alpha tocopherol. Proc Natl Acad Sci USA 1991; 88:1646–1650.

110. Shwaery GT, Vita JA, Keaney JF. Antioxidant protection of LDL by physiologic concentrations of estrogens is specific for 17-beta-estradiol. Atherosclerosis 1998; 138:255–262.

111. Diaz MN, Frei B, Vita JA, Keaney JF. Antioxidants and atherosclerotic heart disease. N Engl J Med 1997; 337:408–416.
112. Teupser D, Thiery J, Seidel D. α-Tocopherol down-regulates scavenger receptor activity in macrophages. Atherosclerosis 1999; 144:109–115.
113. Tasinato A, Boscoboinik D, Bartoli GM, Maroni P, Azzi A. D-alpha-tocopherol inhibition of vascular smooth muscle cell proliferation occurs at physiological concentrations, correlates with protein kinase C inhibition, and is independent of its antioxidant properties. Proc Natl Acad Sci USA 1995; 92:12190–12194.
114. Hennig B, Enoch C, Chow CK. Protection by vitamin E against endothelial cell injury by linoleic acid hydroperoxides. Nutr Res 1987; 7:1253–1260.
115. Belcher JD, Balla J, Balla G. Vitamin E, LDL, and endothelium: brief oral supplementation prevents oxidized LDL-mediated vascular injury in vitro. Arterioscler Thromb 1993; 13:1779–1789.
116. Plane F, Jacobs M, McManus D, Bruckdorfer KR. Probucol and other antioxidants prevent the inhibition of endothelium-dependent relaxation by low density lipoproteins. Atherosclerosis 1993; 103:73–79.
117. Anderson TJ, Meredith IT, Charbonneau F. Endothelium-dependent coronary vasomotion relates to the susceptibility of LDL to oxidation in humans. Circulation 1996; 93:1647–1650.
118. US Department of Health and Human Services. Healthy People 2000: Draft for Public Comment. Government Printing Office, Washington DC, 1998.
119. Tippett KS, Cleveland LE. How current diets stack up: comparisons with dietary guidelines, In: Frazao E, Tippett KS, eds. America's Eating Habits: Changes and Consequences. Agricultural Information Bulletin 750, Washington DC, 1999, pp. 51–70.
120. Block G, Sinha R, Gridley G. Collection of dietary-supplement data and implications for analysis. Am J Clin Nutr 1994; 59:232S–239S.
121. Gey KF. Ten-year retrospective on the antioxidant hypothesis of arteriosclerosis: threshold plasma levels of antioxidant micronutrients related to minimum cardiovascular risk. Nutr Biochem 1995; 6:206–236.
122. Carr AC, Frei B. Toward a new recommended dietary allowance for vitamin C based on antioxidant and health effects in humans. Am J Clin Nutr 1999; 69:1086–1107.
123. Steinberg GD, Parthasarthy S, Carew TE, Khooz JC, and Witztum JL. Beyond cholesterol—modification of low-density lipoprotein that increase its atherogenicity. N Eng J Med 1989, 915–924.

9   Dietary Fat, Blood Lipids, and Coronary Heart Disease Risk

Robert Clarke and Chris Frost

1. INTRODUCTION

Cardiovascular diseases account for about half of all deaths in middle age and a substantial proportion of deaths in old age *(1)*. Elevated blood cholesterol, elevated blood pressure, cigarette smoking, and lack of exercise explain most of these premature deaths. Recent clinical trials that demonstrated that lowering blood total cholesterol is associated with highly significant reductions in coronary heart disease (CHD), stroke, and all-cause mortality *(2–4)*, have prompted a renewed interest in dietary strategies for CHD prevention. Several decades of epidemiological research have established that the amount and type of dietary fat consumed by populations is related to their blood total cholesterol levels and mortality rates from CHD *(5)*. On the basis of this evidence, expert groups have advocated that intake of total fat by the general population should be restricted to 30% of calories, saturated fat restricted to 10% of calories, and dietary cholesterol to less than 300 mg/d *(6)*. Individuals at high risk of coronary disease should restrict saturated fat intake to less than 7% of calories and dietary cholesterol to less than 200 mg/d.

The relevance of these dietary guidelines has been questioned, partly because of the difficulty of achieving compliance with such advice *(7,8)*, but also because of the uncertainty about what should be used to replace saturated fat *(9)*. In the absence of appropriately designed large-scale clinical trials assessing the independent effects of decreasing saturated fat and increasing polyunsaturates or monounsaturates, the debate has centered around the relative importance of restricting total fat intake compared with maintaining total fat while replacing saturated fat with unsaturates. Some of the uncertainty has arisen due to apparently conflicting results from "metabolic ward studies" (in which controlled diets are administered for some weeks to volunteers). These have assessed the effects of

From: *Nutritional Health: Strategies for Disease Prevention*
Edited by: T. Wilson and N. J. Temple © Humana Press Inc., Totowa, NJ

dietary exchanges on blood total cholesterol levels, and more importantly on low-density lipoprotein cholesterol (LDL) and high-density lipoprotein cholesterol (HDL) levels. However, many of these individual metabolic ward studies have been too small to provide reliable information when looked at in isolation. When results of different studies were compared, there was uncertainty about whether the effects of dietary fats on blood total cholesterol levels varied in different age groups or whether the effects of dietary fats on HDL cholesterol levels may have been underestimated if the duration of the experimental diets was too short. Many of these issues have been clarified by a meta-analysis of all the available metabolic ward studies, which provided estimates of the effect of dietary intake of fatty acids and dietary cholesterol on blood cholesterol levels and cholesterol fractions *(10)*.

This chapter assesses the evidence using the data from a previous meta-analysis of the metabolic ward studies in order to (1) provide reliable estimates for the relative effects on blood total cholesterol, LDL cholesterol, and HDL cholesterol levels; (2) examine differences in the effects of intake of dietary lipids on total cholesterol levels when administered in different age groups; (3) assess the effects of dietary lipids on HDL cholesterol levels when the experimental diets were consumed for varying durations; and (4) review some possible exchanges in food intake required to achieve the magnitude of dietary change observed in the metabolic ward studies.

2. META-ANALYSIS OF METABOLIC WARD STUDIES

Published reports of dietary intervention studies conducted under controlled conditions that ensured compliance (metabolic ward studies) with diets administered for at least 2 wk were systematically sought by a MEDLINE search, scanning reference lists, and hand-searching nutrition journals. Details of the studies included in the meta-analysis were provided in the earlier report *(10)*. We excluded studies if the subjects were selected for some disorder (such as diabetes or dyslipidemia), or if the dietary changes were deliberately confounded by other interventions (such as weight reduction or exercise), or if there were no data available about dietary fatty acids or dietary cholesterol. The search strategy did not require data on the availability of changes in body weight. Among the 81 eligible reports identified, we excluded one long-term multicenter study for poor compliance with the experimental diet. Solid food diets were assessed in 72 of these reports among 129 groups of subjects following 395 experimental diets. Details of the major individual saturated fatty acids in 134 experimental diets, and blood concentrations of HDL and LDL cholesterol were available for 226. Liquid formula diets, assessed in 32 experimental diets in eight reports, were excluded from the main analyses because the effects of such diets may differ from those of solid food diets due to physical make-up.

From each publication, we sought information about mean age and weight, the experimental diets (intake of dietary cholesterol, percentage of calories as saturated, polyunsaturated, and monounsaturated fat), and blood cholesterol concentration (total, LDL, and HDL) in plasma or serum at the end of the experiment *(10)*. Fatty acids were classified by carbon chain lengths (with C18, for example, indicating 18 carbons) and by the number of carbon–carbon double bonds (such as C18:1). Saturated fatty acids have no such double bonds, monounsaturated fatty acids have one, and polyunsaturated fatty acids have two or more. Double bonds are *cis* if the two hydrogen atoms at each end are on the same side of the double bond and *trans* if they are on opposite sides.

We used "multilevel" regression analyses (MLN Software, London University Education Institute) that included age, weight, and dietary intake of nutrients, as well as one term per study to ensure that people in any one study were compared directly only with each other. Such analyses appropriately allowed for different sources of variability when combining results: (1) within-group between-experiments, (2) within-study between-matched-groups, (3) within-study between-unmatched-groups, and (4) between studies. A full account of the statistical methods used in the analysis has been described elsewhere *(11)*.

3. RESULTS

3.1. Univariate and Multivariate Analyses for Total Cholesterol

Figure 1 plots the mean dietary saturated fat for each experimental diet against the mean blood total cholesterol concentration at its end in one panel, with a similar display for polyunsaturated fat and monounsaturated fat. Higher intakes of saturated fat are associated with higher blood cholesterol levels and the strength of this association can be summarized by univariate regression equations calculated by a multilevel analysis that takes appropriate account of the variability between and within studies and the variability between and within groups in the same study (*see* Table 1). Increasing the intake of dietary polyunsaturates is associated with decreasing blood total cholesterol levels whereas changing monounsaturates has no significant effect on mean total cholesterol levels. Univariate analyses might be misleading because isocaloric increases in one type of fat in many of the experiments were accompanied by decreases in other dietary fats or in dietary cholesterol. Multivariate analyses were therefore also performed that assessed isocaloric replacement of complex carbohydrates by particular lipids after simultaneous adjustment for the other lipids and dietary cholesterol (and less importantly, for age and initial body weight). Thus, for example, in multivariate analyses effects of saturated fat actually means the effects of replacing carbohydrate isocalorically by saturated fat. The effect of total fat was adjusted for dietary cholesterol (and age and weight) only. Multivariate analyses, with simultaneous adjustment for the other

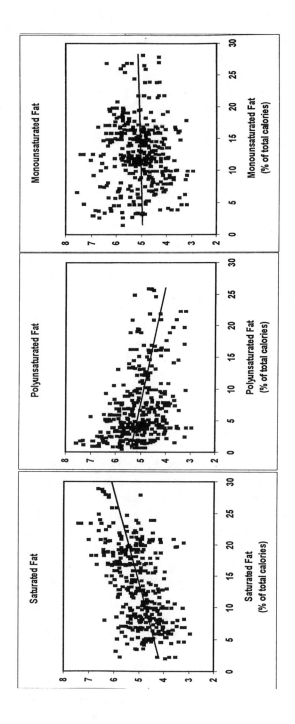

124

Table 1
Comparative Effects of Dietary Fats on Blood Total Cholesterol, LDL Cholesterol,
and HDL Cholesterol Levels[a]

Dietary fat	Univariate analysis for total cholesterol	Multivariate analysis		
		Total cholesterol	LDL	HDL
Saturated fat	0.067	0.052[b]	0.036[b]	0.013[b]
(% of total calories)	(0.003)	(0.003)	(0.005)	(0.002)
Polyunsaturated fat	−0.063	−0.026[b]	−0.022[b]	0.005[b]
(% of total calories)	(0.004)	(0.004)	(0.005)	(0.002)
Monounsaturated fat	0.005	0.005[b]	−0.008[b]	0.006[b]
(% of total calories)	(0.006)	(0.003)	(0.005)	(0.002)
Dietary cholesterol	0.0013	0.0007[b]	0.0005[b]	0.0001[b]
(mg/d)	(0.0002)	(0.0001)	(0.0001)	(0.0001)
Total fat	0.027	0.020[b]	0.012[b]	0.010[b]
(% of total calories)	(0.005)	(0.005)	(0.006)	(0.002)

[a]Regression coefficients (SE) for effects of dietary fats on blood total cholesterol (from 395 solid food experiments) and LDL and HDL concentrations (from 227 solid food experiments).
[b]Change in blood cholesterol per unit change in dietary factor, adjusted for age, weight, all other lipids, and dietary cholesterol.

dietary factors, produced smaller regression coefficients than did the univariate analyses (*see* Table 1).

The effects of saturated fat, polyunsaturated fat, and monounstaurated fat on blood total cholesterol levels were compared in individuals of different age groups (*see* Fig. 2). The top section of Fig. 2 displays the multivariate regression coefficients that describe the apparent effects of saturated fat on blood cholesterol levels after controlling for intake of all other dietary factors, age, and weight. The middle and lower sections of Fig. 2 describe similar analyses of the apparent effects of polyunsaturated fat and of monounsaturated fat on blood total choles-

---

Fig. 1. *(opposite page)* Blood total cholesterol vs dietary intake of saturated fat, polyunsaturated fat, and monounsaturated fat in 395 experimental diets. For each metabolic ward experiment on a group of individuals, a black square indicates the mean values of the dietary saturated fat and of the blood cholesterol at the end of the experimental diet, with no account taken of which experiments were parts of the same study.

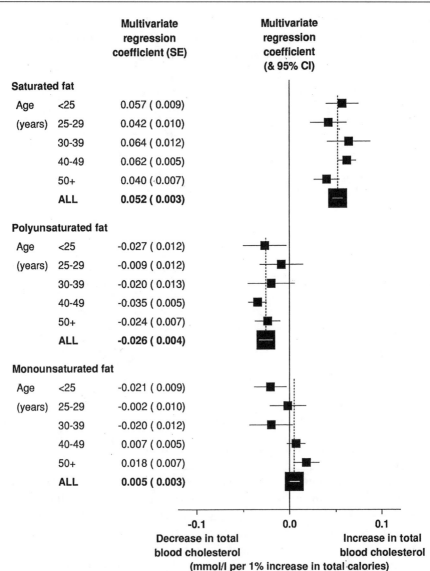

Fig. 2. Comparative effects of intake of saturated, polyunsaturated, and monounsaturated fatty acids on total blood cholesterol levels. Data from 395 experimental diets have been classified by the mean age of the study participants. Multivariate regression coefficients (and their standard errors) from the multilevel regression analyses are given for each group of studies and for the total of all solid food studies. These are plotted as black squares, with 95% confidence intervals (CI) denoted by horizontal lines. The areas of the black squares are proportional to the amount of statistical information contributed by each group of experiments. The multivariate regression coefficients for all 395 experimental diets involving solid food diets after adjustment for other fats, age, and weight are represented here as vertical dotted lines.

terol in each age group. These data show no convincing evidence of any trends with age.

3.2. Multivariate Analyses for LDL and HDL Cholesterol

A subset of 227 of the solid food experiments also reported blood LDL and HDL cholesterol levels. Multivariate analyses indicated that isocaloric increases in saturated fat intake are associated with increases in LDL cholesterol and smaller increases in HDL cholesterol, as are increases in dietary cholesterol (*see* Table 1). Conversely, increases in polyunsaturated fat intake significantly decreases LDL cholesterol and increases HDL cholesterol, whereas monounsaturated fat has no significant effect on LDL cholesterol but does increase HDL cholesterol concentration.

3.3. Effect of Realistic Dietary Changes

The potential importance of differences in intake of individual dietary factors can be illustrated by relating the multivariate regression coefficients to representative nutrient intake data for adult males from the Dietary and Nutritional Survey of British Adults (*see* Table 2) *(12)*. The multivariate analyses indicate that isocaloric replacement of saturated fats equivalent to 10% of dietary calories by complex carbohydrates would typically be associated with a reduction in blood total cholesterol of 0.52 mmol/L (standard error [SE] = 0.03) (*see* Table 2). Conversely, isocaloric replacement by polyunsaturated fat of carbohydrates equivalent to 5% of dietary calories would be expected to reduce blood cholesterol by a further 0.13 mmol/L (SE = 0.02), whereas a similar changes in monounsaturated fat would not be expected to have any material effect on blood cholesterol. A reduction of 200 mg/d in dietary cholesterol would be associated with a further reduction in blood cholesterol of 0.13 mmol/L (SE = 0.02). Together, the estimated effect of these isocaloric dietary changes would reduce blood total cholesterol by 0.76 mmol/L (SE = 0.03, 99% confidence interval [CI] = 0.67 to 0.85), consisting of a reduction in LDL cholesterol of 0.62 (0.04) mmol/L and in HDL cholesterol of 0.10 (0.02) mmol/L (*see* Table 2). Isocaloric replacement of saturated fat by unsaturated fats produced about three times the reduction in blood cholesterol produced by replacement of total fat by complex carbohydrates. Similar associations of blood cholesterol with the intake of saturated fat were observed in men and women, in those with a total caloric intake of over or under 2800 cal/d, in those weighing over or under 70 kg, and in experiments with dietary cholesterol over or under 300 mg/d (data not shown). The effects of these dietary changes on HDL cholesterol levels are achieved rapidly and are consistently observed in dietary experiments of varying duration (*see* Fig. 3).

3.4. Individual Saturated Fatty Acids

Altogether, 134 of the solid food experiments provided information on dietary intake of major individual saturated fatty acids: laurate (C12:0), myristate

Table 2

Mean Daily Intake of Dietary Fats in the Meta-Analysis of Metabolic Ward Experiments Compared with Average UK Adults and Estimated Changes in Blood Lipids for Specified Differences in Intake of Fats

| Dietary fat | Mean daily intake | | Dietary change | Mean (SE) change in blood cholesterol concentration (mmol/L) | | |
	Experimental diets	British diet		Total cholesterol	LDL	HDL
Saturated fat (% of total calories)	14.3	16.5	Replacement of saturated fat by complex carbohydrate (10% of calories)	−0.52 (0.03)	−0.36 (0.05)	−0.13 (0.02)
Polyunsaturated fat (% of total calories)	7.1	6.2	Replacement of complex carbohydrate by polyunsaturated fat (5% of calories)	−0.13 (0.02)	−0.11 (0.03)	0.03 (0.01)
Monounsaturated fat (% of total calories)	12.8	12.4	Replacement of complex carbohydrate by monounsaturated fat (5% of calories)	0.02 (0.03)	−0.04 (0.02)	0.03 (0.01)
Dietary cholesterol (mg/d)	361	390	Reduction in dietary cholesterol by 200 mg/d	−0.13 (0.02)	−0.10 (0.02)	−0.02 (0.01)
			Sum of the above changes	−0.76 (0.03)	−0.62 (0.04)	−0.10 (0.02)
Total fat (% of total calories)	35.0	40.4	Replacement of total fat by complex carbohydrate (10% of calories)	−0.20 (0.05)	−0.12 (0.06)	−0.10 (0.02)

128

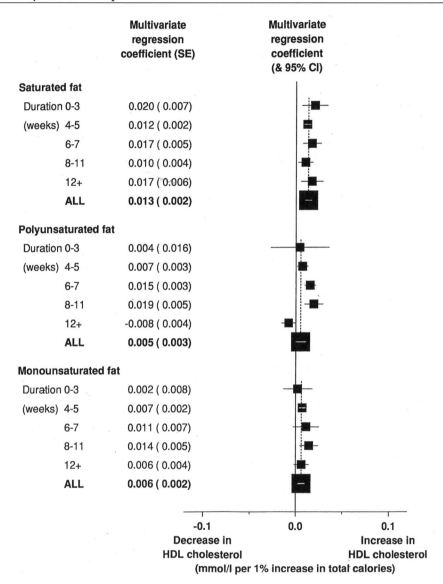

Fig. 3. Comparative effects of dietary saturated, polyunsaturated, and monounsaturated fats on blood HDL cholesterol in 227 experimental diets. Studies were classified by the mean duration of treatment. Multivariate regression coefficients (and their standard errors) from the multilevel regression analyses are given for each group of studies and for the total of all solid food studies. These are plotted as black squares, with 95% confidence intervals (CI) denoted by horizontal lines. The areas of the black squares are proportional to the amount of statistical information contributed by each group of experiments. The multivariate regression coefficients for all 227 experimental diets involving solid food diets after adjustment for other fats, age, and weight are represented here as vertical dotted lines.

Table 3
Estimated Changes in Blood Total Cholesterol (from 134 Solid Food Experiments)
Associated with Halving the Intake of Individual Saturated Fatty Acids Adjusted
for Other Lipids, Age, and Weight

Saturated fatty acid	Mean % of calories in these experiments	Multivariate regression coefficient (SE)	Mean (SE) change in total cholesterol (mmol/L)[a]
Lauric acid (C12:0)	3.7	0.045 (0.008)	–0.08 (0.01)
Myristic acid (C14:0)	1.9	0.071 (0.011)	–0.07 (0.01)
Palmitic acid (C16:0)	6.9	0.053 (0.009)	–0.18 (0.03)
(C12:0-C16:0)	12.5	0.052 (0.007)	–0.32 (0.04)
Stearic acid (C18:0)	3.6	0.015 (0.011)	–0.03 (0.02)

[a]Change from replacing half the intake of particular fatty acid by complex carbohydrate.

(C14:0), palmitate (C16:0), and stearate (C18:0). Intake of the first three were positively related with blood cholesterol, such that a halving of the intake of each with replacement by complex carbohydrates would be expected to reduce blood cholesterol by 0.32 (SE = 0.04) mmol/L (*see* Table 3). The effect of reducing stearic acid (C18:0), however (which accounts for about 25% of all dietary saturated fat) was not statistically significant.

Forty of the solid food experiments provided information on the dietary intake of *trans* monounsaturated fat (mainly *trans* C18:1; elaidate). Multivariate regression coefficients for blood total cholesterol concentration (adjusted for other dietary fats, cholesterol intake, age, and weight) were 0.038 (SE = 0.010), which is similar to 0.047 (SE = 0.008) for saturated fat in the same analyses. *Trans* fatty acids, however, account for only about 2% of calories in the average UK diet *(12)*, so replacing half of the intake of *trans* fatty acids isocalorically by complex carbohydrates would typically be associated with a reduction in total blood cholesterol of only about 0.04 (SE = 0.01) mmol/L.

4. DISCUSSION

This review highlights the quantitative importance of saturated fat, both in terms of its effect on blood cholesterol concentration and of the amount consumed by the general population. There is real need for more work to simplify and communicate dietary advice for health professionals and the general public. For example, Table 4 illustrates a series of possible dietary exchanges in the average consumption of food required to reduce the intake of saturated fatty acids and of saturated fatty acids and *trans* fatty acids by about 10% of calories using data from the Nutritional Survey of British Adults *(12)*. In the absence of full information on food labels, it may be more appropriate to target particular foods that are the chief sources of saturated fat and replace these with foods that are low in saturates. Most of the beneficial effects could be achieved by replacing one type of food by another in each of four food groups: (1) replacing butter and margarine by low-fat spreads, (2) replacing full-fat milk by low-fat milk, (3) replacing cheddar-type cheese by cottage cheese, and (4) replacing average cuts of meat and meat products by lean cuts of meat.

Overall, because of both the strength of the relationship with blood cholesterol and the large amounts present in the Western diet, the factor of greatest relevance was the intake of saturated fats. Among the saturates, those of C12:0, C14:0, or C16:0 chain length are of particular importance, but even if any differences between different saturates are ignored, the average importance of saturated fat intake remains quite substantial. These results indicate that isocaloric replacement of about 60% of the UK dietary intake of saturates by complex carbohydrates would reduce blood cholesterol by about 0.5 mmol/L. Intake of polyunsaturates is also important—in the opposite direction—as that of saturated fat, with effects that are about half as strong. Intake of monounsaturated fat has no significant effect on total cholesterol or LDL cholesterol despite raising HDL cholesterol to the same degree as polyunsaturates. The combined effect of a change in the type, but not in the amount, of dietary fat that involves a 10% reduction in total calories from saturated fat, a 5% increase in total calories from monounsaturates, and a 5% increase in total calories from polyunsaturates, together with a 200 mg reduction in dietary cholesterol, would be about a 0.8 mmol/L reduction in blood cholesterol (with 99% CI 0.7 to 0.9 mmol/L). The reduction in total blood cholesterol produced by these changes in diet chiefly involves a reduction in LDL cholesterol with only a small reduction in HDL cholesterol.

Thus, under isocaloric metabolic ward conditions, replacement of a certain amount of saturated fats by unsaturated fats is likely to lead to a much greater reduction in total blood cholesterol compared with replacement of the equivalent proportion of total fat by complex carbohydrates. Moreover, compliance with advice to replace saturated fat by unsaturated fat (with little reduction in total fat), may be easier to achieve than with advice to replace saturated fat by complex carbohydrate. The magnitude of the reduction in total blood cholesterol levels associated with these relatively modest dietary changes is greater than is sometimes appreciated. The weaker results that have been suggested by dietary studies among free-living individuals may reflect the effects of measurement error and

Table 4

Possible Exchanges in the Average Consumption of Food Required to Reduce the Intake of Saturated Fatty Acids and of Saturated Fatty Acids and *Trans* Fatty Acids Combined by About 10% of Calories in Total

Dietary exchange	Reduction in intake of saturated fat (g/d)	% Calories saving from loss of intake of saturated fat	% Calories saving from loss of intake of saturated and trans fatty acids
Butter and soft margarine by low-fat spreads	3.5	1.5	1.7
Full-fat milk by semiskimmed milk	2.5	1.1	1.1
Cheddar type cheese by cottage cheese	2.9	1.3	1.4
Cream by yogurt	0.6	0.3	0.3
Egg and egg dishes reduced by half	0.6	0.3	0.3
Average cuts of meat and meat products by lean cuts[a]	5.3	2.3	2.6
Poultry and poultry products by poultry without skin	0.3	0.2	0.2
Coated or fried fish by grilled or poached fish	0.4	0.2	0.2
French fries and roast potatoes by baked potatoes	0.9	0.4	0.4
Savory snacks (chips) by fruit	0.5	0.2	0.2
Puddings and ice cream by yogurt	1.2	0.5	0.6
Cake, cookies, and confectionery intake reduced by half and replaced by fruit	3.1	1.4	1.7
Total	21.8	9.7	10.7

[a]Calculations for meat refer here to average portions of ham, bacon, beef, pork, lamb, and veal. Data obtained from the Dietary and Nutritional Survey of British Adults (12).

132

poor compliance with dietary advice in nonmetabolic ward studies. This review took account of the different sources of variability in an appropriately weighted manner in comparing the effects of various diets on blood cholesterol levels. The discrepant results of smaller reviews (and, still more so, of individual trials) reinforce the need for periodically updated systematic reviews of all the available evidence.

Saturated fatty acids with different chain lengths may have quite different effects on blood cholesterol. Stearic acid (C18:0) appears to have little or no effect, and virtually all the cholesterol-raising effects of saturated fatty acids seems to be explained by changes in consumption of the C12:0, C14:0, and C16:0 fatty acids. The standard errors for the separately estimated effects of different saturated fatty acids were large, however, and further direct comparisons are still needed.

Trans isomers of naturally occurring *cis*-unsaturated fatty acids are produced when liquid vegetable oils are chemically hydrogenated to produce hardened fat products. The evidence on the effects of *cis* and *trans* fatty acids is limited, but this review suggests that the *trans* fatty acids studied may raise total cholesterol and LDL cholesterol by about as much as saturated fatty acids do. Despite an equivalent strength of relationship between these types of dietary fat and blood cholesterol, the average intake of *trans* fatty acids in the British diet is so small *(12)* that their overall importance is much less than that of saturated fat (but where individuals consume considerably higher amounts of *trans* fatty acids would be of greater relevance). This review does not produce useful comparisons between one type of *trans* fatty acid and another, and nor can it test the effects of *trans* fatty acids on HDL cholesterol. Additional research carried out after the completion of this meta-analysis has shown that intake of *trans* fatty acids in populations significantly decreases the level of HDL cholesterol *(13)*.

More research is also needed on developing acceptable and effective options for people who want to change their diets to reduce their blood cholesterol and, hence, their cardiac risk. These findings are of some immediate relevance to countries such as the UK, however, where both males and females get 15–17% of dietary calories from saturated fat (chiefly in dairy produce, meat, cooking oils and spreads, egg products, and confectionery) and where the average intake of dietary cholesterol is 280–390 mg/d (chiefly in meat and eggs). Table 2 suggests that changes in dietary intake of fats and cholesterol that many people could find quite practicable would produce about a 0.8 mmol/L reduction in blood cholesterol (equivalent to 10–15% reduction) with large beneficial effects on LDL cholesterol and only small adverse effects HDL cholesterol *(14)*. The effects on vascular disease of a prolonged difference of 0.8 mmol/L in blood cholesterol, with four-fifths of this reduction being in LDL cholesterol concentration, depends on the relative importance at different ages of the benefits of LDL cholesterol and the hazards of decreasing HDL cholesterol, which requires further study.

REFERENCES

1. Peto R, Lopez AD, Boreham J, Thun M, Heath Jr C. Mortality from smoking in developed countries 1950–2000. Oxford University Press, Oxford, 1994.
2. Scandinavian Simvastatin Survival Study Group. Randomised trial of cholesterol lowering in 4444 patients with coronary heart disease: The Scandinavian Simvastatin Study (4S). Lancet 1994; 344:1383–1389.
3. Sacks FM, Pfeffer MA, Moye LA, Rouleau JL, Rutherford JD, Cole TG, et al. The effects of pravastatin on coronary events after myocardial infarction in patients with average cholesterol levels. N Engl J Med 1996; 335:1001–1009.
4. The Long-Term Intervention with Pravastatin in Ischaemic Disease Study Group. Prevention of cardiovascular events and death with pravastatin in patients with coronary heart disease and a broad range of initial cholesterol levels. N Engl J Med 1998; 339:1349–1357.
5. Keys A. Seven Countries: A Multivariate Analysis of Death and Coronary Heart Disease. Harvard University Press, Cambridge, 1980.
6. National Cholesterol Education Program Expert Panel. Report of the National Cholesterol Education Program Expert Panel on detection, evaluation and treatment of high blood cholesterol in adults. Arch Intern Med 1988; 148:36–69.
7. Ramsay LE, Yeo WW, Jackson PR. Dietary reduction of serum cholesterol: time to think again. BMJ 1991; 303:953–957.
8. Tang JL, Armitage JA, Lancaster T, Silagy CA, Fowler GH, Neil HAW. Systematic review of dietary intervention trials to lower blood total cholesterol in free-living subjects. BMJ 1998; 316:1213–1220.
9. Willett W. Nutritional Epidemiology, 2nd ed. Oxford University Press, Oxford, New York, 1998.
10. Clarke R, Frost C, Collins R, Appleby P, Peto R. Dietary lipids and blood cholesterol: quantitative meta-analysis of metabolic ward studies. BMJ 1997; 314:112–117.
11. Frost C, Clarke R, Beacon H. Use of hierarchical models for meta-analysis: experience in the metabolic ward studies of diet and blood cholesterol. Stat Med 1999; 18:1657–1676.
12. Gregory J, Foster K, Tyler H, Wiseman M. The Dietary and Nutritional Survey of British Adults. HMSO, London, 1990.
13. Ascherio A, Katan MB, Zock PL, Stampfer MJ, Willett WC. *Trans* fatty acids and coronary heart disease. N Engl J Med 1999; 340:1994–1998.
14. Law MR, Wald NJ, Wu T, Hackshaw A, Bailey A. Systematic underestimation of association between serum cholesterol concentration and ischaemic heart disease in observational studies: data from the BUPA study. BMJ 1994; 308:363–366.

10 Current Theories Regarding the Influence of Diet and the Control of Obesity

Marie K. Richards, Sahasporn Paeratakul, George A. Bray, and Barry M. Popkin

1. INTRODUCTION

Current theories regarding the role of diet in human obesity have evolved around the macronutrient composition of diet and its effect on weight maintenance. Obesity is the result of long-term positive energy balance caused by intake exceeding expenditure. Fat, protein, and carbohydrate contribute to the total energy intake. Of these, dietary fat is the one most strongly implicated in the development of obesity. In this chapter, we review the role of dietary macronutrient composition, particularly dietary fat content, in the regulation of food intake and body weight. Understanding this role is necessary for answering two important questions: (1) Is the reduction in energy intake through a decrease in fat intake effective in reducing the very high prevalence of obesity in industrialized countries where diet is usually high in fat? (2) Can obesity be prevented in the populations where diet is traditionally low in fat by stopping the progression toward a high-fat diet?

Some researchers argue that fat intake is not associated with body weight independently of total energy intake, and that simply reducing fat intake is not the best solution to prevent or reverse obesity (1,2). Although the focus on fat intake may have been overemphasized at the expense of total energy intake, it is important to place the role of dietary fat in its proper context. Weight maintenance is determined by energy balance, and fat intake must be seen through its effects on total energy intake. For example, it is well known that the high-fat diet is also highly palatable, and this often leads to passive overconsumption of energy. Moreover, high-fat diets are less satiating and the thermic effect of

From: *Nutritional Health: Strategies for Disease Prevention*
Edited by: T. Wilson and N. J. Temple © Humana Press Inc., Totowa, NJ

dietary fat is low. In contrast, a diet rich in complex carbohydrates or protein induces greater satiety and tends to be associated with lower total energy intake. Because the amount as well as composition of food consumed may influence energy intake and hence body weight, the control of energy intake through manipulation of diet composition may be an effective approach to prevent weight gain and obesity.

In this chapter, we first discuss the role of dietary fat in obesity. Current evidence from experimental, clinical, and epidemiologic studies is presented. We then discuss the role of low-fat diets in preventing obesity, and the potential of dietary manipulation as a strategy for obesity treatment. Although the focus of our discussion is on dietary fat, the role of carbohydrate and protein in human obesity is also examined.

2. INCREASING DIETARY FAT ACCELERATES THE DEVELOPMENT OF OBESITY

The human body has the ability to adjust the mix of metabolic fuels it oxidizes so that carbohydrate and protein metabolism is tightly regulated and the body can achieve carbohydrate and protein balance quickly. However, the body has a poor regulatory mechanism for fat utilization and has an almost unlimited ability to store it. There are several ways in which fat intake and the consumption of high-fat diets contribute to the development of obesity. We begin with evidence from animal experiments, clinical studies, and controlled trials and then we discuss results from population studies.

2.1. Animal Experiments

As a rule, experimental animals eating low-fat diets do not become obese. The major exceptions are animals with genetic forms of obesity or neuroendocrine disorders, and animals treated with drugs or certain peptides. Although experimental obesity induced by a low-fat diet is the exception, development of obesity in animals eating high-fat diets is the expected outcome (3,4). Whether the animals are susceptible or resistant to obesity when eating high-fat diets has a strong genetic component. Some strains of mice and rats are exquisitely susceptible to developing obesity when eating high-fat diets or high-fat/high-carbohydrate diets. Other strains of mice (SWR) and rats (S5B/Pl) are resistant to developing obesity when fed similar diets. The observation that genetic susceptibility predisposes one to the development of obesity when exposed to a high-fat diet is also seen in humans.

2.2. Clinical Studies

It is the slow but continual overconsumption of energy relative to daily needs that leads to obesity. As noted above, an increase in dietary fat content increases the tendency to overconsume. When fat intake increases, the body reacts in one of two ways to maintain energy balance. First, the extra fat in the diet can be oxidized by the body. Alternatively, the increased dietary fat can be sensed by the body in such a way that subsequent intake of foods is reduced and the energy balance is maintained.

2.2.1. FAT OXIDATION ON A HIGH-FAT DIET

The possibility that a high-fat diet may stimulate fat oxidation and increase metabolism of excess dietary fat has been tested in several studies. However, results show that when fat is added to a meal, there is no corresponding increase in fat oxidation (5,6). This is in contrast with studies that show that adding carbohydrate to the diet is paralleled by an increase in carbohydrate oxidation. Because fat intake does not stimulate fat oxidation, maintenance of energy balance when consuming a high-fat diet can be achieved only by a reduction in fat intake.

2.2.2. OVERFEEDING STUDIES

The metabolic effect of the transition from a low-fat to a high-fat diet or vice versa in individuals housed in a respiratory chamber has been studied by several investigators (7,8). Overfeeding results in glycogen stores being rapidly filled and, next, to the extent that there is excess dietary protein, the protein stores are also filled. Beyond this point, overfeeding results in metabolism of the available carbohydrate with any excess being converted to fat. Careful overfeeding and underfeeding can also shift energy expenditure: when the body weight of obese volunteers increases after overeating, the energy expenditure increases; when the body weight decreases below baseline weight, energy expenditure decreases (9). In most studies, subjects were in positive energy balance because respiratory chambers restricted their energy expenditure, and thus it was difficult to match energy intake and energy expenditure.

Because obesity may modify the metabolic response to the diet, postobese individuals usually regain weight and are therefore good candidates for studying what forces drive weight upward. Specifically, it appears that postobese subjects are unable to metabolize excess dietary fat and have a smaller rise in energy expenditure when fed a high-fat meal than never-obese control subjects (10). A defect in the ability to oxidize fat by formerly obese individuals and by obese individuals overfed fat while in a respiratory chamber suggests that consistent consumption of a diet high in fat, rather than in carbohydrate, results in the gradual accumulation of fat until the body has reached a new plateau of weight maintenance (11).

2.2.3. PASSIVE OVERCONSUMPTION OF FAT

Unlike protein and carbohydrate, fat stimulates excess energy intake through its oral sensory effects and lack of satiating power (12). Periodic exposure to a high-fat meal, particularly when hungry, may be sufficient to lead to overconsumption of energy that is not compensated (13). Several approaches have been used to examine the effect of macronutrients on satiety and on subsequent food

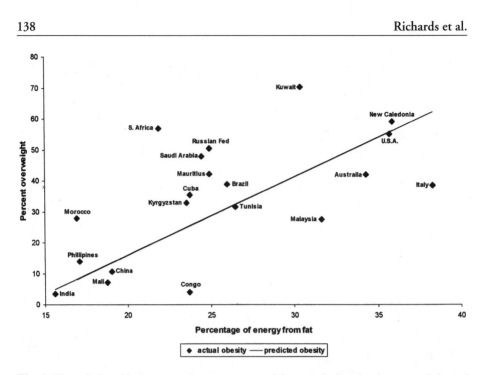

Fig. 1. The relationship between the percentage of the population that is overweight and the porportion of energy intake from fat. Reproduced with permission from © Am J Clin Nutr, American Society for Clinical Nutrition *(34)*.

intake. One question that needs to be answered is whether the degree of reduction in food intake after ingestion of high-fat meals is similar to that after ingestion of meals high in carbohydrate or protein. There is limited understanding of the compensatory mechanisms that link diet composition with total energy intake or energy balance. Overfeeding studies that compare high-fat and high-carbo-hydrate diets indicate that metabolic adaptations to changes in fat in the diet are slow while adjustment to carbohydrate is immediate *(5,8,10,14,15)*. However, it appears that the ability to reduce food intake appropriately to compensate for food eaten earlier is impaired when the food choices are high in fat *(16,17)* and when they are high in both sugar and fat *(18,19)*. These findings point to one reason why sweet, high-fat foods are problematic for obesity: people tend to overconsume them rather than compensate for them.

2.3. Epidemiologic Studies

Ecologic studies are the most basic type of epidemiologic investigation that is useful for raising hypotheses. They do not demonstrate causal relationships, but they do provide an interesting overview of diet and body weight relationships in different populations. Figure 1 shows the results relating the proportion of energy from fat provided by national food balance data to the prevalence of overweight (body mass index [BMI] > 25) in adults using nationally representative surveys from 20 countries. A regression weighted by the population of each country shows a large, significant, positive association between dietary fat consumption and the proportion of the population who are overweight ($P < 0.001$, adjusted $R^2 = 0.78$). These results support the potential role of reducing dietary fat intake as a means of preventing increases in the level of obesity in low- and middle-income countries.

Migration studies have a special place in epidemiology and have been most important in implicating several lifestyle components in the etiology of various chronic diseases. Reanalysis of the famous Ni-Hon-San migration study of Japan examined the role of diet in the etiology of obesity [20]; 8006 Japanese men living in Honolulu were compared with 2183 men living in Hiroshima and Nagasaki. The mean energy intake in men aged 45–64 yr was only slightly greater in Honolulu; however, the percentage of energy from fat was two times greater in Honolulu than in Japan. The mean BMI and subscapular skinfold thicknesses were both greater in the men living in Honolulu. In addition, more of the men living in Honolulu were obese with a BMI > 27.8 (a measure of obesity previously used by the National Center for Health Statistics).

Additional support is provided by the Leeds Fat Study [19]. When the frequency distribution of BMI in individuals who consumed a high-fat diet (>45% of energy) was plotted, the tail was skewed to the right compared with those who ate a diet with less fat (<35% of energy). With a BMI cutoff of 30 to define obesity, there were 19 times as many obese consumers of high-fat diets than of low-fat diets. However, there were still large numbers of individuals eating the high-fat diet whose BMI was normal, suggesting that there are important underlying physiologic factors, probably with a genetic basis, that influence whether a high-fat diet causes an increase in BMI.

Another ecologic approach is to conduct time-trend analyses of the relationship between individuals who are obese and their preceding diet. A study of 377,200 Danish military recruits from the years 1943–1974 related the percentage of energy from fat to obesity (defined as a BMI > 31). There was a marked parallel between the increase in the percentage of energy from fat and the subsequent increase in obesity [21]. A similar set of studies was conducted among Pima Indians in the United States [22] where parallel changes in the proportion of energy from fat and the prevalence of obesity were found. Of course, many other factors may have changed along with diet. For example, the decline in physical activity probably also contributed to the increase in obesity.

Data from a survey that was conducted in China (the China Health and Nutrition Survey) again shows that increases in dietary fat intake lead to increases in body fatness [23,24]. This survey collected detailed dietary, anthropometric, and physical activity data. The results are presented in Table 1. Note that the effect

Table 1
Analysis in Dietary Modification as a Predictor of Change in BMI
Using the China Health and Nutrition Survey[a]

	Adolescents[b] 10–18 yr old (n = 742)	Adults[c] 20–45 yr old (n = 6667)
Predictors	Coefficient ± SE	Coefficient ± SE
Change in energy from fat	0.0005 ± 0.0003^d	0.0001 ± 0.00005^d
Change in energy from nonfat	0.0001 ± 0.0001	0.000007 ± 0.00003
Change in percent energy from fat	0.01 ± 0.008^e	0.003 ± 0.002^e
Change in total energy	0.0002 ± 0.0001^e	0.00002 ± 0.00002

[a]1991 and 1993 survey used for adolescents and 1991, 1992, and 1993 used for adults.
[b]Adjusted for age, gender, and residence.
[c]Adjusted for age, gender, residence, smoking, and physical activity.
[d]$p < 0.05$.
[e]$p < 0.10$.
SE = standard error.

of potential confounders of the diet-BMI relationship (e.g., age, sex, physical activity, and smoking in adults) was taken into account. To test the hypothesis that energy from fat has an independent effect on body fatness, the effect of change in absolute amount of energy from fat was examined while controlling for the effect of change in energy from nonfat sources (i.e., protein and carbohydrate). In a separate regression model, the effect of change in the *percentage* of energy from fat was examined while controlling for the effect of total energy intake. In both cases, a significant independent effect of fat intake on BMI was found. For example, a 100-kcal increase in fat intake was associated with an increase in BMI of about 0.05 and 0.01 unit in adolescents and adults, respectively. In contrast, a 100-kcal increase in protein and carbohydrate intake combined was associated with an increase of only 0.01 and 0.0007 BMI unit in adolescents and adults, respectively. Similar results were seen when fat intake was expressed as the percentage of energy intake. These findings suggest that energy from fat has a greater effect on BMI than energy from nonfat sources or total energy intake. Moreover, they are consistent with the hypothesis that increasing amounts of dietary fat put a significant fraction of the population, who have a genetic susceptibility, at risk of obesity *(3,4,21,25,26)*.

3. CAN A REDUCTION IN DIETARY FAT PREVENT OR REVERSE OBESITY?

3.1. Animal Experiments

Two major findings from animal experiments are noteworthy: first, a high-fat diet induces an increase in the number of fat cells or adipocytes; and second, replacing a high-fat with a low-fat diet may, but not always, reverse obesity. Lemonnier *(27)* was the first to show that feeding mice a high-fat diet will increase the number of adipocytes, with the intraabdominal perirenal depot showing the greatest response. Subsequently, this has been shown in mice and rats by other researchers *(28,29)*. Switching from a high-fat to a low-fat diet might be expected to reverse fat-induced obesity, unless the number of adipocytes increases. In this case, weight reduction may be incomplete. When the mice were switched from a high-fat to a low-fat diet, the number of adipocytes did not dencrease. Thus, when the fat cells returned to normal size, the animals were still obese *(30)*. Rolls and associates *(31)* showed that rats fed a high-fat diet did not return to their baseline weight when switched to a lower-fat diet. In animals switched to a low-fat diet after having been fed a high-fat diet for a short period (4 mo), they reduced their weight to levels similar to that of control animals not eating the high-fat diet *(30)*. However, the animals fed high-fat diet for a longer period (7 mo) failed to reduce their weight to control values. Others also reported that body weight did not return to the level of control animals maintained on a low-fat diet throughout the study *(32,33)*. The extent to which genetic factors are involved in the size or number of fat cells and in this reversal has not yet been determined, but they are likely to play an important role. These data suggest that increased dietary fat may be particularly important in inducing obesity, whereas a reduction in dietary fat has less of an effect on weight loss.

3.2. Effect of Fat Reduction on Weight Loss in Nonobese Subjects

We have reviewed several clinical trials that involved manipulation of diet composition, mostly through the reduction in dietary fat *(34)*. Although weight reduction was not the primary objective of these studies, the subjects who were placed on a low-fat diet nonetheless lost weight *(35–54)*. Typically, greater weight loss was seen in the short-term studies (<6 mo) compared to studies that lasted longer. As observed earlier, the magnitude of weight loss depends on the initial body weight, and patient compliance is the crucial factor in the success of treatment *(55)*. Weight loss maintenance generally declines with long-term interventions *(40,41)*. This may be partially attributed to the fact that weight reduction or weight maintenance was not specifically encouraged in these studies. In any case, decreasing total fat in the diet without intentionally restricting food intake resulted in lower total energy intake in nonobese individuals, and approx 12% of the initial reduction in energy intake was not compensated for by those on low-fat ad libitum regimens.

3.3. Effect of Fat Reduction on Weight Loss in Overweight Subjects

Several intervention trials have examined the effect of a low-fat diet with or without energy restriction in overweight subjects *(48,51,53,56–69)*. The rate of weight loss was generally greater when the low-fat diet was accompanied by reduction in energy intake. These studies show that apart from energy restriction, a low-fat diet is effective in inducing weight loss in overweight subjects, with an observed mean weight loss of about 1.8 kg/mo. Although the rate of weight loss on an ad libitum, low-fat, high-carbohydrate diet may not be as rapid as that induced by energy restriction (calorie counting), that diet has been found to provide greater satiety and, subsequently, the compensation for the decrease in energy content is not complete (i.e., energy intake remains decreased) *(31,55,64,65)*. Even in studies where the goal is to maintain a constant energy intake, the total energy intake is often reduced unintentionally when a low-fat diet is consumed *(57)*. In interventions in obese subjects, about 23% of the initial reduction in total energy intake is not compensated for.

Despite the fact that compliance tends to decrease over time, a low-fat, high-carbohydrate diet is still one of the most effective tools in weight maintenance *(46,55)*. Consumption of reduced-fat products leads to a lower energy consumption, suggesting that a low-fat diet may make it easier to maintain a long-term energy deficit and hence slow down the rate of weight gain or weight regain *(70)*. In at least one study, the ad libitum low-fat, high-carbohydrate diet was shown to be more effective than calorie counting in maintaining weight loss over 1 yr *(55)*. This may be due to the fact that simple energy restriction is often associated with extremely poor compliance *(65)*.

3.4. Effect of Isocaloric Diets on Weight Loss in Obese Subjects

The influence of diet composition on body weight may also be studied by using diets with the same energy content but differing in macronutrient composition, i.e., isocaloric diets. Animal experiments have shown that a low-fat diet is more effective than an isocaloric high-fat diet for inducing weight loss. This has been attributed to the low thermic effect of fat and the high energy cost of converting carbohydrate or protein into body fat. However, the same result has not been clearly shown in humans. In three studies that involved isocaloric diets in obese individuals, there was no significant difference in weight loss induced by low-fat diets and high-fat diets, although all subjects lost weight *(62,71,72)*. Note that in these studies, the subjects were in negative energy balance, and energy deficit was the primary factor responsible for weight loss independent of fat intake. Moreover, these studies may have been confounded by several factors such as physical activity and smoking.

Overall, there is substantial evidence that the macronutrient composition of the diet is an important factor that influences body weight, and that among the macronutrients, dietary fat plays a major role in the development of obesity. At the same time, there is a growing interest in the role of energy density of the diet as it directly contributes to the total energy intake.

Reduction of body weight can be achieved by limiting the total energy intake as well as total fat intake. Although this strategy is only modestly effective in the population, a reduction of a few kilograms in body weight will cause a significant

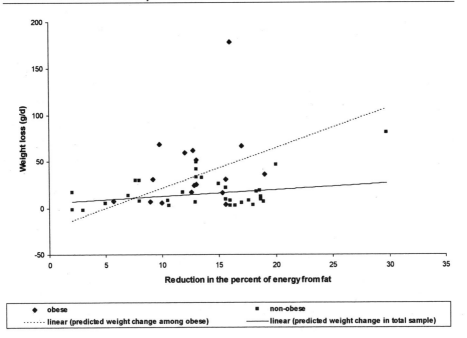

Fig. 2. The effect of a reduction in the percent of energy from fat on grams of weight loss per day.

decrease in the prevalence of obesity and its associated risks *(12)*. We summarize the effect of the reduction of fat intake on body weight in Fig. 2. The data depict the relation between the percentage reduction in energy from fat and the resultant weight change. The predicted weight loss for the entire set of studies of dietary fat reduction and body weight is provided. The main explanatory variable was the change in percentage of energy from fat. Isoenergetic studies were not included. The difference in size of these clinical trials was accounted for. The covariates in the regression model included proportion of men to women, mean initial weight, and mean age of the subjects. The final regression indicated that those with a higher initial weight lost more weight, as was expected. The most important result is shown by the slope of the regression line, which indicates that each additional percentage point reduction in dietary fat produced a weight loss of 0.99 g/d ($p = 0.10$) for all studies. For obese individuals, the reduction in weight was considerably greater at 3.22 g/d ($p = 0.08$). Although these results are borderline significant, they indicate a biologically important relation between the percentage reduction in dietary fat and weight loss. Among the obese a 10% decrease in percent energy from fat (e.g., from 36–26%) translates to a weight loss of 32 g/d. A later very careful meta-analysis of the effect of changes in dietary fat on weight loss found comparable results (Astrup et al., personal communication).

4. EMERGING ROLE OF ENERGY DENSITY
IN WEIGHT REDUCTION

4.1. Fat Substitutes

Fat substitutes such as sucrose polyester (e.g., Olestra) have been used to facilitate research on the degree to which covert changes in energy density alter total energy intake and macronutrient selection. Short-term studies of the substitution of indigestible fat substitutes for fat in the diet show two patterns of adaptation. When 20 or 30 g of Olestra was substituted for fat in a single breakfast meal, there was energy compensation over the next 24–36 h in healthy, young men *(73,74)*. When fat intake was lowered from 40–30% of energy by substituting Olestra for fat in the noon or evening meal, there was no energy compensation over the next 24 h *(75)*. However, when substitution with Olestra lowered the fat intake from 30% to nearly 20% of energy over three meals, healthy subjects felt less satisfied at the end of the substitution and compensated for nearly 75% of the energy deficit over the next day *(76)*.

In longer-term experiments lasting 2 wk or 3 mo, the substitution of Olestra for about one-third of the fat in all meals for a diet containing 40% of energy from fat reduced energy consumption by about 15% for the same weight of food. In each experiment, there was only partial compensation for energy, suggesting that when the energy density of the diet was altered, the subjects continued to eat the same mass of food even though it provided less metabolizable energy. Weight loss in the 2 wk experiment was 1.5 kg and in the 3 mo experiment was nearly 5 kg, which was significantly greater than the amount of weight lost in the control group *(77–79)*.

4.2. Carbohydrate and Water: Role in Reducing Energy Density

The role of complex carbohydrate in weight loss and weight maintenance is well recognized. This may be attributed to the low energy density of high-carbohydrate diets and to the ability of carbohydrate to rapidly induce satiety. Several studies have shown that complex carbohydrate is more satiating than dietary fat *(75,80)*. For example, the isocaloric substitution of fat by carbohydrate results in increased fullness and less desire to eat *(12)*. Conversely, obese subjects overeat when receiving high-fat foods but not when receiving high-carbohydrate foods *(75)*. Intervention trials have shown that replacing fat with complex carbohydrate induces significant weight loss under ad libitum conditions *(64,67,81)*. Ad libitum low-fat, high-carbohydrate diets appear to be particularly effective in maintaining weight loss induced by other means (e.g., drug therapy and calorie counting). In one study, this diet was shown to be more effective than calorie counting in maintaining long-term weight loss of 1 yr or more *(55)*. The mechanism by which a low-fat/high-carbohydrate diet prevents weight regain is not known, but probably involves both reduction in energy intake and increase in energy expenditure *(82,83)*.

There also appears to be a strong role for energy-dilute foods in the prevention and treatment of obesity. Energy density is determined by the water and fat content of foods, of which water accounts for the majority *(84)*. People tend to consume a constant weight or volume of food under ad lib conditions; therefore replacing foods that are high in fat and energy density but lower in weight with those high in water or dietary fiber should lead to lower energy intakes *(84)*. Studies have shown the amount of food consumed more so than its energy content account for short-term satiety and the incomplete compensation for lost calories *(85)*. The ability of a low-energy-dense diet to control energy intake is seen in a study of 18 normal weight healthy women who were each fed three test meals for 2 d *(86)*. The meals did not differ in macronutrient composition, pleasantness, or elicited hunger level. The energy density of the main entree was manipulated through substitution with high water containing foods, but without changing the macronutrient content of the diet. The energy density of the meals did not affect the weight of the food consumed, but significantly more energy was consumed with the diet of higher energy density.

5. CONCLUSIONS

The role of diet composition, particularly dietary fat intake, in the development and control of obesity is complex but becoming better understood. It is difficult for animals and humans to become obese if they consume a low-fat diet. There is strong evidence that the increase in fat intake is associated with an increase in body weight. A high-fat diet produces obesity by increasing the total energy intake and encouraging passive overconsumption. This is especially true when the diet contains a large amount of sweet, high-fat foods. Reduction of fat intake is one of the most practical ways to prevent weight gain, and when coupled with regular exercise, induces a sustainable weight loss. Reduction of fat intake may be accomplished by replacing dietary fat with complex carbohydrate, fruits, and vegetables. Reduction in fat intake alone should not be expected to entirely reverse the development of obesity. Instead, this should be seen as a means to reduce the energy density of the diet and hence the total energy intake. A low-fat diet can be satiating if it contains plenty of complex carbohydrate. This is important because the satiety and palatability of a diet strongly influences its long-term effectiveness and compliance. Note that an increase in consumption of reduced-fat but energy-dense products will not lower the total energy intake and might, in some circumstances, actually mislead individuals into consuming more energy than they would have otherwise.

Epidemiologic evidence shows that excessive fat intake is associated with obesity in the population, especially among population segments with a genetic predisposition to obesity. Populations where diets are traditionally low in fat do not experience rapid increases in obesity. However, when fat intakes increase, the likelihood of obesity also increases in these populations. The increasing prevalence of obesity in many developing countries can be explained in part by the increase in availability of high-fat foods and the adoption of the so-called affluent or Western-style diet. In these countries, limiting further increases in fat intake may be an effective strategy to prevent obesity. In the industrialized countries where fat intake is relatively high, reductions in both fat intake as well as total energy intake may be warranted. In all populations, genetic predisposition has a strong influence on the effect of high-fat diet and subsequent development of obesity. It is likely that some populations or population subgroups are more susceptible to the effect of high-fat diet than others. Therefore, reduction of fat intake may be only modestly effective in preventing or reversing obesity in some individuals. For such individuals the low-fat diet alone may not be effective in inducing weight loss, but nevertheless will be associated with other health benefits such as an improved biochemical profile and reduced cardiovascular risk. We conclude that, at the present time, a diet low in fat and rich in complex carbohydrate, with an energy content that is equal to or less than the energy need, along with an increase in physical activity, appears to be the most prudent recommendation to control obesity in the population.

REFERENCES

1. Willett WC. Is dietary fat a major determinant of body fat? Am J Clin Nutr 1998; 67(Suppl):556S–562S.
2. Katan MB, Grundy SM, Willett WC. Should a low-fat, high-carbohydrate diet be recommended for everyone? Beyond low-fat diets. N Engl J Med 1997; 337:563–566.
3. Bray GA, Fisler JS, York DA. Neuroendocrine control of the development of obesity: understanding gained from studies of experimental animal models. Front Neuroendocrinol 1990; 11:128–181.
4. West DB, York B. Dietary fat, genetic predisposition, and obesity: lessons from animal models. Am J Clin Nutr 1998; 67(Suppl):505S–512S.
5. Flatt JP, Ravussin E, Acheson KJ, Jequier E. Effects of dietary fat on postprandial substrate oxidation and on carbohydrate and fat balances. J Clin Invest 1985; 76:1019–1024.
6. Bennett C, Reed GW, Peters JC, Abumrad NN, Sun M, Hill JO. Short-term effects of dietary-fat ingestion on energy expenditure and nutrient balance. Am J Clin Nutr 1992; 55:1071–1077.
7. Schrauwen P, Lichtenbeit DVM, Saris WHM, Westerterp KR. Adaption of fat oxidation to a high-fat diet. Int J Obes 1996; 20 (Abstr):81.
8. Hill JO, Peters JC, Reed GW, Schlundt DG, Sharp T, Greene HL. Nutrient balance in humans: effects of diet composition. Am J Clin Nutr 1991; 54:10–17.
9. Leibel RL, Rosenbaum M., Hirsch J. Changes in energy expenditure resulting from altered body weight. N Engl J Med 1995; 332:621–628.
10. Astrup A, Buemann B, Christensen NJ, Toubro S. Failure to increase lipid oxidation in response to increasing dietary fat content in formerly obese women. Am J Physiol 1994; 266:E592–E599.
11. Horton TJ, Drougas H, Brachey A, Reed GW, Peters JC, Hill JO. Fat and carbohydrate overfeeding in humans: different effects on energy storage. Am J Clin Nutr 1995; 62:19–29.
12. Astrup A, Toubro S, Raben A, Skov AR. The role of low-fat diet and fat substitutes in body weight management: What have we learned from clinical studies? J Am Diet Assoc 1997; 97(Suppl):S82–S87.

13. Lawton CL, Burley VJ, Wales JK, Blundell JE. Dietary fat and appetite control in obese subjects: weak effects on satiation and satiety. Int J Obes Relat Metab Disord 1993; 17:409–418.

14. Abbott WGH, Howard BV, Christin L, Freymond D, Lillioja S, Boyce VL, et al. Short-term energy balance: relationship with protein, carbohydrate, and fat balances. Am J Physiol 1988; 255:E332–E337.

15. Thomas CD, Peters JC, Reed GW, Abumrad NN, Sun M, Hill, JO. Nutrient balance and energy expenditure during ad libitum feeding of high-fat and high-carbohydrate diets in humans. Am J Clin Nutr 1992; 55:934–942.

16. Sparti A, Windhauser MM, Champagne CM, Bray GA. Effect of an acute reduction in carbohydrate intake on subsequent food intake in healthy men. Am J Clin Nutr 1997; 66:1144–1150.

17. Tremblay A, Lavallde N, Almeras N, Allard L, Despres J-P, Bouchard, C. Nutritional determinants of the increase in energy intake associated with a high-fat diet. Am J Clin Nutr 1991; 53:1134–1137.

18. Green SM. Blundell JE. Effect of fat-and sucrose-containing foods on the size of eating episodes and energy intake in lean dietary restrained and unrestrained females: potential for causing overconsumption. Eur J Clin Nutr 1996; 50:625–635.

19. Blundell JE, Macdiarmid JI. Passive overconsumption. Fat intake and short-term energy balance. Ann NY Acad Sci 1997; 827:392–407.

20. Curb JD, Marcus EB. Body fat and obesity in Japanese Americans. Am J Clin Nutr 1991; 53(Suppl):1552S–1555S.

21. Sonne-Holm S, Sorensen TIA. Post-war course of the prevalence of extreme overweight among Danish young men. J Chronic Dis 1977 30:351–358.

22. Price RA, Charles MA, Pettitt DJ, Knowler WC. Obesity in Pima Indians: large increases among post-World War 11 birth cohorts. Am J Phys Anthropol 1993; 92:473–479.

23. Popkin BM, Paeratakul S, Fengying Z, Keyou G. Dietary and environmental correlates of obesity in a population study in China. Obes Res 1995; 3:135S–143S.

24. Paeratakul S, Popkin BM, Keyou G, Adair LS, Stevens J. Changes in diet and physical activity affect the Body Mass Index of Chinese adults. Intl J Obes 1998; 22: 424–431.

25. Lissner L, Heitmann BL. Dietary fat and obesity: evidence from epidemiology. Eur J Clin Nutr 1995; 49:79–90.

26. Heitmann BL, Lissner L, Sorensen TIA, Bengtsson C. Dietary fat intake and weight gain in women genetically predisposed for obesity. Am J Clin Nutr 1995; 61:1213–1217.

27. Lemonnier D. Effect of age, sex, and site on the cellularity of adipose tissue in mice and rats rendered obese by a high-fat diet. J Clin Invest 1972; 51:2907–2915.

28. Faust IM, Johnson PR, Stem, JS, Hirsch, J. Diet-induced adipocyte number increase in adult rats: a new model of obesity. Am J Physiol 1978; 235:E279–E286.

29. Hill JO. Body weight regulation in obese and obese-reduced rats. Int J Obes 1990; 14:31–47.

30. Hill JO, Lin D, Yakubu F, Peters JC. Development of dietary obesity in rats: influence of amount and composition of dietary fat. Int J Obes Relat Metab Disord 1992; 16:321–333.

31. Rolls DJ, Rowe EA, Turner RC. Persistent obesity in rats following a period of consumption of a mixed, high energy diet. J Physiol (Lond) 1980; 298:415–427.

32. Harris RBS, Kasser TR, Martin RJ. Dynamics of recovery of body composition after overfeeding, food restriction or starvation of mature female rats. J Nutr 1986; 116:2536–2546.

33. Uhley VE, Jen KLC. Changes in feeding efficiency and carcass composition in rats on repeated high-fat feedings. Int J Obes 1989; 3:849–856.

34. Bray GA, Popkin BM. Dietary fat intake does affect obesity. Am J Clin Nutr 1998; 68:1157–1173.

35. Lissner L, Levitsky DA, Strupp BJ, Kalkwarf HJ, Roe DA. Dietary fat and the regulation of energy intake in human subjects. Am J Clin Nutr 1987; 46:886–892.

36. Kendall A, Levitsky DA, Strupp B, Lissner L. Weight loss on a low- fat diet: consequence of the imprecision of the control of food intake in humans. Am J Clin Nutr 1991; 53:1124–1129.

37. Boyar AP, Rose DP, Loughridge JR, Engle A, Palgi A, Laarso K, et al. Response to a diet low in total fat in women with postmenopausal breast cancer: a pilot study. Nutr Cancer 1988; 11:93–99.
38. Lee-Han H, Cousins M, Beaton M, McGuire V, Kiukov V, Chipman M, Boyd N. Compliance in a randomized clinical trial of dietary fat reduction in patients with breast dysplasia. Am J Clin Nutr 1988; 48:575–786.
39. Boyd NF, Cousins M, Beaton M, Kriukov V, Lockwood G, Tritchler D. Quantitative changes in dietary fat intake and serum cholesterol in women: results from a randomized, controlled trial. Am J Clin Nutr 1990; 52:470–476.
40. Bloemberg BPM, Kromhout D, Goddijin HE, Jansen A, Obermann-de Boer GL. The impact of the Guidelines for a Healthy Diet of The Netherlands Nutrition Council on total and high density lipoprotein cholesterol in hypercholesterolemic free-living men. Am J Epidemiol 1991; 134:39–48.
41. Sheppard L, Kristal AR, Kushi LK. Weight loss in women participating in a randomized trial of low-fat diets. Am J Clin Nutr 1991; 54:821–828.
42. Singh RM, Rastogi SS, Verma R, Laxmi B, Singh R, Ghosh S, Niaz MA. Randomized controlled trial of cardioprotective diet in patients with recent acute myocardial infarction: results of one year follow-up. BMJ 1992; 304:1015–1019.
43. Hunninghake DB, Stein EA, Dujovne CA, Harris WS, Feldman EB, Miller VT, et al. The efficacy of intensive dietary therapy alone or combined with lovastatin in out-patients with hypercholesterolemia. N Engl J Med 1992; 328:1213–1219.
44. Kasim SE, Martino S, Kim P, Khilnani S, Boomer A, Depper J, et al. Dietary and anthropometric determinants of plasma lipoproteins during a long-term low-fat diet in healthy women. Am J Clin Nutr 1993; 57:146–153.
45. Schaefer EJ, Lichtenstein AH, Lamon-Fava S, McNamara JR, Scaefer MM, Rasmussen H, Ordovas JM. Body weight and low-density lipoprotein cholesterol changes after consumption of a low-fat ad libitum diet. JAMA. 1995; 274:1450–1455.
46. Westerterp KR, Verboeket-van de Venne WPHG, Westerterp-Plantenga MS, Velthus-te Wierik EJM, de Graaf C, Weststrate JA. Dietary fat and body fat: an intervention study. Int J Obes Relat Metab Disord 1996; 20:1022–1026.
47. Raben A, Jensen ND, Marckmann P, Sandstrom B, Astrup A. Spontaneous weight loss during 11 weeks' ad libitum intake of a low fat/high fiber diet in young, normal weight subjects. Int J Obes Relat Metab Disord 1995; 19:916–923.
48. Prewitt TE, Schmeisser D, Bowen PE, Aye P, Dolcek TA, Langenberg P, et al. Changes in body weight, body composition, and energy intake in women fed high- and low-fat diets. Am J Clin Nutr 1991; 54:304–310.
49. Baer JT. Improved plasma cholesterol levels in men after a nutrition education program at the worksite. J Am Diet Assoc 1993; 93:658–633.
50. Westrate JA, van het Hof KH, van den Berg H, Velthuis-te-Wierik EJ, De Graaf C, Zimmermanns NJ, et al. A comparison of the effect of free access to reduced fat products or their full fat equivalents on food intake, body weight, blood lipids and fat-soluble antioxidants levels and haemostasis variables. Eur J Clin Nutr 1998; 52:389–395
51. Stefanick ML, Mackey S, Sheehan M, Ellsworth N, Haskell WL, Wood PD. Effects of diet and exercise in men and postmenopausal women with low levels of HDL cholesterol and high levels of LDL cholesterol. N Engl J Med 1998; 339:12–20.
52. Thuesen L, Henriksen LB, Engby B. One-year experience with a low-fat, low-cholesterol diet in patients with coronary heart disease. Am J Clin Nutr 1986; 44:212–219.
53. Knopp RH, Walden CE, Retzlaff BM, McCann BS, Dowdy AA, Albers JJ, et al. Long-term cholesterol-lowering effects of 4 fat-restricted diets in hypercholesterolemic and combined hyperlipidemic men: the dietary alternative study. JAMA 1997; 278:1509–1515.

54. Simon MS, Heilbrun LK, Boomer A, Kresge C, Depper J, Kim PN, et al. A randomized trial of a low-fat dietary intervention in women at high risk for breast cancer. Nutr Cancer 1997; 27:136–142.

55. Toubro S, Astrup A. Randomized comparison of diets for maintaining obese subjects' weight after major weight loss: ad lib, low fat, high carbohydrate diet v. fixed energy intake. BMJ 1997; 314:29–34.

56. Buzzard IM, Asp EH, Chlebowski RT, Boyar AP, Jeffery RW, Nixon DW, et al. Diet intervention methods to reduce fat intake: nutrient and food group composition of self-selected low-fat diets. J Am Diet Assoc 1990; 90:42–53.

57. Puska P, Iacono JM, Nissinen A, Korhonen HJ, Vartiainen E, Pietinen P. Controlled, randomized trial of the effect of dietary fat on blood pressure. Lancet 1983; 1:1–5.

58. Hammer, RL, Barrier, CA, Roundy, ES, Bradford, JM, Fisher, AG. Calorie-restricted low-fat diet and exercise in obese women. Am J Clin Nutr 1989; 49:77–85.

59. Rumpler WV, Seale JL, Miles CW, Bodwell CE. Energy-intake restriction and diet-composition effects on energy expenditure in men. Am J Clin Nutr 1991; 53:430–436.

60. Shintani TT, Hughes CK, Beckham S, O'Connor HK. Obesity and cardiovascular risk intervention through the ad libitum feeding of traditional Hawaiian diet. Am J Clin Nutr 1991; 53(Suppl):1647S–1651S.

61. Schlundt DG, Hill JO, Pope-Cordle J, Arnold D, Virts KL, Katahn M. Randomized evaluation of a low fat ad libitum carbohydrate diet for weight reduction. Int J Obes Relat Metab Disord 1993; 17:623–629.

62. Powell JJ, Tucker L, Fisher AG, Wilcox K. The effects of different percentages of dietary fat intake, exercise, and calorie restriction on body composition and body weight in obese females. Am J Health Promot 1994; 8:442–448.

63. Harris JK, French SA, Jeffery RW, McGovern PG, Wing RR. Dietary and physical activity correlates of long-term weight loss. Obes Res 1994; 4:307–313.

64. Shah M, McGovern P, French S, Baxter J. Comparison of a low-fat, ad libitum complex-carbohydrate diet with a low-energy diet in moderately obese women. Am J Clin Nutr 1994; 59:980–984.

65. Jeffery W, Hellerstedt WL, French SA, Baxter JE. A randomized trial of counseling for fat restriction versus calorie restriction in the treatment of obesity. Int J Obes Rel Metab Disord 1995; 19:132–137.

66. Pascale RW, Wing RR, Butler BA, Mullen M, Bononi P. Effects of a behavioral weight loss program stressing caloric restriction versus calorie plus fat restriction in obese individuals with NIDDM or a family history of diabetes. Diabetes Care 1995; 18:1241–1247.

67. Siggaard R, Raben A, Astrup A. Weight loss during 12 week's ad libitum carbohydrate-rich diet in overweight and normal-weight subjects at a Danish work site. Obes Res 1996; 4:347–356.

68. Harvey-Berino J. The efficacy of dietary fat versus total energy restriction for weight loss. Obes Res 1998; 6:202–207.

69. Pritchard JE, Nowson CA, Wark JD. Bone loss accompanying diet-induced or exercised-induced weight loss: a randomized controlled study. Int J Obes 1996; 20:513–520.

70. DeGraaf C, Drijvers JJMM, Zimmermanns NJH. Energy and fat consumption during long-term consumption of reduced fat products. Appetite 1997; 29:305–323.

71. Alford BB, Blankenship AC, Hagen RD. The effects of variations in carbohydrate, protein, and fat content of the diet upon weight loss, blood values, and nutrient intake of adult obese women. J Am Diet Assoc 1990; 90:534–40.

72. Golay A, Allaz AF, Morel Y, de Tonnac N, Tankova S, Reaven G. Similar weight loss with low- or high-carbohydrate diets. Am J Clin Nutr 1996; 63:174–178.

73. Rolls BJ, Pirraglia PA, Jones ME, Peters JC. Effects of olestra, a noncaloric fat substitute, on daily energy and fat intakes in lean men. Am J Clin Nutr 1992; 56:84–92.

74. Burley VJ, Blundell JE. Evaluation of the action of a non- absorbable fat on appetite and energy intake in lean healthy males. In: Ailhaud G, Guy-Grand B, Lafontan M, and Ricquier D, eds. Obesity in Europe. John Libbey, London, 1992, pp 63–65.

75. Cotton JR, Burley VI, Weststrate JA, Blundell JE. Fat substitution and food intake: effect of replacing fat with sucrose polyester at lunch or evening meals. Br J Nutr 1996; 75:545–556.

76. Cotton JR, Weststrate JA, Blundell JE. Replacement of dietary fat with sucrose polyester: effects on energy intake and appetite control in nonobese males. Am J Clin Nutr 1996; 63:891–896.

77. Bray GA, Sparti A, Windhauser MM, York DA. Effect of two weeks fat replacement of olestra on food intake and energy metabolism. FASEB J 1995; 9 (Abstr):A439.

78. Roy J, Lovejoy J, Windhauser M, Bray G. Metabolic effects of fat substitution with olestra. FASEB J. 1997; 11 (Abstr):A358.

79. Astrup A, Raben A. Glucostatic control of intake and obesity. Proc Nutr Soc 1996; 55:485–495.

80. Lawton CL, Burley VJ, Wales JK, Blundell JE. Dietary fat and appetite control in obese subjects: weak effect on satiation and satiety. Int J Obes 1993; 17:409–416.

81. Sheppard L, Kristal AR, Kushi LH. Weight loss in women participating in a randomized trial of low-fat diets. Am J Clin Nutr 1991; 54:821–828.

82. Astrup A, Raben A. Carbohydrate and obesity. Int J Obes 1991; 19 (Suppl 5):S27–S37.

83. Rolls BJ, Bell EA, Castellanos VH, Chow M, Pelkman CL, Thorwart ML. Energy density but not fat content of foods affected energy intake in lean and obese women Am J Clin Nutr 1999; 69:863–871.

84. Drewnowski A. Energy density, palatability, and satiety: implications for weight control. Nutr Rev 1998; 56:347–353.

85. Pi-Sunyer FX. Effect of the composition of diet on energy intake. Nutr Rev 1990; 48:94–105.

86. Bell EA, Castellanos VH, Pelkman CL, Thorwart ML, Rolls BJ. Energy density of foods affects energy intake in normal-weight women. Am J Clin Nutr 1998; 67:412–420.

11 Homocysteine, Diet, and Cardiovascular Disease

Jayne V. Woodside and Ian S. Young

1. INTRODUCTION

This chapter reviews how diet affects the occurrence and severity of hyperhomocysteinemia and coronary heart disease (CHD). The chapter will also provide an update on clinical studies and review the relative importance of this issue for nutritional considerations in health care.

Homocysteine is a sulfur-containing amino acid that is an intermediary product in methionine metabolism *(1)*. In 1969, based on studies of postmortem findings in patients with very high homocysteine levels due to rare genetic defects, McCully proposed that homocysteine may promote the development of vascular lesions *(2)*. More recent investigations have focused on the possibility that moderate elevations may also be associated with increased risk of vascular disease *(3)*. To date, more than 80 clinical and epidemiological studies, including prospective studies, have shown that an elevated total homocysteine level is a common cardiovascular risk factor in the general population *(4)*. This has been shown to be the case for coronary artery disease (CAD), cerebrovascular disease, and peripheral vascular disease.

2. METABOLISM OF HOMOCYSTEINE

Intracellular homocysteine can be (1) remethylated to methionine—the transmethylation pathway, (2) converted to cystathionine—the transsulfuration pathway, or (3) exported from the cells (*see* Fig. 1). Pathway 1 is catalyzed by the enzyme methionine synthase, which requires cobalamin (vitamin B_{12}) as a cofactor and folate (in the form methyltetrahydrofolate) as cosubstrate. The remethylation pathway is favored during relative methionine deficiency, and this recycling and conservation of homocysteine ensures adequate methionine maintenance.

During pathway 2, the vitamin B_6-dependent enzyme cystathionine β-synthase catalyzes the irreversible condensation of homocysteine with serine to

From: *Nutritional Health: Strategies for Disease Prevention*
Edited by: T. Wilson and N. J. Temple © Humana Press Inc., Totowa, NJ

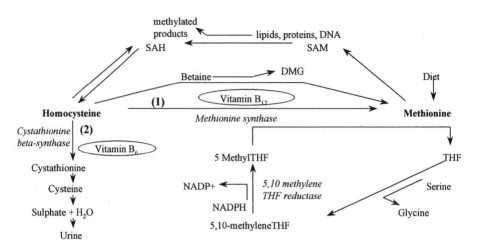

Fig. 1. Methionine cycle: metabolic cycle of homocysteine metabolism. THF = tetra-hydrofolate; DMG = dimethylglycine; SAH = *S*-adenosyl homocysteine; SAM = *S*-adenosyl methionine; NADP+ = nicotinamide adenine dinucleotide phosphate (oxidized form); NADPH = nicotinamide adenine dinucleotide phosphate (reduced form).

form cystathionine, which is then broken down to cysteine and α-ketobutyrate. In the presence of excess methionine, the transsulfuration pathway is favored by the upregulation of cystathionine β-synthase and downregulation of the remethylation pathway.

Release of homocysteine into the extracellular medium represents the third route of homocysteine removal from the cell. Such export is enhanced when production of homocysteine is increased, and reduced when production is inhibited. Thus, the amount of homocysteine in the extracellular media, such as plasma and urine, reflects the balance between intracellular production and utilization *(1,5)*.

2.1. Redox Status of Homocysteine

Homocysteine in plasma exists in different forms, including the major protein-bound fraction (approx 65%), free oxidized fraction (approx 30%), and reduced homocysteine, which is present in only trace amounts (1.5–4%). Because homocysteine in blood is rapidly oxidized, and is associated with plasma proteins, assessment of its redox status and protein binding requires immediate derivatization of the reduced homocysteine and separation of the free and bound forms *(6)*. It is thought that the redox status of homocysteine may differ between patient groups and be linked with its atherogenic effects *(7)*. Reduced homocysteine acts as a pro-oxidant in vitro and may be the atherogenic agent. In patients with early-onset peripheral vascular disease, levels of reduced, oxidized, and protein-bound homocysteine are reportedly elevated *(7)*, whereas in patients with hyperhomocysteinamia because of cobalamin deficiency *(8)*, and in patients infected with human immunodeficiency virus *(9)*, reduced homocysteine concentrations are markedly above normal.

3. MEASUREMENT OF HOMOCYSTEINE

The sum of all homocysteine species in plasma (free plus protein bound) is referred to as total homocysteine (tHcy or homocyst(e)ine). As a marked redistribution between free and bound homocysteine takes place after preparation of plasma, this gives an accurate measurement without the need for exceptionally cautious sample handling and storage *(10)*. The day-to-day variation in fasting tHcy among healthy individuals is small (coefficient of variation 7%), so that a single measurement is viable *(11)*.

The range for total tHcy differs somewhat from one laboratory to another *(12,13)*, but values between 5 and 15 μmol/L are usually considered normal. The variability may be because of different methodologies, differences in sample processing, or the selection of subjects who are under the influence of various factors that affect concentration of homocysteine *(5)*. Because of these differences, a reference range is difficult to define, as are cut-off points for mild and moderate hyperhomocysteinemia *(14)*.

3.1. Food Consumption and Homocysteine

The effect of food consumption on tHcy concentrations is complex. In recent studies, tHcy has been shown to be positively associated with both coffee consumption and dietary protein intake *(15,16)*, although a direct link between methionine content of the diet and tHcy levels has not yet been proven. The routine use of fasting (12 h fast) samples removes this difficulty.

4. CAUSES OF HYPERHOMOCYSTEINEMIA

A number of enzymes, essential cofactors, and the availability of the important cosubstrate methyltetrahydrofolate regulate plasma homocysteine concentrations. Predictably, therefore, the causes of hyperhomocysteinemia are multifactorial.

4.1. Environmental Factors

4.1.1. AGE AND GENDER

Plasma tHcy increases with age in both genders, for reasons that have not been elucidated *(17–20)*. Decreases in cofactor levels *(20,21)* or coexisting renal impairment often seen in older patients may be responsible, and age-dependent reductions in cystathionine β-synthase activity may also play a part *(22)*. In general, men have higher plasma levels than women *(20,23)*. After menopause, fasting tHcy seems to increase *(24,25)* although this has not been confirmed *(20)*, and hormone replacement therapy can lower elevated tHcy levels in postmenopausal women *(26)*. Although gender differences may be explained by the effect of sex hormones on homocysteine metabolism, they may be related to higher creatinine values *(27)* or the greater muscle mass of men than women *(20)*. Homocysteine is decreased by up to 50% during pregnancy, returning to normal 2–4 d postpartum *(28)*. The authors suggest several reasons for this decrease, including the hemodilution known to occur in pregnancy, or an increased demand for methionine by the fetus, leading to increased remethylation of homocysteine *(28)*.

4.1.2. ETHNIC GROUP

Despite a high prevalence of CHD risk factors such as hypertension, obesity, and smoking, CHD incidence rate is much lower among westernized black Africans compared with the white population *(29)*. A group of 27 black men, aged 18–25 yr, had tHcy 46% lower than similarly aged white men *(29)*. By contrast, in a study examining tHcy and B-vitamin levels in American black premenopausal women, who have higher rates of CAD than white women, black women had higher tHcy and lower folate concentrations, largely because of lifestyle factors *(30)*. Another study examined homocysteine and CAD in the Hong Kong Chinese population *(31)*. Although the prevalence of hyperhomocysteinemia was similar to that in white subjects, elevated tHcy was not an independent risk factor, being associated with smoking. Serum vitamin B_{12} did not differ between patients and control subjects. The observation of higher serum folate in those with elevated tHcy does not seem compatible with what is known about tHcy metabolism.

4.1.3. COEXISTENT DISEASE

Elevated homocysteine levels are found in a number of disease states. Impaired renal function is associated with hyperhomocysteinemia *(32–34)*. There is a positive correlation between fasting plasma tHcy and serum creatinine *(20,35)*, although the mechanism is unclear. Markedly elevated homocysteine levels have also been seen in acute lymphoblastic leukemia*(36)*, various carcinomas (including breast, ovary and, pancreas *[37–41]*), severe psoriasis *(18)*, and diabetes mellitus *(42–44)*.

5. HYPERHOMOCYSTEINEMIA AND CORONARY HEART DISEASE

Numerous studies have indicated that mild hyperhomocysteinemia is an independent risk factor for CHD. In the Physicians' Health Study *(45)*, a total of 14,916 US male physicians, aged 40–84 yr, were followed up for 6 yr. Men with homocysteine levels above the 95th percentile (based on control distribution) had a threefold increased risk of myocardial infarction compared with those within the bottom 90%. The findings were also statistically compatible with a graded risk increase across the distribution, a suggestion made by Perry and coworkers *(46)* in a prospective study of stroke in middle-aged British men. Similar findings have been reported for myocardial infarction *(47–49)*, carotid artery thickening *(50)*, and angiographically defined coronary artery stenosis *(51)*. In addition, Selhub and associates *(52)* demonstrated a gradual increase in the prevalence of carotid artery stenosis with increasing levels of homocysteine.

A meta-analysis by Boushey and colleagues *(53)* showed an increase in risk of CAD of about 70% for each 5 μmol/L rise in fasting homocysteine. They concluded that a total of 10% of CAD risk appeared to be attributable to homocysteine. Two recent studies have confirmed the relevance of homocysteine as a risk factor for vascular disease. The first was a multicenter, case-control study where the risk of atherosclerotic vascular disease (cardiac, cerebral, and peripheral) was examined, as well as the association of plasma tHcy with conventional risk factors *(54)*. The subjects comprised 750 cases and 800 controls, both male and female, below 60 yr of age. The relative risk (RR) for vascular disease in the top fifth of the fasting tHcy distribution, when compared with the bottom four-fifths, was 2.2 (95% confidence interval [CI] 1.6–2.9), and a dose-response effect was noted. This level of risk is similar to that observed for hypercholesterolemia and smoking *(54)*. The second study examined the prognostic value of homocysteine in patients with established CAD *(55)*. A total of 587 patients with angiographically confirmed CAD were followed-up for a median period of 4.6 yr. Homocysteine levels were strongly associated with levels of folate and vitamin B_{12}, history of myocardial infarction, the left ventricular ejection fraction, and serum creatinine. A strong, graded relationship was found between plasma tHcy and overall mortality. After 4 yr, 3.8% of patients with tHcy below 9 μmol/L had died compared with 24.7% of those with tHcy greater than 15 μmol/L. The association was not altered significantly when adjusted for other, possibly confounding, factors such as age, sex, serum creatinine, left ventricular ejection fraction, and history of myocardial infarction *(55)*.

However, not all studies examining the effect of homocysteine levels on the incidence of cardiovascular disease (CVD) have shown a positive association, highlighting the need for further investigation. An updated analysis of the Physicians' Health Study data yielded a relative risk for elevated tHcy of only 1.3 (95% CI 0.5–3.1) *(56)*. An analysis of the Multiple Risk Factor Intervention Trial (MRFIT) cohort showed no effect of tHcy after adjustment for other variables (RR = 0.94; 95% CI 0.56–1.56) *(57)*. An analysis of tHcy and CHD in the Caerphilly cohort showed tHcy to be only weakly predictive of CHD events *(58)*. Finally, the ARIC study showed no association between the incidence of CHD and tHcy, although there was a possibility that vitamin B_6 offered independent protection *(59)*, a finding also suggested by others *(60,61)*.

6. MECHANISMS BY WHICH HOMOCYSTEINE MAY LEAD TO VASCULAR DISEASE

Several mechanisms may be involved in the genesis of vascular disease by homocysteine, including effects on connective tissue, smooth-muscle cells,

Table 1
Possible Vascular Damaging Mechanisms of Homocysteine

Endothelial cell injury
       Impaired nitric oxide production
       Overproduction of reactive oxygen species
       Increased von Willebrand factor and thrombomodulin
       Increased tissue factor production
       Decreased antithrombin III production
       Increased smooth muscle cell production
       Increased monocyte adhesion to the vessel wall
Coagulation pathways
       Impaired platelet survival time
       Increased production of thromboxane A2 by platelets and decreased
         production of prostacyclin
       Increased activation of factors V, X, and XII
       Inhibition of antithrombin III and factor C production
       Increased fibrinogen levels
       Enhanced binding of lipoprotein (a) to fibrin
Oxidative stress
       Overproduction of reactive oxygen species
       Decreased plasma antioxidant activities
       Increased lipid peroxidation

platelets, endothelial cells, blood lipids, coagulation factors, and nitric oxide *(62)*—summarized in Table 1. The relative importance of each of these mechanisms is not fully understood *(62–65)*.

Homocysteine is toxic to endothelial cells in vitro, and in vivo. Hyperhomocysteinemia is associated with impaired endothelium-dependent vasodilation and impaired endogenous tissue-type plasminogen activator activity *(63–66)*. Homocysteine promotes increased platelet aggregation as a consequence of increased synthesis of thromboxane A_2 and decreased synthesis of prostaglandin *(63–66)*. Hyperhomocysteinemia is associated with abnormalities of the clotting cascade *(63–66)*. Homocysteine promotes the binding of lipoprotein (a) to fibrin *(67)* and the growth of smooth muscle cells *(68,69)*, and tHcy levels correlate with levels of fibrinogen, an independent risk factor for CVD *(70)*.

It must be noted, however, that many of these effects are not specific to homocysteine; a variety of free thiol-group amino acids, particularly cysteine, show similar tendencies *(63)*. Much of the research into mechanisms has been carried out at millimolar concentrations of homocysteine, which are 100–1000-fold higher than those observed in vivo. In addition, the complex redox reactions involving the various homocysteine forms and their relation to other thiols in vivo are difficult to represent accurately in vitro where a single homocysteine species is used. The complexities of elucidating an atherogenic mechanism are illustrated by the fact that oxidative modification of LDL by tHcy has been demonstrated in vitro *(71,72)* and in animal models *(73)*, but has not been observed in hyperhomocysteinemic patients *(74–77)*. Similarly, supplementation with B-group vitamins, postulated to reduce tHcy and thus inhibit lipid peroxidation, had no effect on the susceptibility of LDL to oxidation*(78)*. Homocysteine's effect on endothelial dysfunction, however, has been confirmed in a clinical setting *(79,80)*. The blocking of the effects of hyperhomocysteinemia on endothelial dysfunction by pretreatment with antioxidant vitamins still suggests the involvement of an oxidative mechanism *(81)*. Similarly, in a cross-sectional study, plasma tHcy was associated strongly ($r = 0.40$, $p < 0.001$) with plasma F-2-isoprostane levels, a marker for in vivo lipid peroxidation *(82)*. The observation by Glueck and associates *(83)* of a higher risk of myocardial infarction in hyperlipidemic patients with hyperhomocysteinemia and low HDL also suggests the possibility of an interaction between these risk factors.

7. EFFECT OF VITAMIN SUPPLEMENTATION AND DIET ON HOMOCYSTEINE

Cross-sectional and experimental evidence suggests that mild hyperhomocysteinemia may be related to subclinical deficiencies of folate, vitamin B_6, and vitamin B_{12}—all cofactors or cosubstrates in homocysteine metabolism *(84–93)*. In a study of vitamin and tHcy levels in an elderly population, Selhub and coauthors *(21)* found a strong inverse correlation between tHcy and plasma folate, and weaker inverse correlations between tHcy and both cobalamin and vitamin B_6 (pyridoxal-5-phosphate). The authors concluded that elevated tHcy levels could, in great part, be due to poor vitamin status, and these results have been confirmed in many other studies.

Many studies have assessed the effects of vitamin supplementation on plasma tHcy. Levels in folate-deficient patients can be reduced by oral folate supplementation *(94)*. In one study, the elevated tHcy in patients with renal failure decreased after only 2 wk of folate therapy *(95)*. Maximal effects may be seen after 4 *(95)* to 6 *(96)* wk of therapy. The lowest effective dose for folate supplementation has not yet been determined. Doses of 5 mg or 10 mg *(97)* alone or 1 mg in conjunction with vitamins B_{12} and B_6 may be effective *(96)*. Ubbink and colleagues *(96)* confirmed by intervention that a daily supplement of folate (1 mg), B_6 (10 mg) and B_{12} (0.4 mg) could normalize elevated tHcy (>16.3 μmol/L, $n = 44$) within 6 wk. Ubbink and colleagues *(98)* then looked at the effect of supplementation with the individual vitamins in 100 men, aged between 20 and 73 yr, with tHcy greater than 16.3 μmol/L, over 6 wk. Folate supplementation (0.65 mg/d) reduced plasma tHcy by 42% whereas a daily vitamin B_{12} supplement (0.4 mg/d) lowered it by 15%. The vitamin B_6 supplement (10 mg/d) had no significant effect. The combination of the three vitamins reduced circulating tHcy by 50% that was not significantly different from the reduction achieved by folate supplementation alone. Brattstrom and coworkers *(99)* noted significantly lower tHcy in middle-aged and elderly subjects taking multivitamins containing doses of folic acid ranging from only 200–400 µg. Homocysteine values increase if vitamin therapy is discontinued *(95,100).*

Ward and colleagues *(101)* carried out an uncontrolled study examining the effect of low-dose folate supplementation in healthy male subjects. Folate supplements were administered daily at doses increasing from 100 µg for 6 wk to 200 µg for 6 wk and then up to 400 µg for 14 wk. A dose of 200 µg/d appeared to be the optimum tHcy-lowering dose as there was no apparent benefit of increasing the dose to 400 µg/d. The subjects had reported a mean dietary folate intake of 281 ± 60 µg/d. Their total folate intake, with the additional 200 µg supplement, therefore corresponds well with the observation by Selhub and colleagues *(21)* that total intakes over 400 µg/d are associated with desirable tHcy in a healthy elderly US population. When the analysis in the former study was carried out by tertiles of baseline tHcy, the lowest tertile group showed no increase in red-cell folate over the 6-mo supplementation period, suggesting that their baseline folate status was optimal to begin with. Ward and associates *(101)* suggests that, although there does not appear to be a threshold in the relationship between elevated tHcy and CVD risk, there may be a threshold of plasma tHcy in terms of ability to respond to folate.

A further randomized placebo-controlled study in healthy women aged 18–40 yr confirmed that both 250 µg and 500 µg folate/d for 4 wk decreased tHcy. Eight weeks after the end of folate supplementation, tHcy had not returned to baseline *(100).*

A meta-analysis of 12 studies using B-group vitamins to lower tHcy has recently been carried out *(102).* The magnitude of tHcy reduction was related to the pretreatment tHcy and folate levels. Folate reduced tHcy by 25% (95% CI 23–28%), and the effects were similar at daily doses ranging from 0.5–5 mg. Vitamin B_{12} yielded a further tHcy reduction of 5–6%, but vitamin B_6 had no significant effect. None of these trials, assessed the effect on tHcy after methionine loading, however, which is determined by the transsulfuration pathway where vitamin B_6 is a cofactor.

The effectiveness of vitamins B_{12} and B_6 in homocysteine-lowering therapies needs further study. Allen and associates *(103)* have shown that folate supplementation will not correct hyperhomocysteinemia that is primarily the result of vitamin B_{12} deficiency, whereas Robinson and colleagues *(104)* found that vitamin B_6 was inversely related to risk of CVD independently of homocysteine, although this may be due to its ability to modulate the homocysteine peak after the oral methionine load test. Administration of vitamin B_6 alone does not lower fasting tHcy *(97,98).* Dose-optimizing studies for these vitamins are also required.

Woodside and colleagues *(105)* have tested the hypothesis that simultaneous administration of antioxidant vitamins may potentiate the effect of B-group vitamins on elevated tHcy. An interaction between antioxidants and folate is conceivable because the latter is susceptible to inactivation by free-radical mediated oxidation, which can be prevented both in vitro and in vivo by vitamin C *(106,107)*. Although B-group vitamins lowered tHcy by roughly 30%, the addition of antioxidant vitamins to the supplement had no effect on this *(105)*.

It is clear from the foregoing evidence above that B-group vitamin supplementation effectively lowers plasma homocysteine. The question therefore arises whether a dietary change in B-vitamin intake or food fortification can achieve similar results. To date, the lowest effective tHcy-lowering supplement was 200 µg folate daily *(101)*. Selhub and coworkers *(21)* found that a total folate intake of 400 µg/d was necessary to prevent elevation of tHcy, and dietary intake approximating this value was only attained by 30–40% of participants in the Framingham study. Boushey and coworkers *(53)* suggested that if the US population were to eat two to three more servings of fruit and vegetables per day, this would lead to a reduction of 4% in CVD deaths per year in the United States through tHcy reduction. Food fortification at 350 µg of folate/100 g of grain products would lead to a reduction in CVD deaths of 8%.

Cuskelly and associates *(108)* looked at the effects of increasing dietary folate on red-cell folate, with a view to preventing neural tube defects. Red-cell folate concentration increased significantly over 3 mo in patients taking folate supplements or food fortified with folate (both given so as to increase consumption by 400 µg/d). There was no increase in those given food naturally rich in folate (again to provide an estimated increase in intake of 400 µg/d) or in those offered dietary advice only. The likely explanation lies in the higher bioavailability of folate supplements compared to food folates. Further investigation is needed using larger numbers of subjects to assess the relative effectiveness of a high-folate diet, food fortification with folate, and folate supplementation on homocysteine.

In 1996, the Food and Drug Administration issued a regulation requiring all enriched grain products to be fortified with folate (140 µg/100 g, providing approximately an additional 70–120 µg folate/d). The main aim of this public health action was to reduce the risk of neural tube defects in newborns. A survey of folate and tHcy in the Framingham Offspring Study cohort before and after fortification showed an increase in folate and decrease in tHcy, and also a reduction in the prevalence of low folate and elevated tHcy, respectively. In this middle-aged and elderly population, fortification has significantly improved folate status and may therefore contribute to reduced CVD prevalence *(109)*. This is in contrast to the findings of Malinow and colleagues *(110)* who, in a crossover trial in 75 subjects, tested the effects of fortified breakfast cereal on plasma tHcy and folate. These researchers found that cereal providing approximately the intake resulting from the FDA enrichment policy only decreased tHcy by 3.7%, a difference that was not statistically significant. Jacques and coworkers *(109)* suggested that several features of this study may have limited its applicability to the general population. The

Table 2
Ongoing Vitamin Supplementation Studies to Lower Homocysteine
and Prevent Cardiovascular Disease

CHD prevention	Number of subjects
NORVIT (Norwegian study of homocysteine lowering with B Vitamins in myocardial infarction; University of Tromso, Norway)	3000
PACIFIC (Prevention with a Combined Inhibitor and Folate in Coronary heart disease; University of Sydney, Australia)	10,000
SEARCH (Study of the Effectiveness of Additional Reductions in Cholesterol and Homocysteine; University of Oxford, England)	12,000
WACS (Women's Antioxidant and Cardiovascular disease Study; Harvard Medical School, USA)	8000
CHAOS-2 (Cambridge Heart Antioxidant Study; University of Cambridge, England)	4000
BERGEN (Bergen Vitamin Study; University of Bergen, Norway)	2000
Stroke prevention	
VISP (Vitamin Intervention for Stroke Prevention; Wake Forest University, USA)	3600
HOPE-2 (Health Outcome and Prevention Evaluation number 2; Canada)	5000

length of the treatment was only 5 wk, which may have not been sufficient time to achieve a new steady-state concentration, while the study was performed in CAD patients who may require higher folate intake to lower tHcy.

8. CLINICAL TRIALS

There is a wealth of epidemiological evidence linking homocysteine with the development of vascular disease, including large prospective cohort studies with confirmation by meta-analysis, and clear evidence that B-group vitamins effectively lower homocysteine. There is presently no clinical trial evidence to show that lowering homocysteine by nutritional or pharmacological intervention will prevent cardiovascular events, however. Such evidence is clearly crucial in providing final confirmation of the homocysteine hypothesis, and a number of large clinical trials will report in the next few years (*see* Table 2).

9. CONCLUSION

In conclusion, there is strong support for tHcy as an independent risk factor for atherosclerosis. Dose-finding studies are required to elucidate the optimum combination of vitamins that will lower tHcy in the general population, whereas further work must be carried out on tHcy's atherogenic mechanism. Intervention studies with clinical endpoints are also required to assess the effect of strategies designed to lower plasma homocysteine, and initial studies suggesting a role for tHcy in other diseases must also be developed.

REFERENCES

1. Finkelstein JD. Methionine metabolism in mammals. J Nutr Biochem 1990; 1:228–237.
2. McCully KS. Vascular pathology of homocysteinemia: implications for the pathogenesis of arteriosclerosis. Am J Pathol 1969; 56:111–128.
3. McCully KS. Homocysteine theory of arteriosclerosis–development and current status. Atheroscler Rev 1983; 11:157–246.
4. Refsum H, Ueland PM, Nygard O, Vollset SE. Homocysteine and cardiovascular disease. Ann Rev Med 1998; 49:31–62.
5. Ueland PM, Refsum H, Stabler SP, Malinow MR, Andersson A, Allen RH. Total homocyst(e)ine in plasma or serum: methods and clinical applications. Clin Chem 1993; 39:1764–1779.
6. Mansoor MA, Svardal AM, Ueland PM. Determination of the in vivo redox status of cysteine, cysteinylglycine, homocysteine and glutathione in human plasma. Anal Biochem 1992; 200:218–229.
7. Mansoor MA, Bergmark C, Svardal AM, Lonning PE, Ueland PM. Redox status and protein binding of plasma homocysteine and other aminothiols in patients with early-onset peripheral vascular disease. Arterioscler Thromb Vasc Biol 1995; 15:232–240.
8. Mansoor MA, Ueland PM, Svardal AM. Redox status and protein binding of plasma homocysteine and other aminothiols in patients with hyperhomocysteinemia due to cobalamin deficiency. Am J Clin Nutr 1994; 59:631–635.
9. Muller, F, Svardal AM, Aukrust P, Berge RK, Ueland PM, Froland SS. Elevated plasma concentration of reduced homocysteine in patients with human immunodeficiency virus infection. Am J Clin Nutr 1996; 63:242–248.
10. Ueland PM, Refsum H. Plasma homocysteine, a risk factor for vascular disease: plasma levels in health, disease and drug therapy. J Lab Clin Med 1989; 114:473–501.
11. Garg UC, Zheng ZJ, Folsom AR. Short-term and long-term variability of plasma homocysteine measurement. Clin Chem 1997; 43:141–145.
12. Rasmussen K, Moller J, Lungbak M. Age- and gender-specific reference intervals for total homocysteine and methylmalonic acid in plasma before and after vitamin supplementation. Clin Chem 1996; 42:630–636.
13. Dudman NPB, Guo XW, Crooks R. Assay of plasma homocysteine: light sensitivity of the fluorescent 7-benzo-2-oxa-1,3-diazo-4-sulfonic acid derivative, and use of appropriate calibrators. Clin Chem 1996; 42:2028-2032.
14. Ubbink JB, Becker PJ, Vermaak WJH, Delport R. Results of a B-vitamin supplementation study used in a prediction model to define a reference range for plasma homocysteine. Clin Chem 1995; 41:1033–1037.
15. Nygard O, Refsum H, Ueland PM, Vollset SE. Major lifestyle determinants of plasma total homocysteine distribution: the Hordaland Homocysteine Study. Am J Clin Nutr 1998; 67:263–270.
16. Stolzenberg-Solomon RZ, Miller ER, Maguire MG, Selhub J, Appel LJ. Association of dietary protein intake and coffee consumption with serum homocysteine concentrations in an older population. Am J Clin Nutr 1999; 69:467–475.
17. Nygard O, Refsum H, Ueland PM, Vollset SE. Major lifestyle determinants of plasma total homocysteine distribution: the Hordaland Homocysteine Study. Am J Clin Nutr 1998; 67:263–270.

18. Ueland PM, Refsum H, Brattstrom L. Plasma homocysteine and cardiovascular disease. In Francis RB, ed. Atherosclerotic Cardiovascular Disease, Hemostasis, and Endothelial Function, Marcel Dekker, New York, pp. 183–236, 1992.
19. Kang SS, Wong PW, Cook HY, Norusis M, Messer JV. Protein-bound homocyst(e)ine. A possible risk factor for coronary artery disease. J Clin Invest 1986; 77:1482–1486.
20. Andersson A, Brattstrom L, Israelsson B, Isaksson A, Amfelt A, Hultberg B. Plasma homocysteine before and after methionine loading with regard to age, gender, and menopausal status. Eur J Clin Invest 1992; 22:79–87.
21. Selhub J, Jacques PF, Wilson PWF, Rush D, Rosenberg IH. Vitamin status and intake as primary determinants of homocysteinemia in an elderly population. JAMA 1993; 270:2693–2698.
22. Nordstrom M, Kjellstrom T. Age dependency of cystathionine beta-synthase activity in human fibroblasts in homocyst(e)inemia and atherosclerotic vascular disease. Atherosclerosis 1992; 94:213–221.
23. Jacobsen DW, Gatautis VJ, Green R, Robinson K, Savon SR, Secic M, et al. Rapid HPLC determination of total homocysteine and other thiols in human serum and plasma: sex differences and correlation with cobalamin and folate concentrations in healthy subjects. Clin Chem 1994; 40:873–881.
24. Boers GH, Smals AG, Trijbels FJ, Leermakers AI, Kloppenborg PW. Unique efficacy of methionine metabolism in premenopausal women may protect vascular disease in the reproductive years. J Clin Invest 72:1971–1976.
25. Wouters MGAJ, Moorrees EC, van der Mooren MJ, Blom HJ, Boers GHJ, Schellekens LA, et al. Plasma homocysteine and menopausal status. Eur J Clin Invest 1995; 25:801–805.
26. Van der Mooren MJ, Wouters MGAJ, Blom HJ, Schellekens LA, Eskes TKAB, Rolland R. Hormone replacement therapy may reduce high serum homocysteine in postmenopausal women. Eur J Clin Invest 1994; 24:733–736.
27. Wu LL, Wu J, Hunt SC, James BC, Vincent GM, Williams RR, Hopkins PN. Plasma homocyst(e)ine as a risk factor for early familial coronary artery disease. Clin Chem 40:552–561.
28. Andersson A, Hultberg B, Brattstrom L, Isaksson A. Decreased serum homocysteine in pregnancy. Eur J Clin Chem 1992; 30:377–379.
29. Vermaak WJH, Ubbink JB, Delport R, Becker PJ, Bissbort SH, Ungerer JPJ. Ethnic immunity to coronary heart disease? Atherosclerosis 1991; 89:155–162.
30. Gerhard GT, Malinow MR, DeLoughery TG, Evans AJ, Sexton G, Connor SL, et al. Higher total homocysteine concentrations and lower folate concentrations in premenopausal black women than in premenopausal white women. Am J Clin Nutr 1999; 70:252–260.
31. Lolin YI, Sanderson JE, Cheng SK, Chan CF, Pang CP, Woo KS, Masarei JRL. Hyperhomocysteinaemia and premature coronary artery disease in the Chinese. Heart 1996; 76:117–122.
32. Wilcken DEL, Gupta VJ. Sulfur containing amino acids in chronic renal failure with particular reference to homocystine and cysteine-homocysteine mixed disulfide. Eur J Clin Invest 1979; 9:301–307.
33. Soria C, Chadefaux B, Coude M, Gaillard O, Kamoun P. Concentrations of total homocysteine in plasma in chronic renal failure. Clin Chem 1990; 36:2137–2138.
34. Woodside JV, Fogarty DG, Lightbody JH, Loughrey CM, Yarnell JWG, Maxwell AP, Young IS. Homocysteine and B-group vitamins in renal transplant patients. Clin Chim Acta 1999; 282:157–166.
35. Brattstrom L, Lindgren A, Israelsson B, Malinow MR, Norrving B, Upson B, Hamfelt A. Hyperhomocysteinemia in stroke: prevalence, cause, and relationships to type of stroke and stroke risk factors. Eur J Clin Invest 1992; 22:214–221.
36. Refsum H, Wesenberg F, Ueland PM. Plasma homocysteine in children with acute lymphoblastic leukemia: changes during a chemotherapeutic regimen including methotrexate. Cancer Res 1991; 51:828–835.

37. Wu JT, Wu L, Wilson W. Increased levels of plasma homocysteine in patients with various carcinomas (Abstract). Ir J Med Sci 1995; 164:29A.
38. Stolzenberg-Solomon RZ, Albanes D, Nieto FJ, Hartman TJ, Tangrea JA, Rautalahti M, et al. Pancreatic cancer risk and nutrition-related methyl group availability indicators in male smokers. J Natl Cancer Inst 1999; 91:535–541.
39. Zhang S, Hunter DJ, Hankinson SE, Giovannucci EL, Rosner BA, Colditz GA, et al. A prospective study of folate intake and the risk of breast cancer. JAMA 1999; 281:1632–1637.
40. Kato I, Dnistrian AM, Schwartz M, Toniolo P, Koenig K, Shore RE, et al. Serum folate, homocysteine and colorectal cancer risk in women: a nested case-control study. Br J Cancer 1999; 79:1917–1921.
41. Wu KN, Helzlsouer KJ, Comstock GW, Hoffman SC, Nadeau MR, Selhub J. A prospective study on folate, B12 and pyridoxal 5-phosphate (B6) and breast cancer. Cancer Epidemiol Biomarker Prev 1999; 8:209–217.
42. Hultberg B, Agardh E, Andersson A, Brattstom L, Isaksson A, Israelsson B, Agardh CD. Increased levels of plasma homocysteine are associated with nephropathy, but not severe retinopathy in type I diabetes mellitus. Scand J Clin Lab Invest 1991; 51:277–282.
43. Araki A, Sako Y, Ito H. Plasma homocysteine concentrations in Japanese patients with non-insulin-dependent diabetes mellitus: effect of parenteral methylcobalamin treatment. Atherosclerosis 1993; 103:149–157.
44. Vaccaro O, Ingrosso D, Rivellese A, Greco G, Riccardi G. Moderate hyperhomocysteinaemia and retinopathy in insulin-dependent diabetes. Lancet 1997; 349:1102–1103.
45. Stampfer MJ, Malinow MR, Willett WC, Newcomer LM, Upson B, Ullmann D, et al. A prospective study of plasma homocyst(e)ine and risk of myocardial infarction in US physicians. JAMA 1992; 268:877–881.
46. Perry IJ, Refsum H, Morris RW, Ebrahim SB, Ueland PM, Shaper AG. Prospective study of serum total homocysteine concentration and risk of stroke in middle-aged British men. Lancet 1995; 346:1395–1398.
47. Arnesen E, Refsum H, Bonaa KH, Ueland PM, Forde OH, Nordrehaug JE. Serum total homocysteine and coronary heart disease. Int J Epidemiol 1995; 24:704–709.
48. Wald NJ, Watt HC, Law MR, Weir DG, McPartlin J, Scott JM. Homocysteine and ischaemic heart disease. Results of a prospective study with implications regarding prevention. Arch Intern Med 1998; 158:862–867.
49. Ridker PM, Manson JE, Buring JE, Shih J, Matias M, Hennekens CH. Homocysteine and risk of cardiovascular disease among postmenopausal women. JAMA 281:1817–1821.
50. Malinow MR, Nieto FJ, Szklo M, Chambless LE, Bond G. Carotid artery intimal-medial wall thickening and plasma homocyst(e)ine in asymptomatic adults: the Atherosclerosis Risk in Communities Study. Circulation 1993; 87:1107–1113.
51. Genest JJ, McNamara JR, Salem DN, Wilson PWF, Schaefer EJ, Malinow MR. Plasma homocyst(e)ine levels in men with premature coronary artery disease. J Am Coll Cardiol 1990; 16:1114–1119.
52. Selhub J, Jacques PF, Boston AG, D'Agostino RB, Wilson PWF, Belanger AJ, et al. Association between plasma homocysteine concentrations and extracranial carotid-artery stenosis. N Engl J Med 1995; 332:286–291.
53. Boushey CJ, Beresford SAA, Omenn GS, Motulsky AG. A quantitative assessment of plasma homocysteine as a risk factor for vascular disease. Probable benefits of increasing folic acid intakes. JAMA 1995; 274:1049–1057.
54. Graham IM, Daly LE, Refsum HM, Robinson K, Brattstrom L, Ueland PM, et al. Plasma homocysteine as a risk factor for vascular disease. The European Concerted Action Project. JAMA 1997; 277:1775–1781.
55. Nygard O, Nordrehaug JE, Refsum H, Ueland PM, Farstad M, Vollset SE. Plasma homocysteine levels and mortality in patients with coronary artery disease. N Engl J Med 1997; 337:230–236.

56. Chasan-Taber L, Selhub J, Rosenberg IH, Malinow MR, Terry P, Tishler PV, et al. A prospective study of folate and vitamin B6 and risk of myocardial infarction in US physicians. J Am Coll Nutr 1996; 15:136–143.

57. Evans RW, Shaten BJ, Hempel JD, Cutler JA, Kuller LH. Homocyst(e)ine and risk of cardiovascular disease in the Multiple Risk Factor Intervention Trial. Arterioscler Thromb Vasc Biol 1997; 17:1947–1953.

58. Ubbink JB, Fehily AM, Pickering J, Elwood PC, Vermaak WJH. Homocysteine and ischaemic heart disease in the Caerphilly cohort. Atherosclerosis 1998; 140:349–356.

59. Folsom AR, Nieto FJ, McGovern PG, Tsai MY, Malinow MR, Eckfeldt JH, et al. Prospective study of coronary heart disease incidence in relation to fasting total homocysteine, related genetic polymorphisms, and B vitamins. The Atherosclerosis Risk in Communities (ARIC) Study. Circulation 1998; 98:204–210.

60. Robinson K, Arheart K, Refsum H, Brattstrom L, Boers G, Ueland P, et al. Low circulating folate and vitamin B6 concentrations. Risk factors for stroke, peripheral vascular disease, and coronary artery disease. Circulation 1998; 97:437–443.

61. Rimm EB, Willett WC, Hu FB, Sampson L, Colditz GA, Manson JE, et al. Folate and vitamin B6 from diet and supplements in relation to risk of coronary heart disease among women. JAMA 1998; 279:359–364.

62. Refsum H, Ueland PM, Nygard O, Vollset SE. Homocysteine and cardiovascular disease. Ann Rev Med 1998; 49:31–62.

63. Rees MM, Rodgers GM. Homocysteinemia: association of a metabolic disorder with vascular disease and thrombosis. Thromb Res 1993; 71:337–359.

64. Moghadasian MH, McManus BM, Frohlich JJ. Homocysteine and coronary artery disease. Clinical evidence and genetic and metabolic background. Arch Intern Med 1997; 157:2299–2308.

65. Welch GN, Loscalzo J. Homocysteine and atherothrombosis. N Engl J Med 1998; 338:1042–1050.

66. Stein JH, McBride PE. Hyperhomocysteinemia and atherosclerotic vascular disease. Pathophysiology, screening and treatment. Arch Intern Med 1998; 158:1301–1306.

67. Harpel PC, Chang VT, Borth W. Homocysteine and other sulfhydryl compounds enhance the binding of lipoprotein(a) to fibrin: a potential biochemical link between thrombosis, atherogenesis, and sulfhydryl compound metabolism. Proc Natl Acad Sci USA 1992; 89:10,193–10,197.

68. Tsai JC, Perrella MA, Yoshizumi M, Hsieh CM, Haber E, Schlegel R, Lee ME. Promotion of vascular smooth muscle cell growth by homocysteine: a link to atherosclerosis. Proc Natl Acad Sci USA 1994; 91:6369–6373.

69. Tang L, Mamotte CDS, van Bockxmeer FMV, Taylor RR. The effect of homocysteine on DNA synthesis in cultured human vascular smooth muscle. Atherosclerosis 1998; 136:169–173.

70. Von Eckardstein A, Malinow MR, Upson B, Heinrich J, Schulte H, Schonfeld R, et al. Effects of age, lipoproteins and hemostatic parameters on the role of homocyst(e)inemia as a cardiovascular risk factor in men. Arterioscler Thromb 1994; 14:960–964.

71. Heinecke JW, Rosen H, Suzuki LA, Chait A. The role of sulphur-containing amino acids in superoxide production and modification of low density lipoprotein by arterial smooth muscle cells. J Biol Chem 1987; 262:10,098–10,103.

72. Parthasarathy S. Oxidation of low density lipoprotein by thiol compounds leads to its recognition by the acetyl LDL receptor. Biochem Biophys Acta 1987; 917:337–340.

73. Young PB, Kennedy S, Molloy AM, Scott JM, Weir DG, Kennedy DG. Lipid peroxidation induced in vivo by hyperhomocysteinaemia in pigs. Atherosclerosis 1997; 129:67–71.

74. Halvorsen B, Brude I, Drevon CA, Nysom J, Ose L, Christiansen EN, Nenseter MS. Effect of homocysteine on copper ion-catalysed, azo compound-initiated, and mononuclear cell-mediated oxidative modification of low density lipoprotein. J Lipid Res 1996; 37:1591–1600.

75. Clarke R, Naughten E, Cahalane S, O'Sullivan K, Mathias P, McCall T, Graham I. The role of free radicals as mediators of endothelial cell injury in hyperhomocysteinaemia. Ir J Med Sci 1992; 161:561–564.

76. Cordoba-Porras A, Sanchez-Quesada JL, Gonzales-Sastre F, Ordonez-Llanos J, Blanco-Vaca F. Susceptibility of plasma low- and high-density lipoproteins to oxidation in patients with severe hyperhomocysteinemia. J Mol Med 1996; 74:771–776.

77. Blom HJ, Kleinvel HA, Boers GHJ, Demacker PNM, Haklemmers HLM, Tepoelepothoff MTWB, Trijbels JMF. Lipid peroxidation and susceptibility of low-density-lipoprotein to in-vitro oxidation in hyperhomocysteinaemia. Eur J Clin Invest 1995; 25:149–154.

78. Woodside JV, Yarnell JWG, McMaster D, Young IS, Roxborough HE, McCrum EE, et al. Antioxidants, but not B-group vitamins increase the susceptibility of LDL to oxidation: a randomised, factorial design, placebo-controlled trial. Atherosclerosis 1999; 144:419–427.

79. Woo KS, Chook P, Lolin YI, Cheung ASP, Chan LT, Sun YY, et al. Hyperhomocysteinemia is a risk factor for arterial endothelial dysfunction in humans. Circulation 1997; 96:2542–2544.

80. Van den Berg M, Boers GHJ, Franken DG, Blom HJ, van Kamp GJ, Jakobs C, et al. Hyperhomocysteinaemia and endothelial dysfunction in young patients with peripheral arterial occlusive disease. Eur J Clin Invest 1995; 25:176–181.

81. Nappo F, de Rosa N, Marfella R, de Lucia D, Ingrosso D, Perna AF, et al. Impairment of endothelial functions by acute hyperhomocysteinemia and reversal by antioxidant vitamins. JAMA 1999; 281:2113–2118.

82. Voutilainen S, Morrow JD, Roberts LJ, Alfthan G, Alho H, Nyyssonen K, Salonen JT. Enhanced in vivo lipid peroxidation at elevated plasma total homocysteine levels. Arterioscler Thromb Vasc Biol 1999; 19:1263–1266.

83. Glueck CJ, Shaw P, Lang J, Tracy T, Seive–Smith L, Wang Y. Evidence that homocysteine is an independent risk factor for atherosclerosis in hyperlipidaemic patients. Am J Cardiol 1995; 75:132–136.

84. Brattstrom L, Israelsson B, Lindgarde F, Hultberg B. Higher total plasma homocysteine in vitamin B12 deficiency than in heterozygosity for homocystinuria due to cystathionine b-synthase deficiency. Metabolism 1988; 37:175–178.

85. Stabler SP, Marcell PD, Podell ER, Allen RH, Savage DG, Lindenbaum J. Elevation of total homocysteine in serum of patients with cobalamin or folate deficiency detected by capillary gas chromatography-mass spectrometry. J Clin Invest 1988; 81:466–474.

86. Lindenbaum J, Healton EB, Savage DG, Brust JCM, Garrett TJ, Podell ER, et al. Neuropsychiatric disorders caused by cobalamin deficiency in the absence of anemia or macrocytosis. N Engl J Med 1988; 318:1720–1728.

87. Kang SS, Wong PWK, Norusis M. Homocysteinemia due to folate deficiency. Metabolism 1987; 36:458–462.

88. Park KY, Linkswiler H. Effect of vitamin B6 depletion in adult man on the excretion of cystathionine and other methionine metabolites. J Nutr 1970; 100:110–116.

89. Slavik M, Smith KJ, Blanc O. Decrease of serum pyridoxal phosphate levels and homocystinemia after administration of 6-azauridine triacetate and their prevention by administration of pyridoxine. Biochem Pharmacol 1982; 31:4089–4092.

90. Smolin LA, Crenshaw TD, Kurtycz D, Benevenga NJ. Homocysteine accumulation in pigs fed diets deficient in vitamin B-6: relationship to atherosclerosis. J Nutr 1983; 113:2022–2033.

91. Smolin LA, Benevenga NJ. Accumulation of homocyst(e)ine in vitamin B6 deficiency: A model for the study of cystathionine b-synthase deficiency. J Nutr 1982; 112:1264–1272.

92. Miller JW, Ribaya-Mercado JD, Russell RM, Shepard DC, Morrow FD, Cochary EF, et al. Effect of vitamin B6 deficiency on fasting plasma homocysteine concentrations. Am J Clin Nutr 1992; 55:1154–1160.

93. Lussier-Cacan S, Xhignesse M, Piolot A, Selhub J, Davignon J, Genest J. Plasma total homocysteine in healthy subjects: sex-specific relation with biological traits. Am J Clin Nutr 1996; 64:587–593.

94. Stabler SP, Marcell PD, Podell ER, Allen RH, Savage DG, Lindenbaum J. Elevation of total homocysteine in serum of patients with cobalamin or folate deficiency detected by capillary gas chromatography-mass spectrometry. J Clin Invest 1988; 81:466–474.

95. Wilcken DEL, Gupta VJ, Betts AK. Homocysteine in the plasma of renal transplant recipients: effects of cofactors for methionine metabolism. Clin Sci 1981; 61:743-749.

96. Ubbink JB, Vermaak WJH, van der Merwe A, Becker PJ. Vitamin B12, vitamin B6, and folate nutritional status in men with hyperhomocysteinemia. Am J Clin Nutr 1993; 57:47–53.

97. Brattstrom L, Israelsson B, Norrving B, Bergqvist D, Thorne J, Hultberg B, Hamfelt A. Impaired homocysteine metabolism in early-onset cerebral and peripheral occlusive arterial disease: effects of pyridoxine and folic acid treatment. Atherosclerosis 1990; 81:51–60.

98. Ubbink JB, Vermaak WJH, Van der Merwe A, Becker PJ, Delport R, Potgieter HC. Vitamin requirements for the treatment of hyperhomocysteinemia in humans. J Nutr 1994; 124:1927–1933.

99. Brattstrom L, Lindgren A, Israelsson B, Andersson A, Hultberg B. Homocysteine and cysteine: determinants of plasma levels in middle-aged and elderly subjects. J Intern Med 1994; 236:633–641.

100. Brouwer IA, van Dusseldorp M, Thomas CMG, Duran M, Hautvast JGAJ, Eskes T, et al. Low-dose folic acid supplementation decreases plasma homocysteine concentrations: a randomized trial. Am J Clin Nutr 1999; 69:99–104.

101. Ward M, McNulty H, McPartlin J, Strain JJ, Weir DG, Scott JM. Plasma homocysteine, a risk factor for cardiovascular disease, is lowered by physiological doses of folic acid. Q J Med 1997; 90:519–524.

102. Brattstrom L, Landgren F, Israelsson B, Lindgren A, Hultberg B, Andersson A, et al. Homocysteine Lowering Trialists Collaboration. Lowering blood homocysteine with folic acid-based supplements: meta-analysis of randomized trials. BMJ 1998; 316:894–898.

103. Allen RH, Stabler SP, Savage DG, Lindenbaum J. Diagnosis of cobalamin deficiency 1: Usefulness of serum methylmalonic acid and total homocysteine concentrations. Am J Haematol 1990; 34:90–98.

104. Robinson K, Mayer EL, Miller DP, Green R, Vanlente F, Gupta A, et al. Hyperhomocysteinemia and low pyridoxal phosphate. Common and independent reversible risk factors for coronary artery disease. Circulation 1995; 92:2825–2830.

105. Woodside JV, Yarnell JWG, McMaster D, Young IS, Harmon DL, McCrum EE, et al. Effect of B-group vitamins and antioxidant vitamins on hyperhomocysteinemia: a double-blind, randomized, factorial-design, controlled trial. Am J Clin Nutr 1998; 67:858–866.

106. Jacob RA, Otradovec CL, Russell RM, Munro HN, Hartz SC, McGandy RB, et al. Vitamin C status and nutrient interactions in a healthy elderly population. Am J Clin Nutr 1988; 48:1436–1442.

107. Jacob RA, Kelley DS, Pianalto FS, Swendeid ME, Henning SM, Zhang JZ, et al. Immunocompetence and oxidant defense during ascorbate depletion of healthy men. Am J Clin Nutr 1991; 54:1302S–1309S.

108. Cuskelly GJ, McNulty H, Scott JM. Effect of increasing dietary folate on red-cell folate: Implications for prevention of neural tube defects. Lancet 1996; 347:657–659.

109. Jacques PF, Selhub J, Bostom AG, Wilson PWF, Rosenberg IH. The effect of folic acid fortification on plasma folate and total homocysteine concentrations. N Engl J Med 1999; 340:1449–1454.

110. Malinow MR, Duell PB, Hess DL, Anderson PH, Kruger WD, Phillipson BE, et al. Reduction of plasma homocysteine levels by breakfast cereal fortified with folic acid in patients with coronary heart disease. N Engl J Med 1998; 338:1009–1015.

12 Medical Nutrition Therapy for Diabetes

What Are the Unanswered Questions?

Marion J. Franz

I. INTRODUCTION

There has been a steady increase in prevalence of diabetes over the past 40 years. In 1998, approx 5.9% of the US population, 15.7 million Americans, were reported to have diabetes *(1)*. Of that total, 10.3 million people have been diagnosed, and another 5.4 million people have diabetes but are not aware of it. This is in contrast to 1958, when it was reported that approx 1.5 million Americans had diabetes. Diabetes is most prevalent in the middle-aged and elderly population, affecting approx 18.4% of people age 65 or older. Ethnic populations that have a two- to fivefold increased risk of diabetes include Native-Americans, Hispanic-Americans (Latino or Mexican origin), African-Americans, Asian-Americans, and Pacific Islanders, and Alaska natives *(1)*.

Medical costs are three times more for persons with diabetes. The medical cost for the person with diabetes is reported to be $10,071/yr, compared to $2669/yr for the person without diabetes. Furthermore, two-thirds of these costs are borne by the elderly *(2)*. Delaying the onset or slowing the progression of diabetes has tremendous potential to reduce medical costs.

2. CLASSIFICATION OF DIABETES MELLITUS

The classification of diabetes is now based on its etiology. With the previous classification system it was often assumed that if an individual required insulin for glycemic control, they had insulin-dependent or type 1 diabetes and if they did not require insulin, they had non-insulin-dependent or type 2 diabetes. Genetic factors play a role in both types of diabetes, but are more prominent in the development of type 2 diabetes where the concordance among identical twins is close to 100%.

From: *Nutritional Health: Strategies for Disease Prevention*
Edited by: T. Wilson and N. J. Temple © Humana Press Inc., Totowa, NJ

Table 1
Diagnostic Criteria for Diabetes[a]

Stage of glycemia	Fasting plasma glucose (FPG)	75 g Oral glucose tolerance test (OGTT) at 2 h	Casual plasma glucose
Normal	<6.1 mmol/L (<110 mg/dL)	<7.8 mmol/dL (<140 mg/dL)	
Impaired fasting glucose (IFG)	≥6.1 and <7.0 mmol/L (≥110 and <126 mg/dL)		
Impaired glucose tolerance (IGT)		≥7.8 and <11.1 mmol/L (≥140 and <200 mg/dL)	
Diabetes	≥7.0 mmol/L (≥126 mg/dL)	≥11.1 mmol/L (≥200 mg/dL)	≥11.1 mmol/L (≥200 mg/dL) plus symptoms (polyuria, polydipsia, and unexplained weight loss)

[a]Although there are three methods by which diabetes can be diagnosed, the FPG test is preferred. One of the three tests should be used on a different day to confirm diagnosis. Previously, a FPG 7.8 mmol/L (>140 mg/dL) had been used to make the diagnosis of diabetes. At this time, HbA1c, a measure of average blood glucose levels during the past 6–8 wk, is not recommended for diagnosis.
    From ref. 4.

In type 1 diabetes, by contrast, the concordance among identical twins is only 30–50% (3). Normal fasting plasma glucose values are listed in Table 1 (4).

2.1. Type 1 Diabetes Mellitus

Type 1 diabetes, previously referred to as insulin-dependent diabetes mellitus or IDDM, accounts for approx 5–10% of all known cases in the United States. Individuals are usually lean at diagnosis and are dependent on exogenous insulin to prevent ketoacidosis and death. It may occur at any age, even in the eighth and ninth decade, however, approx 75% of cases develop before 30 yr of age (3). Genetic predisposition to an immunologic destruction of the islet cells results in an insulin deficiency. Antibodies associated with the risk of developing type 1 diabetes include: autoantibodies to islet cell antigens (ICA), insulin autoantibodies (IAA) (which occur in persons who have never received insulin therapy), and autoantibodies to glutamic acid decarboxylase (GAD) (a protein on the surface of the beta cell). GAD autoantibodies appear to provoke an attack by the T-cells (killer T-lymphocytes), which may be what destroys the beta cells (4).

2.2. Type 2 Diabetes Mellitus

Type 2 diabetes, previously referred to as non-insulin-dependent diabetes mellitus or NIDDM, accounts for 90–95% of all known cases of diabetes. Although approx 50% of men and 70% of women are obese at the time of diagnosis, type 2 diabetes can also occur in nonobese individuals, especially in the elderly *(3)*. Initially, insulin resistance (decreased cell sensitivity or responsiveness to insulin) may be the primary cause, but as the disease progresses, insulin deficiency becomes more of a factor.

Type 2 diabetes is associated with defects in both insulin secretion and insulin action. Endogenous insulin may be normal, depressed, or elevated. However, insulin levels are inadequate to overcome coexisting insulin resistance. Insulin is released by the pancreas in two phases, and persons with type 2 diabetes lose the initial sharp acute release of insulin (first phase insulin release). As a result, insulin levels may be normal, but the effectiveness of insulin is decreased. Resistance to insulin may result from either a postreceptor or a cellular receptor defect in peripheral tissues and occurs early in the disease process. At the cellular level, there is a decrease in glucose uptake and utilization, which is reflected by an increase in postprandial glucose levels.

There may also be an increase in hepatic glucose production, especially in the early morning. Hepatic release of glucose is the primary determinant of fasting glucose levels. Fasting hyperglycemia appears to occur somewhat later in the progression of diabetes.

Initially, type 2 diabetes may be well controlled by medical nutrition therapy alone, but as the disease progresses from insulin resistance to insulin deficiency, medications are needed in addition to medical nutrition therapy. Oral medications may be prescribed as monotherapy or in combination, however, after approx 10 yr, 40–50% of the individuals with type 2 diabetes will require exogenous insulin for adequate glycemic control and to prevent complications of diabetes *(3)*. Diagnostic criteria for diabetes are listed in Table 1 *(4)*.

2.3. Other Classifications

2.3.1. GESTATIONAL DIABETES MELLITUS

Gestational diabetes mellitus (GDM) is defined as any degree of glucose intolerance with onset or first recognition during pregnancy. It occurs in about 4% of pregnancies, resulting in approx 135,000 cases annually *(5)*. It is usually diagnosed during the second or third trimester, at which point insulin-antagonist hormones increase and insulin resistance occurs. In the majority of cases, blood glucose levels return to normal when the pregnancy is over. The major concerns for the fetus are macrosomia (>4 kg [9 lb] at term or >90th percentile in weight for gestational age), hypoglycemia at birth, and increased incidence of obesity. Women who have had GDM are at increased risk for later development of type 2 diabetes.

2.3.2. IMPAIRED GLUCOSE HOMEOSTASIS

Impaired glucose homeostasis is a newly described stage and includes impaired fasting glucose (IFG) and impaired glucose tolerance (IGT). IFG is defined as a fasting plasma glucose (FPG) between 6.1 and 7.0 mmol/L (110 and 126 mg/dL). Approximately 7% of the population (13.4 million persons) is estimated to have IFG. IGT is defined as an oral glucose tolerance test value between 7.8 and 11.1 mmol/L (140 and 200 mg/dL). Both IFG and IGT are risk factors for future diabetes and cardiovascular disease (4).

2.4. Screening Recommendations for Diabetes

Early detection and treatment has the potential to reduce the burden of diabetes. The American Diabetes Association suggests testing for diabetes at age 45 yr and, if normal, repeat at 3-yr intervals. There is little likelihood of developing any of the complications of diabetes within a 3-yr interval of a negative test. Testing should be considered at a younger age, or be done more frequently, in individuals who are obese ($\geq$120% desirable body weight or a body mass index [BMI] $\geq$30 kg/m^2, have a first-degree relative with diabetes, are members of a high-risk ethnic population, have delivered a baby weighing >4 kg (9 lb) or have been diagnosed with GDM, have a high-density lipoprotein-cholesterol $\leq$0.9 mmol/L ($\leq$35 mg/dL) and/or a triglyceride level $\geq$2.0 mmol/L ($\geq$250 mg/dL), or on previous testing had IGT or IFG (4). Early treatment strategies include medical nutrition therapy (MNT) and an increase in physical activity.

3. IMPORTANCE OF METABOLIC CONTROL

3.1. Type 1 Diabetes

The Diabetes Control and Complications Trial (DCCT) demonstrated beyond doubt a clear link between glycemic control and the development of complications in type 1 diabetes and that any improvement in glycemic control reduces the chances of developing complications (6). The DCCT, sponsored by the National Institutes of Health, was a long-term, prospective, randomized, controlled multicenter trial that studied approx 1400 young persons (age 13–39) with type 1 diabetes treated with intensive insulin therapy (multiple injections of insulin or use of insulin infusion pumps guided by blood glucose monitoring), nutrition therapy, and frequent interventions with the health-care team. The conventional group received insulin therapy (one or two insulin injections per day), self-monitoring of urine or blood glucose, and nutrition education as requested by the participants. Average HbA1c, a test that reflects the previous 6–8 wk of glycemic control, for the intensively treated group was 7.2% and for the conventional treated group 9.1% (normal 4–5.8%). The intensive therapy group experienced a 50–75% reduction in the risk of developing progression of retinopathy, neuropathy, and nephropathy.

Side effects of intensive therapy included weight gain and hypoglycemia. Individuals in the intensive therapy group experienced on average a gain of approx 4.5 kg (10 lb) during the first year of the trial *(7)*. Weight gain was related to (1) fewer calories being lost as glycosuria, (2) euglycemia promoting rehydration, which can add 0.9–2.3 kg (2–5 lb) of weight, and (3) need for frequent treatment, as well as overtreatment, of hypoglycemia. Therefore, it is essential that patients have a general concept of total calories needed as well as carbohydrate choices. Intensive therapy was accompanied by a threefold increase in severe hypoglycemia of which approx 50% occurred overnight *(8)*. Individuals also did better if they consistently ate a bedtime snack to prevent overnight hypoglycemia *(9)*.

3.2. Type 2 Diabetes

The United Kingdom Prospective Diabetes Study (UKPDS) demonstrated that elevated blood glucose levels cause long-term complications in type 2 diabetes, just as in type 1 diabetes *(10,11)*. The UKPDS recruited 5102 newly diagnosed individuals with type 2 diabetes in 23 centers within the UK between 1977 and 1991. A significant reduction in microvascular complications was achieved with intensive therapy that lowered HbA1c to an average of 7.0% over 10 yr compared to 7.9% in the conventional therapy group. Cardiovascular outcomes were also consistently associated with hyperglycemia. Aggressive treatment of even mild-to-moderate hypertension had a similar benefit to glycemic control in reducing diabetic complications *(12,13)*.

The UKPDS also demonstrated the progressive nature of type 2 diabetes and the need to provide follow-up and aggressive treatment *(10)*. Both treatment groups received intensive diet intervention at the start of the study. The trend toward loss of glycemic control was extended over the 10-yr follow-up in both groups and confirmed that type 2 diabetes worsens over time. The ability to prevent or at least slow this rise may be facilitated by newer glucose-lowering drugs that were not available to the UKPDS.

4. GLUCOSE, LIPID, AND BLOOD PRESSURE GOALS

Persons with diabetes need to know their target blood glucose, lipid, and blood pressure goals. Self-monitoring of blood glucose (SMBG) is used on a day-to-day basis to fine tune treatment regimens because it reflects day-to-day glycemia. Glycohemoglobin can be assayed by several methods and is expressed as a percentage of hemoglobin that has glucose attached. HbA1 is an evaluation of a combination of all fractions of the hemoglobin molecule. HbA1c is a measurement of the glycation of the "c" fraction and the values are lower because only one fraction is measured.

Other parameters besides glucose that must be regularly monitored are lipids and blood pressure. *See* Tables 2 and 3 for glucose and lipid indicators *(14,15)*. The blood pressure goal for adults is <130/85 mm Hg. If lifestyle modifica-

Table 2
Indicators of Glycemic Control

Indicator	Normal	Goal	Action suggested
Premeal or fasting plasma glucose	<6.1 mmol/L (<110 mg/dL)	<5.0–8.3 mmol/L (90–130 mg/dL)	<5.0 or >7.2 mmol/L (<90 or >150 mg/dL)
Postprandial plasma glucose[a]	<7.8 mmol/dL (<140 mg/dL)	<8.9 mmol/L (<160 mg/dL)	>10 mmol/L (>180 mg/dL)
Bedtime plasma glucose	<6.7 mmol/L (<120 mg/dL)	6.1–8.3 mmol/L (110–150 mg/dL)	<6.1 or >10.0 mmol/L (<110 or >180 mg/dL)
HbA1c[b]	<6%	<7%	>8%

[a]Not in the American Diabetes Association's Standards of Care, but values listed are generally accepted.
[b]HbA1c is referenced to a nondiabetic range of 4.0 to 6.0%.
From ref. 14.

Table 3
Coronary Heart Disease Risk by Lipoprotein Levels for Adults

Risk	Cholesterol	LDL-Cholesterol[a]	HDL-Cholesterol[b]	Triglycerides
High	>240 mg/dL (>6.2 mmol/L)	≥130 mg/dL (≥3.3 mmol/L)	<35 mg/dL (<0.9 mmol/L)	≥400 mg/dL (≥4.5 mmol/L)
Borderline	200–239 mg/dL (5.2–6.2 mmol/L)	100–129 mg/dL (2.6–3.3 mmol/L)	35–45 mg/dL (0.9–1.2 mmol/L)	200–399 mg/dL (2.3–4.5 mmol/L)
Low	<200 mg/dL (<5.2 mmol/L)	<100 mg/dL (<2.6 mmol/L)	>45 mg/dL (>1.2 mmol/L)	<200 mg/dL (<2.3 mmol/L)

[a]Medical nutrition therapy is initiated in adults when LDL-cholesterol is >100 mg/dL with a LDL goal <100 mg/dL. Drug therapy should be initiated when LDL-cholesterol level is >130 mg/dL, and with coronary heart disease, peripheral vascular disease, or cardiovascular disease, drug therapy should be initiated when LDL-cholesterol level is >100 mg/dL. In both cases, the LDL goals are <100 mg/dL.
[b]For women, the HDL-cholesterol value should be increased by 10 mg/dL.
From ref. 15.

tions—moderate weight loss, exercise, reduction of dietary sodium, and limited ingestion of alcohol—do not achieve these goals, medications should be added in a stepwise fashion until blood pressure goals are met (14).

Table 4
Insulin Therapy

Type of insulin	Onset of action	Monitor effect at:
Premeal Insulins (Bolus)		
Lispro/Aspart	5–15 min	2 h
Regular	30–60 min	4 h (next meal)
Background Insulins (Basal)		
NPH/Lente	2–4 h	8–10 h
Ultralente	3–5 h	10–12 h
Glargine (24 h insulin)	30 min	

Urine testing, however, remains the only practical way to detect ketones. Testing for ketonuria should be done regularly during illness and when blood glucose levels are consistently >13 mmol/L (240 mg/dL). The presence of urine ketones, along with elevated blood glucose levels, requires immediate insulin adjustments. Persons with type 2 diabetes rarely have ketosis.

5. MEDICATIONS

5.1. Oral Medications for Type 2 Diabetes

Many individuals will do well initially with MNT alone; however, as the disease progresses, oral medications alone or in combination will be needed along with nutrition therapy. There are now six classes of pharmacological agents approved for use in the United States for treatment of diabetes: sulfonylureas, meglitinide, biguanide, α-glucosidase inhibitors, and thiazolidinediones. Each class has a different site and mechanism of action; therefore, for optimal control they can be used as monotherapy or in combination.

5.2. Insulins

Persons with type 1 diabetes are dependent on insulin by injection for survival. However, after approx 10 yr, 40–60% of individuals with type 2 diabetes will also require insulin to achieve adequate metabolic control *(3)*. Today, with the many options available for insulin regimens, if an individual's usual eating patterns are known, insulin regimens can be integrated into lifestyle. Therefore, it is essential that lifestyle information be shared with the professional planning the insulin regimen. Table 4 lists the types of insulin, onset, and approximate duration of action.

6. MEDICAL NUTRITION THERAPY: WHAT DO WE KNOW AND WHAT ARE THE UNANSWERED QUESTIONS?

Based on outcome research, it is evident that MNT is integral to and essential for successful diabetes management *(16,17)*. However, there is also recognition that nutrition therapy is challenging for persons with diabetes and for professionals *(18,19)*. In the past, research attempted to find the "ideal diet" that would apply to all persons with diabetes. This was usually assumed to be some ideal percentage of macronutrients—carbohydrate, protein, and fat. The emphasis today is on determining the goals of MNT for diabetes and the nutrition-related strategies shown to achieve these goals *(20–22)*. Just as there is no longer one insulin regimen that applies to all persons who require insulin therapy, there is also no one nutrition prescription that applies to all persons with diabetes.

6.1. Goals and Strategies for Medical Nutrition Therapy for Diabetes

The primary goal of nutrition self-management in persons with diabetes is to assist with maintenance of near-normal glucose levels to prevent both acute and long-term complications. This is done by balancing food with insulin, either endogenous or exogenous, and physical activity. There is a two- to fourfold increase in the prevalence of macrovascular diseases in persons with diabetes *(15)*. Therefore, it is also important for persons with diabetes to achieve optimal lipid levels and MNT plays an essential role in achieving these goals.

Another goal is to provide adequate calories for maintanance of a reasonable body weight. A reasonable body weight is defined as that level of weight acknowledged by both patient and professionals as achievable and maintainable both short term and long term. For children and adolescents with diabetes, it is essential that calories be prescribed to provide for normal growth and development. The meal plan is not a restriction of calories, but is intended to ensure a reasonably consistent food intake and nutritional balanced diet. Insulin regimens are then designed to cover the amount of food children and adolescents are hungry for. During pregnancy and lactation women generally require an increase in calories. Monitoring blood glucose levels, urine ketones, appetite, and weight gain allows for the making of appropriate calorie adjustments.

Improving health though optimal nutrition is another goal. The First Step in Diabetes Meal Planning, which includes the Food Guide Pyramid, outlines and illustrates nutrition guidelines and nutrient needs for all healthy Americans and can be used for persons with diabetes and their family members *(23)*. Food and meal planning flexibility for individuals with diabetes requires individualization and nutrition education.

6.1.1. NUTRITION-RELATED STRATEGIES FOR INSULIN USERS

By determining usual food and exercise habits, insulin regimens can be integrated into an individual's lifestyle habits. Two types of insulin therapy were defined during the DCCT: conventional and intensive. Conventional therapy usually consists of injections of regular (or rapid-acting) and NPH given before breakfast and the evening meal. If fasting blood glucose values are not adequately controlled with this regimen, the next step is to move the pre-evening meal NPH to bedtime. The meal plan is based on the food and nutrition assessment. Consistency in food intake and timing is critical, then blood glucose monitoring results can be used to determine basic insulin doses. Based on blood glucose patterns, insulin doses and/or insulin regimens can then be further adjusted.

Intensive therapy provides increased flexibility in the timing and consistency of meals, amount of carbohydrate eaten at meals, and timing of physical activity. Intensive therapy consists of three or more insulin injections per day or insulin pump therapy. Generally, NPH or ultralente insulin is used as background (basal) insulin and rapid-acting or regular insulin is used premeal (bolus). The differences in onset, duration of action, and peak times make it possible to tailor therapy to individual needs. By knowing how much carbohydrate is eaten at meals, a carbohydrate-to-insulin ratio can be determined (*see* Section 7.3.). Adjustments can then be made in the premeal insulin dose to accommodate changes from the usual carbohydrate intake and to compensate for premeal blood glucose values that are not in the target goal range *(24)*.

After a mixed meal, the blood glucose rise is essentially determined by the amount of carbohydrate in the meal and insulin requirements should be proportional to the carbohydrate content of the meal. Patients are taught to count the carbohydrate content (or choices) of their meals and to adjust insulin doses accordingly. Compared with the traditional meal plan based on food exchanges, carbohydrate counting is more precise, easier to teach, more flexible, and can facilitate better glycemic control. Rabasa-Lhoret and associates *(25)* validated this concept. They studied the effects of high- (55%) and low- (40%) carbohydrate diets on insulin requirements treated intensively with ultralente as background insulin and regular insulin as premeal insulin adjusted to the carbohydrate content of the meal. When premeal insulin was prescribed in units of premeal insulin per 10 g of carbohydrate, the postmeal glycemic control remained constant over a range of carbohydrate ingested. Furthermore, the premeal insulin dose was not affected by the glycemic index, fiber, fat, and caloric content of the meal.

6.1.2. NUTRITION-RELATED STRATEGIES FOR TYPE 2 DIABETES

Traditional dietary advice for people with type 2 diabetes focused on avoiding sugar and losing weight. MNT now focuses on lifestyle strategies that can contribute to improvements in metabolic control. Although there are a number of lifestyle changes that have been shown to improve glycemic control, there is no clear answer regarding which of these should be the first priority. The strategy is to individualize therapy and set goals based on what the person with diabetes chooses to focus on *(26)*. The field trial of nutrition practice guidelines for type 2 diabetes showed evidence of the effectiveness of lifestyle changes by 6 wk–3 mo. At this point, it can be determined if lifestyle changes alone will maintain metabolic control or if changes in medication(s) will also be needed *(16)*.

Caloric restriction is an independent factor for improved glycemic control. Several research studies indicate that glycemic control improves within 24 h of caloric restriction and before any weight loss occurs *(27,28)*. Energy restriction results in changes in macronutrient intake, especially a reduced carbohydrate intake. This appears to deplete liver glycogen stores and as a result fasting blood glucose levels improve *(29)*.

Moderate weight loss results in later improvements in glycemia and insulin sensitivity and is related to reduction in abdominal fat, which also improves lipid profiles *(30)*. Metabolic changes responsible for improved glycemic control have been demonstrated with moderate weight losses of 4.5–9.1 kg (10–20 lb) *(31,32)*. Watts and colleagues *(32)* reported, however, that if blood glucose levels are not less than 10 mmol/L (180 mg/dL) after a weight loss of 4.5 kg (10 lb), additional weight loss is not likely to be helpful. Because of a slowed first phase insulin release, spacing meals and distributing food intake throughout the day may also be beneficial *(33,34)*.

Carbohydrate is the macronutrient with the greatest impact on blood glucose levels. Individuals with type 2 diabetes need to be provided with the basic guidelines for the amount of carbohydrate to eat at meals and snacks, e.g., 60 g (four carbohydrate choices) per meal plus or minus 15 g (one carbohydrate choice), and 15–30 g of carbohydrate (one to two carbohydrate choices) at snacks. Testing blood glucose postprandially provides tangible information to assist the person to take a more active role in evaluating food choices and understanding the carbohydrate load tolerable for them at a particular meal.

The benefits of physical activity are well documented *(35)*. It enhances blood glucose uptake by muscle during or shortly after activity and improves insulin sensitivity. It is recommended that individuals adopt a lifetime activity model, an approach developed by the Centers for Disease Control and the American College of Sports Medicine, which states that all Americans need to accumulate 30 min daily of moderate intensity physical activity *(36)*.

6.2. Macronutrients and Metabolic Control

The American Diabetes Association for many years has been stressing the need for individualized nutrition prescriptions and therapy *(20,21)*. What we do know is that glycemic control is possible with varying percentages of macronutrients *(25,37)*. There is no one nutrition prescription or so-called "ADA diet" that can be recommended for all persons with diabetes. Instead, the macronutrient distribution is based on individual preferences and treatment goals.

Multiple factors influence the postmeal glycemic response with the amount of glucose absorbed being the key determinant. However, persons with diabetes need to be reminded of the other variables which affect blood glucose and that food is not always the reason for variance. Also affecting glycemic response is the premeal glucose level, gastric emptying rate, intestinal motility, and other factors that affect glucose removal from the circulation such as insulin resistance. For example, gastric emptying is known to be enhanced with hypoglycemia and inhibited with hyperglycemia *(38,39)*.

6.2.1. CARBOHYDRATE: WHAT IS KNOWN

Carbohydrate is the nutrient that determines the amount of glucose absorbed from a meal and is the primary determinant of the blood glucose response. The increase in blood glucose depends on the rate and completeness of digestion of starch. Because starch is composed of glucose molecules, starchy foods raise blood glucose concentration more than sugars found in sucrose, fruit, or milk. Fructose and galactose (half of the sucrose and lactose molecule, respectively) have a minimal effect on blood glucose levels as they both appear to be stored in the liver as glycogen and, therefore, do not enter directly into the general circulation *(40)*. Although sugars in general have a lower glycemic response than starches, and individual starches do have differing glycemic responses, clinically the total amount of carbohydrate ingested will be more important than the type of carbohydrate *(20)*.

6.2.1.1. SUCROSE

Numerous research studies have reported that traditional dogma restricting sugars in the diet of persons with diabetes cannot be justified based on scientific evidence *(41–44)*. The belief that sucrose must be restricted is based on the assumption that sucrose is more rapidly digested and absorbed than starches and, thereby, aggravates hyperglycemia. However, at least 12–15 studies, in which sucrose was substituted for other carbohydrates, found no adverse effect of sucrose or foods containing sucrose on glycemia compared to foods containing starch. Therefore, sucrose and sucrose-containing foods can be substituted for other carbohydrates in the meal plan. The primary concern with sugar-containing foods is that often they contain significant amounts of total carbohydrate, fat, and calories and should be eaten within the context of a healthful diet.

6.2.1.2. FIBER

Although important for the prevention of other disease processes, dietary fiber has a minimal effect on glycemia *(45)*. Large amounts of guar gum and other viscous nonstarch polysaccharides have been shown to reduce the postprandial glucose response *(46)*; however, when eaten in amounts that are likely to be tolerable to most patients, fiber appears to be of minor importance in postmeal glucose control *(47)*. Fiber-rich foods (whole grains, vegetables, and fruits) are, however, good sources of important micronutrients, such as vitamin B_6, folate,

Table 5
Nonnutritive Sweeteners, Acceptable Daily Intake (ADI),
and Amounts in Soda and Sweeteners

Sweetener	ADI (mg/kg body weight)	12-Oz can soda (mg)	# Can = ADI[a]	1 Pkg sweetener (mg)	# Pkg = ADI[a]
Acesulfame K	15	40[b]	25[b]	50	18
Aspartame	50	200	15	35	86
Saccharin	5	140	2	40	7.5
Sucralose	5	70	4.5	5	60

[a]For a 60 kg (132 lb) person.
[b]Fountain drinks may have different amounts as they may contain a sweetener blend.
Adapted from ref. 48.

β-carotene, and phytochemicals, and in combination with a low-fat diet may have beneficial effects on plasma cholestrol levels.

6.2.1.3. Nonnutritive Sweeteners

The advantage of nonnutritive sweeteners over nutritive sweeteners for persons with diabetes is that they have the potential to help control total carbohydrate intake. There are currently four nonnutritive sweeteners available: aspartame, acesulfame K, saccharin, and sucralose. They were all rigorously tested and the safety data scrutinized by the Food and Drug Administration (FDA) before being approved and marketed for human use (20,48). The FDA determines an acceptable daily intake (ADI) for products it approves, which is defined as a safe amount for daily consumption over a lifetime. The ADI includes a 100-fold safety factor and greatly exceeds average consumption levels. For example, aspartame consumption (14-d average) in persons with diabetes is 2–4 mg/kg/d, well below the ADI of 50 mg/kg/d (49). Table 5 lists the ADI for nonnutritive sweeteners, the amount found in soft drinks and sweeteners, and the amounts needed to reach the ADI (48). All FDA-approved nonnutritive sweeteners can be used by individuals with diabetes, including pregnant women (because saccharin can cross the placenta, other sweeteners are better choices) (20).

6.2.2. Carbohydrate: What Are the Unanswered Questions?

6.2.2.1. Glycemic Index

The role of the glycemic index in food and meal planning for diabetes continues to be debated (50,51). Although the glycemic index is useful as an indicator of the general order of glucose responses to food, its accuracy has been questioned and its overall utility remains undetermined (40). It remains to be shown that using the glycemic index over the long term improves not only postprandial blood glucose values (expressed as percentages), but also glycosylated hemoglobin values. Percentage change is misleading and actual significant changes in blood glucose and HbA1c values need to be demonstrated. For now, it is suggested that individuals determine their own glycemic index based on self-monitoring of blood glucose. Furthermore, the glycemic differences of unprocessed versus processed foods have not been well defined.

Would the glycemic index of foods be helpful for women with gestational diabetes? Breakfast postprandial glucose levels are often a problem for these women. Therefore, selecting carbohydrates with a low glycemic index may be helpful.

6.2.2.2. RESISTANT STARCH

Starch may be categorized as readily digestible, slowly digestible, or resistant starch. For example, 94% of the starch in Rice Krispies is readily digested, whereas in beans and legumes 27–60% of it is resistant starch. Although bars containing resistant starch are widely advertised as preventing hypoglycemia in persons with type 1 diabetes, they have not been well studied.

6.2.3. PROTEIN: WHAT IS KNOWN

For the general public the average intake of protein is between 10% and 20% of calories and there is no evidence suggesting that persons with diabetes require more or less protein than this, or that a high-protein diet contributes to the development of nephropathy (52). Therefore, it is recommended that prior to the onset of renal disease, protein intake for the person with diabetes be similar to the protein intake of the general public (20). However, with the onset of nephropathy (macroalbuminuria), protein restriction is beneficial (53,54). It is recommended that protein intake be reduced to 10% of calories or 0.8 g/kg of body weight (20). An unresolved issue is the type of protein to restrict. Preliminary studies suggest that only animal proteins and not plant proteins may need to be restricted with nephropathy (55,56).

Protein, as well as carbohydrate and fat, requires insulin for metabolism, and the effect on blood glucose level is dependent on insulin availability. Without adequate insulin, gluconeogenesis occurs rapidly and protein can contribute to the resultant elevation in glycemia. However, with adequate insulin, protein appears to have minimal, if any, effect on blood glucose levels, despite the fact, that in theory, 50–60% of protein ingested can be deaminated and converted to glucose (57).

6.2.3.1. TYPE 2 DIABETES

Studies by Nuttall and associates (58) reveal that blood glucose concentrations do not increase in subjects with type 2 diabetes following the ingestion of

50 g protein. However, the insulin response to 50 g protein and 50 g glucose is similar, and the insulin response to 50 g protein and 50 g glucose combined is approx double the individual response. The peak blood glucose response to 50 g protein and 50 g glucose combined is similar to that from 50 g glucose alone, but the glucose response from 2 to 5 h may be slightly lower with protein added. This may be because of the increased insulin response to glucose and protein when combined. It is of interest to note that the insulin response to protein is greater in persons with type 2 diabetes than in persons without diabetes *(57)*.

6.2.3.2. TYPE 1 DIABETES

Although not well studied, if blood glucose is well controlled, protein appears to have a minimal effect on blood glucose level. Peters and Davidson *(59)* fed euglycemic subjects with type 1 diabetes a control lunch with and without an extra 200 calories (50 g) from protein or fat. The postprandial glucose response (2–5 h) to the meal with the added protein was slightly higher, but at 5 h the glucose response was similar for all three meals. The peak glucose response was similar for the control and added protein meals but delayed for the fat added meal.

Gray and coworkers *(60)* compared the ability of carbohydrate or carbohydrate plus protein to treat and to prevent subsequent hypoglycemia in patients with type 1 diabetes whose blood glucose levels were lowered to 2.8 mmol/L (50 mg/dL). Treatment responses were similar and subjects became hypoglycemic again at identical rates. The investigators concluded that adding protein to the treatment of hypoglycemia only added unnecessary and often unwanted calories.

6.2.4. PROTEIN: UNANSWERED QUESTIONS

What percentage of protein is metabolized to glucose and why doesn't protein affect blood glucose levels? A 50–60% conversion figure was theorized in 1915 by Janney from a calculation based on the amount of nitrogen excreted in the urine following a beef protein meal *(57)*. However, since that time it has been observed that the amount of glucose that is produced from protein may be considerably less. The small amount of glucose released into the circulation appears to be matched by an equal increase in glucose utilization provided that adequate insulin is available. Another theory suggests that if 50–60% of ingested protein is converted to glucose, it is being stored as liver or muscle glycogen and, therefore, has no immediate effect on glycemia.

As noted, protein stimulates insulin release in mild type 2 diabetes. However, it has been suggested that elevated levels of circulating endogenous insulin, which are often found in individuals with type 2 diabetes and insulin resistance, are atherogenic. Is it, therefore, beneficial that protein stimulates insulin concentration because of the potential to improve postprandial blood glucose levels? Or conversely, is protein detrimental because of the concern related to atherogenesis? What are the benefits or detriments of high-protein diets? At various times in history population subgroups have reportedly consumed high-protein diets of 35, 45, or even 80% calories out of necessity *(57)*. However, anecdotal reports suggest that high-protein diets are not well tolerated for any long period of time. Limited data are available regarding the long-term effect or benefit of high-protein diets for diabetes.

What are the differences between plant and animal protein in renal disease? When compared to animal protein, plant-based proteins appear to have different renal effects which are comparable to those seen by reducing total protein intake *(61)*. There is no evidence of any detrimental effects of plant-based protein in renal disease to date, but the mechanism of the beneficial effects of plant-based diets is unclear.

6.2.5. FAT: WHAT IS KNOWN

The amount of dietary fat in the nutrition prescription is based on the nutrition assessment and treatment goals. Persons who are at a healthy weight and have normal lipid levels are encouraged to follow the guidelines recommended for all Americans, that is, to limit fat to 30% of calories and saturated fat to 10% of calories. For those who need to lose weight, the emphasis is placed on reducing total fat amounts. If cholesterol or LDL-cholesterol levels are elevated, the National Cholesterol Education Program Step II diet should be implemented *(20)*. If triglyceride levels are elevated, improved blood glucose control, moderate weight loss, exercise, eliminating excess alcohol, and a more moderate fat and carbohydrate diet can be tried. Added fats should, however, be monounsaturated and not saturated fats. Another option for persons in these situations is a low-fat, low-calorie diet *(62)*.

6.2.5.1. SATURATED FATS

Saturated fats are known to increase risk for cardiovascular disease. Reduced intake of saturated fat has the potential to lower LDL-cholesterol levels by 15–25 mg/dL (0.39–0.65 mmol/L). Replacing dietary saturated fat with either carbohydrate or monounsaturated fat has been found to improve lipid levels in patients with diabetes *(62–65)*. Dietary cholesterol should be less than 300 mg/d *(20)*. These restrictions have been found to have a beneficial effect on lipid levels and insulin sensitivity in those with diabetes.

6.2.5.2. TOTAL FAT

In type 2 diabetes, it remains advisable to limit total fat intake to prevent weight gain that may adversely affect lipids and glycemic control. Fat replacers may help decrease fat and calorie intake if eaten in the same portion as regular foods *(66,67)*.

6.2.6. Fat: Unanswered Questions

Preliminary evidence from several studies indicates that total fat intake may contribute to insulin resistance *(68,69)* and inhibit glucose uptake *(70)*. However, is it total fat intake or does the type of dietary fat make a difference? Two epidemiological studies of individuals with type 2 diabetes found higher reported intake of total dietary fat (not the type of fat) was related to increased LDL-cholesterol levels. Higher intake of carbohydrate was related to increased triglyceride levels only in individuals with previously undiagnosed diabetes or among individuals who gained weight during the previous year *(71)*.

Which is more harmful: saturated fat or *trans* fatty acids? Both types of fat have been shown to increase serum total cholesterol and LDL-cholesterol. *Trans* fatty acids may also lower HDL-cholesterol levels (*see* Chapter 9 by Clarke and Frost). However, none of these studies have been conducted in persons with diabetes. Should monounsaturated or polyunsaturated fats be substituted for saturated and *trans* fatty acids? Several small studies comparing monounsaturated to polyunsaturated fat have not provided conclusive evidence regarding the superiority of one over the other *(72)*.

What is the influence of carbohydrate vs monounsaturated fats and/or calories on prevention and/or treatment for hypertriglyceridemia? When calories are kept at a level to prevent weight loss, high-carbohydrate diets compared to a high monounsaturated fat diet have been shown to elevate triglyceride levels *(63)*. However, a low-calorie, low-fat diet (high carbohydrate) has been shown to have no detrimental effects on lipids *(62)*. Furthermore, it is suggested that the triglycerides formed from a high-carbohydrate diet are the large, foamy types that are not as atherogenic as are the small dense endogenous VLDL particles *(72)*.

Are omega-3 fatty acids of value in controlling lipids in persons with diabetes? Epidemiological studies show that individuals who consume diets rich in omega-3 fatty acids have lower rates of cardiovascular disease (*see* Chapter 13 by de Deckere). However, several studies have reported that supplements of these fats increase LDL-cholesterol levels *(73)*. Nutrition advice to increase fish consumption versus the more saturated fat protein sources remains valid. If use of fish oil supplements is considered as a therapy for hypertriglyceridemia, LDL-cholesterol should be monitored closely.

6.2.7. Alcohol: What Is Known

Alcohol is not metabolized to glucose and does not require insulin for metabolism. It is oxidized in the liver by alcohol dehydrogenase to acetaldehyde and acetate, and used as an energy source. Other consequences of alcohol oxidation include impaired gluconeogenesis and potentially an increased production of triglycerides *(74)*.

With usual food intake, blood glucose and insulin levels are not affected by moderate amounts of alcohol. Koivisto and coworkers *(75)* carried out a study in persons taking their usual insulin doses or in persons with type 2 diabetes. They reported no effect on glucose and insulin responses during the 15 h following consumption of alcoholic beverages with the usual evening meal. However, in persons receiving insulin and in the fasting state, hypoglycemia can occur at blood alcohol levels that do not exceed mild intoxication *(74)*.

The same precautions that apply to the consumption of alcohol by the general population apply to persons with diabetes. Daily intake of no more than one drink for women and two drinks for men is recommended. Twelve ounces (355 mL) of beer, 5 oz (148 mL) of wine, or 1 1/2 oz (44 mL) distilled spirits are considered to be one alcoholic beverage. If desired, alcoholic beverages should be consumed with and in addition to the regular meal plan. Because of the possibility of alcohol-induced hypoglycemia, it is advisable that no food be omitted. Persons with inadequate glucose control, elevated triglycerides, neuropathy, or pancreatitis, and pregnant women should avoid consumption of alcohol *(20)*.

6.2.8. ALCOHOL: UNANSWERED QUESTIONS

An overall beneficial effect of alcohol consumption in decreasing risk of death due to coronary heart disease has been reported in people with type 2 diabetes *(76)*. Moderate amounts of alcohol have also been reported to decrease insulin resistance. Light-to-moderate drinkers (10–30 g/d) are reported to be relatively more insulin sensitive and to have lower plasma insulin levels than do nondrinkers *(77)*. The mechanism by which this occurs remains to be determined. Furthermore, it remains to be determined if long-term moderate consumption of alcohol can prevent or delay the onset of type 2 diabetes by decreasing insulin resistance, and, if so, how. Also unanswered is the question as to the types of alcoholic beverages and their effect on insulin resistance and coronary heart disease, i.e., is there a difference if the alcoholic beverage is wine, beer, or distilled spirits?

6.2.9. MICRONUTRIENTS: WHAT IS KNOWN

Micronutrients play an integral role in carbohydrate and glucose metabolism, as well as in insulin release and sensitivity. Therefore, it is understandable that the public hears recommendations for micronutrients and diabetes far beyond what existing research has proven to be of benefit. Well-controlled studies examining the role of micronutrients and carbohydrate intolerance are usually not done in humans, and, therefore, animal studies are often extrapolated to humans. There are challenges to obtaining reliable data in humans: (1) trace mineral and water soluble vitamin losses in the urine are increased with uncontrolled hyperglycemia and glycosuria, (2) the degree of the response to supplementation may be dependent on the level of glucose intolerance, and (3) it is often unknown what amount of the micronutrient being studied has been eaten in the diet. To further confuse the role of micronutrients and diabetes, serum or tissue content of certain elements—copper, manganese, iron, and selenium—are reported to be higher in people with diabetes than in nondiabetic control subjects. On the other hand, serum ascorbic acid, the B vitamin group, and vitamin D are reported to be in lower in individuals with diabetes, whereas vitamins A and E are reported to be normal or increased *(78)*.

Supplementation recommendations for persons with diabetes are the same as for the general population. Deficiency should be diagnosed by clinical and laboratory data. Those at greatest risk for deficiency include the following: older adults, low-calorie dieters, persons with poor diabetes metabolic control, critically ill patients, pregnant or lactating women, vegans, and those with renal disease *(79)*.

6.2.9.1. SODIUM

Hypertension is twice as common in persons with diabetes, whereas those with type 2 diabetes are reported to be more sodium sensitive than the average nondiabetic person *(80,81)*. For persons with diabetes, guidelines for sodium are similar to those for the general population: less than 3000 mg/d and for those with mild to moderate hypertension, less than 2400 mg/d *(20)*.

6.2.9.2. MAGNESIUM

Individuals with diabetes who may be at high risk for magnesium deficiency include the elderly and those with chronic hyperglycemia. Those at risk should have their status assessed and receive supplementation with oral magnesium chloride if a deficiency is identified *(82)*.

6.2.9.3. CALCIUM

Persons with diabetes, especially type 1 diabetes, have been identified as being at greater risk for decreased bone density *(83)*. The specific causes of low bone mineral density are unknown. Supplementation with elemental calcium is appropriate for many adults, especially women, regardless of whether or not diabetes is present (*see* Chapter 3 by Heaney). The National Institute of Health Osteoporosis Consensus Conference recommends a total daily intake of 1000 mg for women on hormone replacement therapy and 1500 mg for women not on this therapy *(84)*. Prevention of long bone fractures is a proactive treatment for maintaining physical activity (and vice versa).

6.2.9.4. VITAMIN E

Individuals with diabetes may have higher requirements for antioxidants than the general population. For those with cardiovascular disease, the benefits of taking up to 400 IU of vitamin E per day probably outweigh the risks, although this remains to be proven *(78)*. Paolisso and associates *(85)* reported that subjects with type 2 diabetes given a vitamin E supplement of 900 mg/d showed lower plasma glucose, HbA1c, and lipids compared to a control group. However, it is unclear whether sufficient levels of vitamin E can be given to affect oxidized

LDL-cholesterol and reduce their atherogenic potential, without negative long-term effects on the liver and kidney. Although observational epidemiological studies have shown a correlation between dietary or supplemental consumption of vitamins and clinical outcomes, the large scale, placebo-controlled interventional studies have failed to show a beneficial outcome. Of particular interest is The Heart Outcomes Prevention Evaluation (HOPE) trial that included 9541 subjects, of whom 38% had diabetes (86). In this trial, supplementation of vitamin E (400 IU/d) for 4.5 yr did not result in any significant beneficial outcomes.

6.2.10. MICRONUTRIENTS: UNANSWERED QUESTIONS

Are there any micronutrients that are beneficial for people with diabetes? The reader is referred to references 78 and 79 for a review of the current literature. Of particular interest is the role of micronutrients, such as folic acid, and their effect on cardiovascular disease risk reduction. In another chapter, Woodside and Young discuss whether folate lowers homocysteine levels and reduces risk for coronary heart and vessel disease. The relevance of this to persons with diabetes is not known (87).

Does vitamin C have particular efficacy for persons with diabetes? Tissue stores are known to be depleted by chronic hyperglycemia. Vitamin C may inhibit protein glycosylation by competing with glucose for binding to proteins (88). Supplementation with 500 mg/d has been shown to have no effect on blood glucose levels, and larger doses have the potential to interfere with blood glucose monitoring results and/or increase plasma glucose (89).

Is there a role for chromium supplementation? Chromium is well distributed in the food supply and no methods are currently available to identify individuals who may be chromium deficient. Chromium picolinate appears to be the chromium supplement that is best absorbed because it incorporates picolinic acid, a natural mineral transporter produced in the liver and kidney. Anderson and associates (90) reported that in subjects fed chromium-deficient diets, supplementation with 200 mg/d was beneficial to individuals with impaired glucose tolerance but had no effect on blood glucose levels in those with diabetes. Anderson and associates (91) studied subjects with type 2 diabetes in China divided into three groups: supplementation with 200 μg or 1000 μg/d of chromium picolinate or placebo. Supplementation reduced HbA1c, fasting and 2-h glucose concentration, whereas total cholesterol also decreased in the group receiving the 1000 μg supplement. However, before recommending chromium supplementation in the United States, well-controlled studies in people with diabetes with known intake of chromium are needed.

Can nicotinamide prevent or delay the onset of type 1 diabetes? In animal studies, nicotinamide has been shown to offer protection to pancreatic beta cells against a variety of toxic or immune-mediated insults. A trial, called the European–Canadian Nicotinamide Diabetes Intervention Trial (ENDIT) is testing the hypothesis that the rate of type 1 diabetes can be substantially reduced with the use of pharmacological doses of nicotinamide *(92)*.

7. APPLYING NUTRITION SCIENCE TO CLINICAL PRACTICE

It is clear that there can be no one nutrition prescription that applies to everyone with diabetes. The nutrition prescription for patients with diabetes should not be based on a predetermined calorie level with set percentages for carbohydrate, protein, and fat. Instead, it should focus on the goals of therapy and known strategies to achieve these goals. Furthermore, it must be based on an assessment of what the individual with diabetes is willing and able to implement.

Applying nutrition recommendations requires professionals with a high level of clinical skills and knowledge, not only about medical nutrition therapy, but who also know how to integrate nutrition therapy into the overall management of diabetes. As a result, the role of dietitians has changed:

- From the traditional role of limiting food choices to teaching flexibility in food choices and problem solving to achieve metabolic control;
- From restricting macronutrients to emphasizing to persons with diabetes relationships between food intake and glucose, lipid, and blood pressure outcomes;
- From teaching specific nutrition recommendations to teaching behavior-change skills so persons with diabetes can achieve their own nutritional goals;
- From working independently to being team members;
- From only assessment and implementation to implementing a system that promotes evaluation and actions related to the outcomes of nutrition therapy.

The nutrition prescription and meal/food plan is a modification of usual food intake, individualized to meet treatment goals. Appropriate educational materials are selected that meet the client's needs. Traditionally, all persons with diabetes were taught the use of exchange lists for meal planning. Although the exchange lists are still of value in assisting the dietitian in assessing caloric and macronutrient percentages of usual and modified food intake, many clients will do better with a more simplified method of meal planning based on the Food Guide Pyramid *(23)* or with carbohydrate counting *(93,94)*.

Measurement and documentation of outcomes is essential. This requires a system of planned follow-up and ongoing education and support. If expected outcomes are not being met by lifestyle changes, there will be a need for changes in medications. As the disease progresses, rarely can individuals be controlled by nutrition therapy alone. Today, the management of diabetes often requires lifestyle modifications along with medications

7.1. Carbohydrate Counting

Carbohydrate counting is a useful system of food and meal planning for all people with diabetes. Instead of grouping foods into six lists as in the exchange

Table 6
Carbohydrate Choices or Servings[a]

Starch	Milk
1 slice bread	1 cup skim/low-fat milk
1/2 cup cooked pasta	3/4 cup fruited yogurt sweetened
3/4 cup dry cereal	with nonnutritive sweetener
4–6 crackers	
1/3 cup cooked rice	
Fruit	Desserts/Other
1 small piece	2 small cookies
1/2 cup fruit juice	1 tablespoon jam, honey, syrup
	1/2 cup ice cream, frozen yogurt

[a]One serving contains 15 g of carbohydrate.

system, it groups foods into only three food groups: carbohydrate, meat and meat substitutes, and fat. The carbohydrate list is composed of starches, fruits, milk, and sweets, and one serving is the amount of food that supplies 15 g of carbohydrate. Table 6 lists some examples of a carbohydrate serving. Carbohydrate counting does not mean that meat and fat portions can be ignored. Individuals with diabetes must also know the approximate number of meat and fat servings they should select for meals and snacks. Weight control is important, as is the maintenance of a healthy balance of food choices.

Learning how to use the Nutrient Facts on food labels is useful to individuals with diabetes. First, they should take note of the serving size and the total amount (grams) of carbohydrate in that serving size. They should ignore the grams of sugar as they are included in the total grams of carbohydrate. If there are more than 5 g of fiber in a serving, the grams of fiber can be subtracted from the total grams of carbohydrate (95).

Women with type 2 diabetes often do well with three to four carbohydrate servings per meal and one to two between meals. Men with type 2 diabetes may need four to five carbohydrate servings per meal and one to two between meals. Food records along with blood glucose monitoring data can then be used to evaluate if treatment goals are being met or if there is a need for additional lifestyle and/or medication changes.

7.2. Carbohydrate-To-Insulin Ratios

Carbohydrate-to-insulin ratios are used to determine the premeal short or rapid-acting insulin doses. Individuals must be consistent in their carbohydrate intake and the premeal insulin is adjusted to cover that amount of carbohydrate. The grams of carbohydrate per meal are divided by the premeal insulin dose to determine how many units of insulin are needed to cover the grams of carbohydrate. For example, if an individual usually eats 75 g of carbohydrate for dinner and takes 5 units of rapid acting insulin premeal, the carbohydrate-to-insulin ratio is 15:1. Individuals can then adjust their premeal insulin based on the amount of meal carbohydrate they plan to eat *(96)*.

8. SUMMARY

In the past, nutrition recommendations for diabetes were rigid and allowed for little flexibility. However, there is no longer one set of guidelines that apply to all persons with diabetes. By individualizing treatment and focusing on metabolic outcomes, healthcare professionals can facilitate lifestyle changes needed to achieve the patient's metabolic and behavioral goals. Clinical nutrition recommendations are based on the answers research has provided. However, many questions still remain and, hopefully, research will continue to answer these questions.

REFERENCES

1. Centers for Disease Control and Prevention. National Diabetes Fact Sheet: National estimates and general information on diabetes in the United States. U.S. Department of Health and Human Services, Centers for Disease Control and Prevention, Atlanta, GA, 1997.
2. American Diabetes Association. Economic consequences of diabetes mellitus in the U.S. in 1997. Diabetes Care 1998; 21:296–309.
3. National Institutes of Health. National Institute of Diabetes and Digestive and Kidney Disease. Diabetes in America. 2nd edition. NIH Publication No. 1995; 95–1468.
4. American Diabetes Association. Report of the Expert Committee on the Diagnosis and Classification of Diabetes Mellitus. Diabetes Care 2000; 23(Suppl 1):S4–S19.
5. American Diabetes Association. Gestational diabetes mellitus (Position Statement) Diabetes Care 2000; 23(Suppl 1):S77–S79.
6. Diabetes Control and Complications Trial Research Group. The effect of intensive treatment of diabetes on the development and progression of long-term complications in insulin-dependent diabetes mellitus. N Engl J Med 1993; 329:997–986.
7. Diabetes Control and Complications Trial Research Group. Weight gain associated with intensive therapy in the Diabetes Control and Complications Trial. Diabetes Care, 1988; 11:567–573.
8. Diabetes Control and Complications Trial Research Group. Epidemiology of severe hypoglycemia in the Diabetes Control and Complications Trial. Am J Med 1991; 90:450–459.
9. Delahanty LM, Halford BN. The role of diet behaviors in achieving improved glycemic control in intensively treated patients in the Diabetes Control and Complications Trial. Diabetes Care 1993; 16:1453–1458.
10. UK Prospective Diabetes Study (UKPDS) Group. Intensive blood-glucose control with sulphonylureas or insulin compared with conventional treatment and risk of complications in patients with type 2 diabetes (UKPDS 33). Lancet 1998; 352:837–853.
11. UK Prospective Diabetes Study (UKPDS) Group. Effect of intensive blood-glucose control with metformin on complications in overweight patients with type 2 diabetes (UKPDS 34). Lancet 1998; 352:854–865.
12. UKPDS Study Group. Tight blood pressure control and risk of macrovascular and microvascular complications in type 2 diabetes: UKPDS 38. BMJ 1998; 317:703–713.

13. UK Prospective Diabetes Study. Efficacy of atenolol and captopril in reducing risk of macrovascular and microvascular complications in type II diabetes. UKPDS 39. BMJ 1998; 317:713–720.

14. American Diabetes Association. Standards of medical care for patients with diabetes mellitus. Diabetes Care 2000; 23(Suppl 1):S32–S42.

15. American Diabetes Association. Management of dyslipidemia in adults with diabetes. Diabetes Care 2000; 23(Suppl 1):S57–S60.

16. Franz MJ, Monk A, Barry B, McClain K, Weaver T, Cooper N, et al. Effectiveness of medical nutrition therapy provided by dietitians in the management of non-insulin-dependent diabetes mellitus: a randomized, controlled clinical trial. J Am Diet Assoc 1995; 95:1009–1017.

17. Kulkarni K, Castle G, Gregory R, Holmes A, Leontos C, Powers M., et al. for the Diabetes Care and Education Dietetic Practice Group. Nutrition practice guidelines for type 1 diabetes mellitus positively affect dietitian practices and patient outcomes. J Am Diet Assoc 1998; 98:62–70.

18. Lockwood D, Prey M, Galadish N, Hiss R. The biggest problem in diabetes. Diabetes Educator 1986; 12:30–33.

19. Ary DV, Toobert D, Wilson W, Glasgow RE. Patient perspective on factors contributing to nonadherence to diabetes regimen. Diabetes Educator 1986; 9:168–172.

20. American Diabetes Association. Nutrition recommendations and principles for people with diabetes mellitus (Position Statement). Diabetes Care 2000; 23(Suppl 1):S43–S46.

21. Franz MJ, Horton ES Sr, Bantle J P, Beebe CA, Brunzell JD, Coulston AM, et al. Nutrition principles for the management of diabetes and related complications (Technical Review). Diabetes Care 1994;17:490–518.

22. Franz MJ, Bantle JP, eds. The American Diabetes Association Guide to Medical Nutrition Therapy for Diabetes. American Diabetes Association, Alexandria, VA, 1999.

23. American Diabetes Association and The American Dietetic Association. The First Step in Diabetes Meal Planning. American Diabetes Association, Alexandria, VA, 1995.

24. Kulkarni K, Franz, MJ. Nutrition therapy for type 1 diabetes. In: Franz MJ, Bantle JP, eds., The American Association Guide to Medical Nutrition Therapy for Diabetes, American Diabetes Association, Alexandria, VA, 1999, pp. 26–45.

25. Rabasa-Lhoret R, Garon J, Longelier H, Poisson D, Chiasson J. Effects of meal carbohydrate content on insulin requirements in type 1 diabetic patients treated intensively with the basal-bolus (ultralente-regular) insulin regimen. Diabetes Care 1999; 22:667–673.

26. Beebe CA. Nutrition therapy for type 2 diabetes. In: Franz MJ, Bantle JP, eds., The American Association Guide to Medical Nutrition Therapy for Diabetes, American Diabetes Association, Alexandria, VA, 1999, pp. 46–68.

27. Wing RR, Blair EH, Bononi P, Marcus MD, Watanabe R, Bergman RN. Caloric restriction per se is a significant factor in improvements in glycemic control and insulin sensitivity during weight loss in obese NIDDM patients. Diabetes Care 1994; 17:30–36.

28. Kelly DE, Wing R, Buonocore P, Sturis J, Polonsky K, Fitzsimmons M. Relative effects of calorie restriction and weight loss in noninsulin-dependent diabetes mellitus. J Clin Endocrinol Metab 1993; 77:1287–1293.

29. Markovic TP, Jenkins AB, Campbell LV, Furler SM, Kraegen EW, Chisholm DJ. The determinants of glycemic responses to diet restriction and weight loss in obesity and NIDDM. Diabetes Care 1998; 21:687–694.

30. Markovic TP, Campbell LV, Balasubramanian S, Jenkins AB, Fleury AC, Simons LA, Chisholm DJ. Beneficial effect on average lipid levels from energy restriction and fat loss in obese individuals with or without type 2 diabetes. Diabetes Care 1998; 21:695–700.

31. Wing, RR, Koeske R, Epstein LH, Nowalk MP, Gooding W, Becker D. Long-term effects of modest weight loss in type II diabetic patients. Arch Intern Med 1987; 147:1749–53.

32. Watts NB, Spanheimer RG, DiGirolamo M, Gebhart SS, Musey VC, Siddiq K, Phillips LS. Prediction of glucose response to weight loss in patients with non-insulin-dependent diabetes mellitus. Arch Intern Med 1990; 150:803–806.

33. Jenkins DJA, Ocana A, Jenkins A, Wolever TMS, Vuksan V, Katzman L, et al. Metabolic advantages of spreading the nutrient load: effects of increased meal frequency in non-insulin-dependent diabetes. Am J Clin Nutr 1992; 55:461–467.

34. Bertelsen J, Christiansen C, Thomsen C, Poulsen PL, Vestergaard S, Steinov A, et al. Effect of meal frequency on blood glucose, insulin, and free fatty acids in NIDDM subjects. Diabetes Care 1993; 16:3–7.

35. Barlow CE, Kohl HW, Gibbons LW, Blair SN. Physical fitness, mortality and obesity. Int J Obesity 1995; 19(Suppl 4):S41–S44.

36. Pate RR, Pratt M, Blair SN, Haskell WL, Macera CA, Bouchard C, et al. Physical activity and public health. a recommendation from the Centers for Disease Control and Prevention and the American College of Sports Medicine. JAMA 1995; 273:402–407.

37. Milne RM, Mann JI, Chisholm AW, Williams SM. Long-term comparison of three dietary prescriptions in the treatment of NIDDM. Diabetes Care 1994; 17:74–80.

38. Fraser RJ, Horowitz M, Maddox AF, Harding PE, Chatterton BE, Dent J.Hyperglycemia slows gastric emptying in type 1 (insulin-dependent) diabetes mellitus. Diabetologia 1990; 33:675-680.

39. Schvarcz E, Palmer M, Aman J, Lindkvist B, Beckman K-W. Hypoglycaemia increases gastric emptying rate in patients with type 1 diabetes mellitus. Diabet Med 1993; 10:660–663.

40. Nuttall FQ, Gannon MC. Carbohydratrates and diabetes, In: Franz, M.J. and Bantle, J.P, eds. The American Association Guide to Medical Nutrition Therapy for Diabetes American, Diabetes Association, Alexandria, VA, 1999, pp. 85–106.

41. Wise JE, Keim KS, Huisinga JL, Willmann PA. Effect of sucrose-containing snacks on blood glucose control. Diabetes Care 1989; 12:423–426.

42. Bantle JP, Swanson JE, Thomas W, Laine DC. Metabolic effects of dietary sucrose in type II diabetic subjects. Diabetes Care 1993; 16:1301–1305.

43. Peterson DB, Lambert J, Gerrig S, Darling P, Carter RD, Jelfs R, Mann JI. Sucrose in the diet of diabetic patients - just another carbohydrate? Diabetologia 1986; 29:216–20.

44. Rickard KA, Loghmani E, Cleveland JL, Fineberg NS, Greidenberg GR. Lower glycemic response to sucrose in the diets of children with type 1 diabetes. J Pediatr 1998; 133:429–432.

45. Nuttall FQ. Dietary fiber in the management of diabetes. Diabetes 1993; 42:503–508.

46. Simpson HCR, Simpson RW, Lously S, Carter RD, Geekie M, Hockaday TDR, Mann JI. A high carbohydrate leguminous fibre diet improves all aspects of diabetic control. Lancet 1981; 3:1–5.

47. Hollenbeck CB, Coulston AM, Reaven GM. To what extent does increased dietary fiber improve glucose and lipid metabolism in patients with noninsulin-dependent diabetes mellitus. Am J Clin Nutr 1986; 43:16–24.

48. Powers M. Sugar alternatives and fat replacers. In: Franz MJ, Bantle JP, eds., The American Association Guide to Medical Nutrition Therapy for Diabetes, American Diabetes Association, Alexandria, VA, 1999, pp. 148–164.

49. Butchko HH, Kotsonis FN. Acceptable intake vs actual intake: the aspartame example. J Am Coll Nutr 1991; 10:258–266.

50. Coulston AM, Reaven GM. Much ado about (almost) nothing. Diabetes Care 1999; 20:241–243.

51. Franz MJ. In defense of the American Diabetes Association's recommendations on the glycemic index. Nutr Today 1999; 34:78–81.

52. Henry RR. Protein content of the diabetic diet (Technical Review). Diabetes Care 1994; 17:1502–1513.

53. Zeller KR, Whittaker E, Sullivan L, Raskin P, Jacobson HR. Effect of restricting dietary protein on the progression of renal disease in patients with insulin-dependent diabetes mellitus. N Engl J Med 1991; 324:78–84.

54. Pedrini MT, Levey AS, Lau J, Chalmers TC, Wang PH. The effect of dietary protein restriction on the progression of diabetic and nondiabetic renal disease: a meta-analysis. Ann Intern Med 1996; 124:627–632.

55. Jibani MM, Bloodworth LL, Foden E, Griffiths KD, Galpin OP. Predominantly vegetarian diet in patients with incipient and early clinical diabetic nephropathy: effects on albumin excretion rate and nutritional status. Diabet Med 1991; 8:949–53.

56. Nakamura H, Ito S, Ebe N, Shibata A. Renal effects of different types of protein in healthy volunteer subjects and diabetic patients. Diabetes Care 1993; 16:1071–1075.

57. Gannon MC, Nuttall FQ. Protein and diabetes. In: Franz MJ, Bantle JP, eds. The American Association Guide to Medical Nutrition Therapy for Diabetes, American Diabetes Association, Alexandria, VA, 1999, pp. 107–125.

58. Nuttall FQ, Mooradian AD, Gannon MC, Billington C, Krezowski P. Effect of protein ingestion on the glucose and insulin response to a standardized oral glucose load. Diabetes Care 1984; 7:465–470.

59. Peters AL, Davidson MB. Protein and fat effects on glucose response and insulin requirements in subjects with insulin-dependent diabetes mellitus. Am J Clin Nutr 1993; 58:555–600.

60. Gray RO, Butler PC, Beers TR, Kryshak EJ, Rizza RA. Comparison of the ability of bread versus bread plus meat to treat and prevent subsequent hypoglycemia in patients with insulin-dependent diabetes mellitus. J Clin Endocrinol Metab 1996; 81:1508–1511.

61. Wheeler ML. Nephropathy and medical nutrition therapy, In: Franz MJ, Bantle JP, eds. The American Association Guide to Medical Nutrition Therapy for Diabetes, American Diabetes Association, Alexandria, VA, 1999, pp. 312–329.

62. Heilbronn L, Noakes M. Clifton P. Effect of energy restriction, weight loss, and diet composition on plasma lipids and glucose in patients with type 2 diabetes. Diabetes Care 1999; 22:889–895.

63. Garg A, Bantle JP, Henry RR, Coulston AM, Griver KA, Raatz SK, et al. Effects of varying carbohydrate content of diet in patients with non-insulin dependent diabetes mellitus. JAMA 1994; 271:1421–1428.

64. Parillo M, Rivellese AA, Ciardullo AV, Capaldo B, Giacco A, Genovese S, Riccardi G. A high-monounsaturated-fat/low carbohydrate diet improves peripheral insulin sensitivity in non-insulin-dependent diabetic patients. Metabolism 1992; 41:1371–1378.

65. Abbott WGH, Boyce VL, Grundy SM, Howard BV. Effects of replacing saturated fat with complex carbohydrate in diets with of subjects with NIDDM. Diabetes Care 1989; 12:102–107.

66. Warshaw HS, Franz MJ, Powers MA, Wheeler ML. Fat replacers: their use in foods and role in diabetes medical nutrition therapy (Technical Review). Diabetes Care 1996; 19:1294–1301.

67. American Diabetes Association. Role of fat replacers in diabetes medical nutrition therapy (Position Statement). Diabetes Care 2000; 23(Suppl 1):S96–S97.

68. Mayer-Davis EJ, Monacoe JH, Hoen HM. Dietary fat and insulin sensitivity in a triethnic population: the role of obesity. The Insulin Resistance Atherosclerosis Study (IRAS). Am J Clin Nutr 1997; 65:79–87.

69. Feskens EJM, Loeber JG, Kromhout D. Diet and physical activity as determinants of hyperinsulinemia: The Zutphen Elderly Study. Am J Epidemiol 1994; 140:354–360.

70. Boden G, Chen X. Effects of fat on glucose uptake and utilization in patients with non-insulin dependent diabetes. J Clin Invest 1995; 96:1261–1267.

71. Mayer-Davis EJ, Levin S, Marshall JA. Heterogeneity in association between macronutrient intake and lipoprotein profile in individuals with type 2 diabetes. Diabetes Care 1999; 22:1632–1639.

72. Purnell JQ, Brunzell JD. Food fats and dyslipidemia, In: Franz, MJ and Bantle, JP, eds. The American Association Guide to Medical Nutrition Therapy for Diabetes. American Diabetes Association, Alexandria, VA, 1999, pp. 126–147.

73. Fridberg CE, Janssen MJF, Heine RJ, Grobbee DE. Fish oil and glycemic control in diabetes. Diabetes Care 1998; 21:494–500.

74. Franz MJ. Alcohol and diabetes. In: Franz MJ, Bantle JP, eds. The American Association Guide to Medical Nutrition Therapy for Diabetes. American Diabetes Association, Alexandria, VA, 1999, pp. 192–208.

75. Koivisto VA, Tulokas S, Toivonen M, Haapa E, Pelkonen R. Alcohol with a meal has no adverse effects on postprandial glucose homeostasis in diabetic patients. Diabetes Care 1993; 16:1612–1614.

76. Valmadrid CT, Klein R, Moss SE, Klein BE, Cruickshanks KJ. Alcohol intake and the risk of coronary heart disease mortality in persons with older-onset diabetes mellitus. JAMA 1999; 282:239–246.

77. Facchini F, Chen Y-D, Reaven GM. Light-to-moderate alcohol intake is associated with enhanced insulin sensitivity. Diabetes Care 1994; 17:115–119.

78. Franz MJ. Micronutrients and diabetes. In: The American Association Guide to Medical Nutrition Therapy for Diabetes, Franz MJ, Bantle JP, eds., American Diabetes Association, Alexandria, VA, 1999, pp. 165–191.

79. Mooradian AD, Failla M, Hoogwerf B, Isaac R, Maryniuk M, Wylie-Rosett J. Selected vitamins and minerals in diabetes mellitus (Technical Review). Diabetes Care 1994; 17:464–479.

80. Tuck M, Corry D, Trujillo A. Salt-sensitive blood pressure and exaggerated vascular reactivity in the hypertension of diabetes mellitus. 1990; Am J Med 88: 210–216.

81. Dodson PM, Beevers M, Hallworth R, Webberley MJ, Fletcher RD, Taylor KG. Sodium restriction and blood pressure in hypertensive type II diabetics: randomized blind controlled and cross over studies of moderate sodium restriction and sodium supplementation. Br Med J 1989; 298:226–230.

82. American Diabetes Association. Magnesium supplementation in the treatment of diabetes (Consensus Statement). Diabetes Care 1992; 15:1065–1067.

83. Tuominen, J.T., Impivaara, O., Puukka, P., Ronnemaa, T. Bone mineral density in patients with type 1 and type 2 diabetes. Diabetes Care 1999; 22:1196–1200.

84. National Institutes of Health. Optimal Calcium Intake. NIH Consensus Statement. 1994; 12(4):1–24.

85. Paolisso G, D'Amore A, Galzerano D, Balbi V, Giogliano D, Varricchio M, D'Onofrio F. Daily viatmin E supplements improve metabolic control but not insulin secretion in elderly type II diabetic patients. Diabetes Care 1993; 16:1433–1437.

86. Yusuf S, Dagenais G, Pogue J, Bosch J, Sleight P. Vitamin E supplementation and cardiovascular events in high-risk patients. The Heart Outcomes Prevention Evaluation Study Investigators. N Engl J Med 2000; 342:154–160.

87. Okada E, Oida K, Tada H, Asazuma K, Eguchi K, Tohda G, et al. Hyperhomocysteinemia is a risk factor for coronary arteriosclerosis in Japanese patients with type 2 diabetes. Diabetes Care 1999; 22:484–490.

88. Davie SJ, Gould EJ, Yudkin JS. Effect of vitamin C on glycosylation of protein. Diabetes 1992; 41:1671–1673.

89. Branch DR. High-dose vitamin C supplementation increases plasma glucose. Diabetes Care 1999; 22:1218–1219.

90. Anderson RA, Polansky MM, Bryden NA, Canary JJ. Supplemental-chromium effects on glucose, insulin, glucagon, and urinary chromium losses in subjects consuming controlled low-chromium diets. Am J Clin Nutr 1991; 54:909–916.

91. Anderson RA, Cheng N, Bryden NA, Polansky MM, Cheng N, Chi J, Feng J. Elevated intakes of supplemental chromium improve glucose and insulin variables in individuals with type 2 diabetes. Diabetes 1997; 46:1786–1791.

92. Pozzilli P, Browne PD, Kolb H. The Nicotinamide Trialist. Meta-analysis of nicotinamide treatment in patients with recent-onset IDDM. Diabetes Care 1996; 19:1357–1363.

93. American Diabetes Association and The American Dietetic Association. Carbohydrate Counting: Getting Started, Moving On, Using Carbohydrate/Insulin Ratios. American Diabetes Association, Alexandria, VA, 1995.

94. International Diabetes Center. My Food Plan. IDC Publishing, Minneapolis, MN, 1996.
95. Wheeler M.L., Franz, M., Barrier, P., Holler, H., Cronmiller, N., Delahanty, L.M. Macronutrient and energy database for the 1995 Exchange Lists for Meal Planning: a rationale for clinical practice decisions. J Am Diet Assoc 1996; 96:1167–1171.
96. Gillespie SJ, Kulkarni K. Using carbohydrate counting in diabetes clinical practice. J Am Diet Assoc 1998; 98:897–905.

13 Health Aspects of Fish and n-3 Polyunsaturated Fatty Acids from Plant and Marine Origin

Emile A. M. de Deckere

1. INTRODUCTION

Ischemic or coronary heart disease (CHD) is the main cause of deaths in the United States (32% of total deaths in 1994) and other Western countries where it is associated with a high (saturated) fat intake. However, Greenland Eskimos (Inuit) on their traditional diet, which is rich in fat (40% of calories) and cholesterol, did not have such a high incidence of CHD and also much less atherosclerosis (1,2). This has been ascribed to the high amount of very long chain n-3 polyunsaturated fatty acids (VLC n-3 PUFA; approx 14 g/d) in their diet derived from fish and marine mammals (3). The VLC n-3 PUFA comprise mainly eicosapentaenoic acid (EPA, C20:5 n-3) and docosahexaenoic acid (DHA, C22:6 n-3) (see Fig. 1). Recently, less atherosclerosis and CHD have also been found in native Alaskans whose diet is also rich in marine fish and mammals (4). In addition, certain types of cancer, such as breast cancer, were found to be rare in Eskimos and Alaskan natives (5), which has also been ascribed to VLC n-3 PUFA.

The aforementioned findings have led to an avalanche of studies and discussions on health aspects of VLC n-3 PUFA and, because humans can synthesize these fatty acids from α-linolenic acid (C18:3 n-3), this has also been the case for α-linolenic acid. This chapter is based on a broad discussion by various experts on health aspects of fish and the n-3 PUFA from plant (α-linolenic acid) and marine origin (VLC n-3 PUFA) (6).

2. INTAKE OF n-3 PUFA

Daily average intake of α-linolenic acid in population groups in industrialized countries ranges from 1.0–2.2 g (7–9). In a considerable part of these popula-

From: *Nutritional Health: Strategies for Disease Prevention*
Edited by: T. Wilson and N. J. Temple © Humana Press Inc., Totowa, NJ

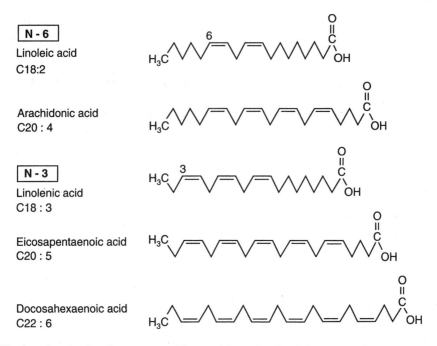

Fig. 1. n-6 and n-3 polyunsaturated fatty acids. n-6 and n-3 denote the first double bond from the methyl end ($-CH_3$) of the molecule. Humans can only insert double bonds into unsaturated fatty acid molecules between the last double bond counting from the methyl end and the carboxyl group, resulting in n-6 and n-3 families of fatty acids.

tions, intake is less than 1 g per day which might be too low *(6,9)*. The main dietary sources are products containing unhardened or partially hardened soybean and rapeseed (canola) oil. α-Linolenic acid is also present in chloroplasts of green leafy vegetables, but because chloroplasts are difficult to digest, the bioavailabilitiy of α-linolenic acid from this source is poor.

Estimates of the average intake of VLC n-3 PUFA in US population groups ranged from 117 to 177 mg/d *(7,10)*. In an epidemiological study by Ascherio and associates *(11)*, the median intake ranged from 70 mg/d for the lowest intake group to 580 mg/d for the highest. Fatty fish (mackerel, salmon, herring, trout, tuna), in which the fat is stored in the muscles, is the main source of VLC n-3 PUFA. White fish (cod, pollock, hake, haddock), in which the fat is stored in the liver, contains much less VLC n-3 PUFA. The VLC n-3 PUFA in fish are mainly derived from phytoplankton, microalgae, and bacteria. Lean beef and poultry (due to the use of feed containing fish meal) are also sources of VLC n-3 PUFA.

In addition to n-3 PUFA, our diet also contains n-6 PUFA; mainly linoleic acid (C18:2 n-6) from which arachidonic acid is synthesized (C20:4 n-6) *(see* Fig. 1). The dietary ratio of n-6 PUFA over n-3 PUFA is often used in discussions on the adequacy of the intake of n-3 PUFA because a ratio between 5 and 10 is recommended. However, the ratio in the diet in industrialized countries (and also in mother's milk) lies between 6.3 and 13 (7,8), which is, in fact, not very different from the recommended ratio. The use of this ratio is arguably not very helpful because the fatty acids involved (linoleic acid, α-linolenic acid, VLC n-3 PUFA) have different physiological effects and the effects of VLC n-3 PUFA (which can also be formed in the body from α-linolenic acid, see section 3) cannot be fully reproduced by α-linolenic acid, even in high doses (12).

α-Linolenic acid, like linoleic acid, is an essential fatty acid which means that the body cannot synthesize it. The minimal requirement is 0.2–0.3% of energy intake. Symptoms of α-linolenic acid deficiency are learning difficulties and impaired visual acuity. However, diseases resulting from α-linolenic acid deficiency have only be detected in patients on long-term gastric-tube feeding (13).

3. METABOLISM OF n-3 PUFA

Dietary α-linolenic acid is converted into VLC n-3 PUFA (e.g., in brain, liver, testes) which are incorporated into phospholipids of cell membranes, in particular in brain and retina. In rats it has been found that when the dietary level of α-linolenic acid is between zero and 0.3% of calories, DHA rises sharply in liver total fatty acids whereas above 0.3% of calories of α-linolenic acid, DHA hardly increases further. This will probably be similar in humans and may be the reason that dietary supplementation with α-linolenic acid (10 g/d or more) hardly affects the DHA levels (14), suggesting that the (average) habitual intake of α-linolenic acid is sufficient for the body requirement of DHA. EPA is an intermediate in the synthesis of DHA. The amount of EPA in cell membrane phospholipids is very low and the efficacy of α-linolenic acid in raising EPA in lipids is low. For every 10 g of dietary α-linolenic acid in the diet, 0.5 to 1 g EPA has been found to be incorporated into plasma and cell membrane phospholipids (15,16).

Enhanced dietary EPA and DHA consumption can increase the incorporation of these fatty acids into phospholipids. The effect on DHA levels is small, but the effect on EPA levels can be substantial. Then, EPA partly replaces arachidonic acid in the cell membrane phospholipids. This can lead to physiological effects, because eicosanoids are formed from arachidonic acid which has important physiological functions. Eicosanoids can also be formed from EPA, but these are generally less active. In addition, both EPA and DHA can inhibit eicosanoid synthesis.

4. CORONARY HEART DISEASE

4.1. Findings on Fish Consumption and α-Linolenic Acid

Epidemiological studies have shown that one serving of fish weekly may decrease the risk of fatal CHD by approx 40% relative to no fish (11,17–19). Higher intakes do not provide greater protection. The prospective studies had a comparable methodology; they compared either fish with no fish, or low doses of VLC n-3 PUFA with no VLC n-3 PUFA, and give a consistent picture. Recently, the inverse relationship between fish consumption and mortality from CHD was confirmed in an ecological study of 36 countries (20) and in a meta-analysis of prospective cohort studies (21). However, in the latter study the inverse relationship was only found for high-risk groups and not for low-risk groups.

No inverse association between fish intake and fatal CHD has been found in a number of other epidemiological studies. This was probably due to the fact that the lowest intake groups were already consuming a protective amount of fish (22,23). These studies do not contradict the hypothesis of the beneficial effects of one serving of fish per week. They do strengthen the conclusion that larger amounts of fish are not associated with increased benefits however.

Much of the fish consumed in the epidemiological studies was probably lean white fish. Combining data on the consumption of fish and the effects on CHD-risk parameters with insights on mechanisms make it plausible, but not certain, that the VLC n-3 PUFA were the fish components responsible for the decrease in the risk of fatal CHD (10,24). The reduction in risk, however, might be greater with fish than with VLC n-3 PUFA supplements.

The reduction in mortality by fish (fatty fish) and VLC n-3 PUFA has been confirmed in two clinical trials in patients who had myocardial infarction(25,26). In the study on fish (25), two weekly portions of fatty fish decreased all-cause mortality by 29% and in the study on VLC n-3 PUFA supplement (26) 1 g daily decreased cardiovascular death by 17%.

Epidemiological studies (7,9,27) and one clinical trial (28) suggest that intake of α-linolenic acid-rich food can decrease the risk of myocardial infarction and death. In the clinical trial with patients who had a first myocardial infarction, a "Mediterranean-type" of diet with more fish and vegetables, in which an α-linolenic acid-rich margarine replaced butter, was compared with the habitual diet. The margarine increased the intake of α-linolenic acid from 0.7 g/d to 1.8 g/d. Conversion of α-linolenic acid into EPA might play a role in the protection against CHD. This conversion, however, is low (see Section 3).

A relative deficiency of n-3 PUFA may be present in a large proportion of the population and might be a factor in CHD. In the Health Professional Follow-up Study (27) and the Nurses' Health Study (9) lower relative risks of fatal CHD were only found at the highest daily intakes of α-linolenic acid (1.5 and 1.12–1.36 g/d, respectively). Daily intake of α-linolenic acid in the lower intake groups was less than 1 g, which is below the recommended intake value (1–2 g/d).

4.2. Experimental Findings on VLC n-3 PUFA and α-Linolenic Acid

4.2.1. BLOOD LIPIDS

A high plasma triglyceride level is now recognized as an independent risk factor for CHD *(29)*. Dietary α-linolenic acid does not affect blood triglycerides, even at high intakes, and it lowers LDL cholesterol probably only when it replaces saturated fatty acids. However, plasma triglycerides can be decreased by VLC n-3 PUFA, which is the most characteristic effect of these fatty acids. VLC n-3 PUFA in doses of up to 7 g/d (average 3–4 g/d) lower fasting plasma triglycerides (mainly VLDL triglycerides) by approx 25%; somewhat more in normal subjects than in hypertriglyceridemic subjects *(12)*. There is evidence of a dose-response relation. The postprandial plasma triglyceride level is also lowered by VLC n-3 PUFA *(30)*. DHA and EPA may be equally effective in lowering triglyceride levels *(31)*.

After consuming VLC n-3 PUFA, LDL cholesterol increases by 4% in healthy subjects and by 7% in hypertriglyceridemic patients. HDL cholesterol increases by 3% in healthy people, but not in hypertriglyceridemic patients *(12)*. There are no indications for a modulating effect of linoleic acid on the effects of VLC n-3 PUFA on blood lipids.

4.2.2. BLOOD PRESSURE

Intake of VLC n-3 PUFA can moderately reduce blood pressure in hypertensive subjects, but less commonly in normotensive subjects. A minimum daily amount of 3 g may be needed for a significant reduction *(32,33)*. Typically, 5–6 g n-3 PUFA daily reduces systolic and diastolic blood pressure by 3.4 and 2.0 mm Hg, respectively, which can be expected to reduce risk for both stroke and CHD. However, this represents about 300 g of fatty fish or about 1500 g of white fish daily, which is a large amount to consume. Not surprisingly, therefore, no relation in epidemiological studies could be detected between fish intake and blood pressure. The limited data on α-linolenic acid show variable effects *(34,35)*.

4.2.3. THROMBOSIS/HEMOSTASIS

Because direct effects on arterial thrombosis cannot be measured, surrogate endpoints have to be used to estimate effects on thrombotic risk. In endothelial cells (in vitro studies), VLC n-3 PUFA reduced the levels of mRNA coding for adhesion molecules and increased prostacyclin synthesis, whereas effects on nitric oxide release were inconsistent. Data on effects of VLC n-3 PUFA and α-linolenic acid on coagulation and fibrinolysis are incomplete and inconsistent. VLC n-3 PUFA, but not α-linolenic acid, have been suggested to reduce the level of circulating platelet aggregates, although this has not been conclusively demonstrated. In vegetarians an additional amount of α-linolenic acid did not affect thrombotic risk factors *(36)*. In summary, there are insufficient data on the extent to which the anti-CHD effects of VLC n-3 PUFA and α-linolenic acid are mediated by changes in hemostasis *(37)*.

The relationship between fish and VLC n-3 PUFA intake and stroke incidence and mortality is also inconsistent. A reason might be that there are two types of stroke, thrombotic and hemorrhagic types, which are affected by VLC n-3 PUFA differently.

4.2.4. Arrhythmia

Sudden cardiac death is a major cause of death in industrialized countries. Mortality statistics from the United States indicate that up to 80% of sudden cardiac deaths are due to ventricular fibrillation, which is the most common arrhythmia *(38)*. Studies in cell cultures and animal models, observational evidence, and human trials all show that fatty acids can be involved in fatal arrhythmia *(38,39)*. In animal models, α-linolenic acid, EPA, DHA, and other PUFA reduced the susceptibility to ventricular fibrillation and in cardiac myocytes they had antiarrhythmic activity *(38,40)*. Epidemiological and clinical studies also suggest antiarrhythmic effects (e.g., decrease in heart rate variability and ventricular ectopic beats) from the consumption of fish and VLC n-3 PUFA *(10,24)*. These effects may well contribute to lower death rates in patients at high risk of cardiac arrhythmias.

4.2.5. Vascular Effects

A clinical trial suggests that VLC n-3 PUFA may mitigate coronary atherosclerosis *(41)*, but there is no solid evidence for a reduction in restenosis after coronary angioplasty. In addition to atherosclerosis, arterial spasm or vasoconstriction may also impair blood flow. VLC n-3 PUFA may affect vascular tone of blood vessels by decreasing the release of the vasoconstrictor compound thromboxane, whereas the release of vasodilators such as prostacyclin and nitric oxide, is not affected or may be increased. Higher arterial elasticity has been found in people who consume fish frequently, in comparison with nonfish eaters *(42)*, and by an α-linolenic acid-rich diet *(35)*. An increase in arterial elasticity might decrease the workload of the heart, contributing in this way to a reduced risk of CHD.

5. CANCER

Animal studies show that high doses of VLC n-3 PUFA inhibit the development of chemically induced breast and colorectal cancers in the promotion phase, but probably not in the initiation phase. Human data suggest that an increase in the consumption of fish and VLC n-3 PUFA may lead to lower breast and colorectal cancer risks *(43)*. A recent epidemiological study suggests an interaction between animal fat and fish, from which might be hypothesized that VLC n-3 PUFA protect against the effect of animal fat on risk of colorectal cancer *(44)*. In trials with patients prone to development of colorectal adenomas, VLC n-3 PUFA have been found to "normalize" hyperproliferation of mucosal crypt cells *(45)*. The effects of dietary VLC n-3 PUFA on cancer are described more fully in Chapter 5 by Clifford and McDonald.

Data on α-linolenic acid and cancer in humans are scarce *(7),* and the results of animal studies are conflicting. In some epidemiological studies, increased intake of α-linolenic acid was associated with increased prostate cancer incidence *(46).* Other studies do not suggest an effect of α-linolenic acid intake on cancer mortality *(47).*

6. NEURAL DEVELOPMENT

Both VLC n-3 and n-6 PUFA are necessary for proper neural development. Infants, as well as preterm infants, can synthesize VLC n-3 and n-6 PUFA from α-linolenic and linoleic acid, respectively *(48–50).* An important controversial issue that remains is the adequacy of α-linolenic acid in infant formulas as a precursor for DHA and the need of DHA in formulas for optimal development, in particular for preterm infants *(51).* Plasma and red blood cell levels of DHA are positively affected by dietary DHA. Although DHA levels in brain autopsy tissue from babies fed formulas have been found to be lower than in breast-fed babies, it is not clear whether supplementation of formulas with VLC n-3 PUFA has beneficial effects on brain development, in particular with respect to learning ability and memory *(52).*

DHA is a main component of the retina and a shortage of DHA might affect visual development. However, there are too many uncertainties in the studies with infants for a solid conclusion on the use of VLC n-3 PUFA in infant formulas, in particular for term infants *(53).* In preterm infants, formulas enriched with DHA were found to improve visual acuity (a validated measure of visual function development) in the first half of the first year *(54,55).* This effect might be transient *(54).* Nevertheless, in some countries all preterm formulas are supplemented with DHA (and arachidonic acid).

The question of whether the addition of DHA alone or in combination with arachidonic acid to (term) infant formulas confers a physiological benefit to the infant has not yet been clarified. A major reason is the low number of infants in the studies *(56),* but results of larger studies will be available soon. The same holds true for supplementation with α-linolenic acid at realistic doses to pregnant or lactating mothers in relation to the health of the newborn *(57).* It is also uncertain to what extent the ratio of linoleic acid to α-linolenic acid and/or the absolute amounts of linoleic acid and α-linolenic acid in the mothers' diet are of relevance to the health status of the fetus and breast-fed infant.

7. IMMUNE FUNCTION AND INFLAMMATION

VLC n-3 PUFA have been found to exert beneficial effects in rheumatoid arthritis, renal immunological disorders, and inflammatory bowel disease. In rheumatoid arthritis, VLC n-3 PUFA moderately, but reproducibly, decrease pain and morning stiffness and can reduce the need for concomitant medication *(58)*. Apparently, VLC n-3 PUFA have an analgesic effect and are therefore of value in other diseases with chronic pain. In renal immunological disorders, beneficial effects have been reported in immunoglobulin A nephropathy and renal transplantation *(59)*. Here, the therapeutic use of VLC n-3 PUFA can lead to a slowing in the loss of renal function. In inflammatory bowel disease, clinical and histological improvements and reduction in concurrent medication have been reported *(60)* and VLC n-3 PUFA might be used as an adjuvant to drug therapy in ulcerative colitis *(61)*.

There is no solid evidence that VLC n-3 PUFA are effective in asthma and only weak evidence in psoriasis. There are no epidemiological data for fish consumption effects on rheumatoid arthritis; there is only one study on α-linolenic acid and rheumatoid arthritis, which indicates that it is ineffective. Because of the effects of n-3 PUFA on immune and inflammation mediators, an increased intake of EPA might lead to a suppression of immune and inflammation responses, and consequently, to a decrease in host resistance to infections. However, no adverse effects of VLC n-3 PUFA on infection in humans have been reported.

8. POSSIBLE ADVERSE EFFECTS OF n-3 PUFA

8.1. Lipid Oxidation

Oxidized LDL has been implicated in atherosclerosis and is discussed in Chapter 8 by Woodside and Young. Oxidizability of LDL is measured in vitro, but this parameter might not reliably reflect oxidation sensitivity of LDL in vivo. Inconsistent results have been published with respect to the effect of α-linolenic and VLC n-3 PUFA on this parameter. However, since consumption of n-3 PUFA can be associated with a higher susceptibility to in vitro oxidizability of LDL, this should be accompanied by adequate amounts of antioxidants such as α-tocopherol *(62)*. The established beneficial effects of n-3 PUFA on other risk factors for CHD likely outweigh any increased risk from oxidative changes. While Greenland Eskimos and Alaskan natives with a habitual high consumption of VLC n-3 PUFA had a low incidence of atherosclerosis *(63)*, the oxidizability of their LDL has not been investigated.

8.2. Bleeding Time

High doses of VLC n-3 PUFA (as in the original Eskimo diet) seem to modestly prolong skin bleeding time and may also increase the tendency for nosebleeding. However, daily intake of 3 g or less of EPA + DHA does not appreciably increase bleeding time. Moreover, no clinically significant bleeding has been found in clinical trials with more than 3 g EPA + DHA daily *(64)*. Recently, menhaden oil containing 25% VLC n-3 PUFA is generally recognized as safe (GRAS) as a direct human food ingredient if less than 3 g EPA + DHA daily is consumed *(65)*.

8.3. Diabetes

Some studies suggest unfavorable effects of VLC n-3 PUFA in diabetics *(66)*. However, the effects of VLC n-3 PUFA on CHD risk factors in non-insulin-dependent diabetics are not much different from those in nondiabetics *(67)*. Moderate doses of VLC n-3 PUFA and fish consumption can be beneficial in diabetes by decreasing plasma triglycerides, but the use of large doses of VLC n-3 PUFA should not be encouraged. The Food and Drug Administration *(65)* have concluded that consumption of 3 g EPA + DHA daily by diabetics is safe with respect to glycemic control. Further dietary recommendations for the treatment of diabetes are discussed in Chapter 12 by Franz.

9. CONCLUSIONS

There is sufficient evidence to support the view that VLC n-3 PUFA can be beneficial for health, especially for those at high risk for CHD. It is generally advised to eat fish at least once a week. Fatty fish is preferable because of its high content of VLC n-3 PUFA. People who do not eat fish could consider taking VLC n-3 PUFA supplements, e.g., 200 mg EPA + DHA daily, which is equivalent to 10–40 g of fatty fish per day. Pregnant women and neonates may require, in addition to linoleic acid and α-linolenic acid, some intake of VLC n-3 PUFA to cover the needs for optimal growth and development. The recommended daily intake of α-linolenic acid is 1–2 g. Separate recommendations for VLC n-3 PUFA and α-linolenic acid (in addition to that for linoleic acid) are needed due to their dissimilar physiological effects. The n-6/n-3 PUFA ratio should not be used.

REFERENCES

1. Dyerberg J, Bang HO. Haemostatic function and platelet polyunsaturated fatty acids in Eskimos. Lancet 1979; 2:433–435.
2. Kromann N, Green A. Epidemiological studies in the Upernavik district, Greenland. Incidence of some chronic diseases 1950–1974. Acta Med Scand 1980; 208:401–406.
3. Dyerberg J. Linolenate-derived polyunsaturated fatty acids and prevention of atherosclerosis. Nutr Rev 1986; 44:125–134.
4. Middaugh JP. Cardiovascular deaths among Alaskan Natives. Am J Public Health 1990; 80:282–285.
5. Nielsen NH, Hansen JPH. Breast cancer in Greenland: selected epidemiological, clinical, and histological features. J Cancer Res Clin Oncol 1980; 98:287–299.
6. De Deckere EAM, Korver O, Verschuren PM, Katan MB. Health aspects of fish and n-3 polyunsaturated fatty acids from plant and marine origin. Eur J Clin Nutr 1998; 52:749–753.
7. Dolecek TA. Epidemiological evidence of relationships between dietary polyunsaturated fatty acids and mortality in the multiple risk factor intervention trial. Proc Soc Exptl Biol Med 1992; 200:177–182.
8. De Vries JHM, Jansen A, Kromhout D, Bovenkamp P, Van Staveren W, Mensink RP, Katan MB. The fatty acid and sterol content of food composites of middle aged men in seven countries. J Fd Comp Anal 1997; 10:115–141.

9. Hu FB, Stampfer MJ, Manson JE, Rimm EB, Wolk A, Colditz GA, et al. Dietary intake of a-linolenic acid and risk of fatal ischemic heart disease among women. Am J Clin Nutr 1999; 69:890–897.
10. Siscovick DS, Raghunathan TE, King I, Weinmann S, WicklundKG, Albright J, et al. Dietary intake and cell membrane levels of long chain n-3 polyunsaturated fatty acids and the risk of primary cardiac arrest. JAMA 1995; 274:1363–1367.
11. Ascherio A, Rimm EB, Stampfer MJ, Giovannucci EL, Willett WC. Dietary intake of marine n-3 fatty acids, fish intake, and the risk of coronary disease among men. N Engl J Med 1995; 332:977–982.
12. Harris WS. n-3 Fatty acids and serum lipoproteins: human studies. Am J Clin Nutr 1997; 65:1645S–1654S.
13. Bjerve KS, Løvold Mostad I, Thoresen L. Alpha-linolenic acid deficiency in patients on long-term gastric-tube feeding: estimation of linolenic acid and long-chain unsaturated n-3 fatty acid requirement in man. Am J Clin Nutr 1987; 45:66–77.
14. Mantzioris E, James MJ, Gibson RA, Cleland LG. Dietary substitution with an a-linolenic acid-rich vegetable oil increases eicosapentaenoic acid concentrations in tissue. Am J Clin Nutr 1994; 59:1304–1309.
15. Emken EA, Adlof RO, Rakoff H, Rohwedder WK, Gulley RM. Metabolism in vivo of deuterium-labeled linolenic and linoleic acid in humans. Biochem Soc Trans 1990; 18:766–769.
16. Valsta LM, Salminen I, Aro A, Mutanen M. Alpha-linolenic acid in rapeseed oil partly compensates for the effect of fish restriction on plasma long chain n-3 fatty acids. Eur J Clin Nutr 1996; 50:229–235.
17. Gillum RF, Mussolino ME, Madans JH. The relationship between fish consumption and stroke incidence. The NHANES I Epidemiologic Follow-up Study. Arch Intern Med 1996; 156:537–542.
18. Daviglus ML, Stamler J, Orencia AJ, Dyer AR, Liu K, Greenland P, et al. Fish consumption and the 30-year risk of fatal myocardial-infarction. N Engl J Med 1997; 336:1046–1053.
19. Albert CM, Hennekens CH, O'Donnell CJ, Ajani UA, Carey VJ, Willett WC, et al. Fish consumption and risk of sudden cardiac death. JAMA. 1998; 279:23–28.
20. Zhang J, Sasaki S, Amano K, Kestelot H. Fish consumption and mortality from all causes, ischemic heart disease, and stroke: an ecological study. Prev Med 1999; 28:520–529.
21. Marckmann P, Gronbaek M. Fish consumption and coronary heart disease mortality. A systematic review of prospective cohort studies. Eur J Clin Nutr 1999; 53:585–590.
22. Lapidus L, Andersson H, Bengtsson C, Bosaeus I. Dietary habits in relation to incidence of cardiovascular disease and death in women: a 12-year follow-up of participants in the population study of women in Gothenburg, Sweden. Am J Clin Nutr 1986; 44:444–448.
23. Morris MC, Manson JE, Rosner B, Buring JE, Willett WC, Hennekens CH. Fish consumption and cardiovascular disease in the Physicians Health Study: a prospective study. Am J Epidemiol 1995; 142:166–175.
24. Singh RB, Niaz MA, Sharma JP, Kumar R, Rastogi V, Moshiri M. Randomized, double blind placebo controlled trial of fish oil and mustard oil in patients with suspected acute myocardial infarction: The Indian Experiment of Infarct Survival-4. Cardiovasc Drugs Ther 1997; 11:485–491.
25. Burr ML, Fehily AM, Gilbert JF, Rogers S, Holliday RM, Sweetnam PM, et al. Effects of changes in fat, fish and fibre intakes on death and myocardial reinfarction: diet and reinfarction trial (DART). Lancet 1989; 2:757–761.
26. GISSI Prevenzione Investigators. Dietary supplementation with n-3 polyunsaturated fatty acids and vitamin E after myocardial infarction: results of the GISSI-Prevenzione trial. Lancet. 1999; 354:447–455.
27. Ascherio A, Rimm EB, Giovannucci EL, Spiegelman D, Stampfer MJ, Willett WC. Dietary fat and risk of coronary heart disease in men: cohort follow up study in the United States. BMJ 1996; 313:84–90.

28. de Lorgeril M, Salen P, Martin J-L, Monjaud I, Delaye J, Mamelle N. Mediterranean diet, traditional risk factors, and the rate of cardiovascular compliance after myocardial infarction. Final report of the Lyon Diet Heart Study. Circulation 1999; 99:779–785.

29. Austin MA, Hokanson JE, Edwards KL. Hypertriglyceridemia as a cardiovascular risk factor. Am J Cardiol 1998; 81(4A):7B–12B.

30. Zampelas A, Peel AS, Gould BJ, Wright J, Williams CM. Polyunsaturated fatty acids of the n-6 and n-3 series: effects on postprandial lipid and lipoprotein levels in healthy men. Eur J Clin Nutr 1994; 48:842–848.

31. Grimsgaard S, Bønaa KH, Hansen J-B, Nordøy A. Highly purified eicosapentaenoic acid and docosahexaenoic acid in humans have similar triacylglycerol-lowering effects but divergent effects on serum fatty acids. Am J Clin Nutr 1997; 66:649–659.

32. Appel LJ, Miller ER, Seidler AJ, Whelton PK. Does supplementation of diet with fish oil reduce blood pressure? A meta-analysis of controlled clinical trials. Arch Intern Med 1993; 153:429–438.

33. Morris MC, Sacks F, Rosner B. Does fish oil lower blood pressure? A meta-analysis of controlled trials. Circulation 1993; 88:523–533.

34. Salonen JT. Dietary fats, antioxidants and blood pressure. Ann Med 1991; 23:295–298.

35. Nestel PJ, Pomeroy SE, Sasahara T, Yamashita T, Liang YL, Dart AM, et al. Arterial compliance in obese subjects is improved with dietary plant n-3 fatty acid from flaxseed oil despite increased LDL oxidizability. Arterioscler Thromb Vasc Biol 1997; 17:1163–1170.

36. Li D, Sinclair A, Wilson A, Nakkote S, Kelly F, Abedin L, et al. Effect of dietary alpha-linolenic acid on thrombotic risk factors in vegetarian men. Am J Clin Nutr 1999; 69:872–882.

37. Knapp H. Dietary fatty acids in human thrombosis and hemostasis. Am J Clin Nutr 1997; 65:S1687–S1698.

38. Charnock JS. Lipids and cardiac arrhythmia. Prog Lipid Res 1994; 33:355–385.

39. Nair SSD, Leitch JW, Falconer J, Garg ML. Prevention of cardiac arrhythmia by dietary (n-3) polyunsaturated fatty acids and their mechanism of action. J Nutr 1997; 127:383–393.

40. Leaf A, Kang JX. ω3 Fatty acids and cardiovascular diseases. World Rev Nutr Diet 1998; 83:24–37.

41. Von Schacky C, Angerer P, Kothny W, Theisen K, Mudra, H. The effect of dietary w-3 fatty acids on coronary atherosclerosis. Ann Int Med 1999; 130:554–562.

42. Wahlqvist ML, Lo CS, Meyers KA. Fish intake and arterial wall characteristics in healthy people and diabetic patients. Lancet 1989; 2:944–946.

43. De Deckere EAM. Possible beneficial effect of fish and fish n-3 polyunsaturated fatty acids in breast and colorectal cancer. Eur J Cancer Prev 1999; 8:213–221.

44. Caygill CPJ, Charlett A, Hill MJ. Fat, fish, fish oil and cancer. Br J Cancer 1996; 74:159–164.

45. Anti M, Marra G, Armelao F, Percesepe A, Gentiloni N. Modulating effect of omega-3 fatty acids on proliferative pattern of human colorectal mucosa. Adv Exp Med Biol 1997; 400B:605–610.

46. Harvei S, Bjerve KS, Tretli S, Jellum E, Robsahm TE, Vatten L. Prediagnostic level of fatty acids in serum phospholipids: omega-3 and omega-6 fatty acids and the risk of prostate cancer. Int J Cancer 1997; 71:545–551.

47. Kolonel LN, Yoshizawa CN, Hankin JH. Diet and prostatic cancer: a case-control study in Hawaii. Am J Epidemiol 1988; 127:999–1012.

48. Carnielli VP, Wattimena DJL, Luijendijk IHT, Boerlage A, Degenhart HJ, Sauer PJ. The very low birth weight premature infant is capable of synthesising arachidonic and docosahexaenoic acids from linoleic and linolenic acids. Pediatr Res 40; 1996:169–174.

49. Salem N, Wegher B, Mena P, Uauy R. Arachidonic acid and docosahexaenoic acids are biosynthesized from their 18-carbon precursors in human infants. Proc Natl Acad Sci USA 1996; 93:49–54.

50. Sauerwald TU, Hachey DL, Jensen SL, Heird WC. New insights into the metabolism of long chain polyunsaturated fatty acids during infancy. Eur J Med Res 1997; 2:88–92.

51. Crawford MA, Costeloe K, Ghebremeskel K, Phylactos A. The inadequacy of the essential fatty acid content of present preterm feeds. Eur J Pediatr 1998; 157(Suppl. 1):S23–S27.

52. Carlson SE, Neuringer M. Polyunsaturated fatty acid status and neurodevelopment: a summary and critical analysis of the literature. Lipids 1999; 34:171–178.

53. Gibson R, Makrides M. Polyunsaturated fatty acids and infant visual development: a critical appraisal of randomized clinical trials. Lipids 1999; 34:179–184.

54. Carlson SE, Werkman SH, Rhodes PG, Tolley EA. Visual-acuity development in healthy preterm infants: effect of marine-oil supplementation. Am J Clin Nutr 1993; 58:35–42.

55. Uauy R, Peirano P, Hoffman D, Mena P, Birch D, Birch E. Role of essential fatty acids in the function of the developing nervous system. Lipids 1996; 31:S167–S176.

56. Morley R. Nutrition and cognitive development. Nutrition 1998; 14:752–754.

57. Al MDM, Van Houwelingen AC, Hornstra G. Relation between birth order and the maternal and neonatal docosahexaenoic acid status. Eur J Clin Nutr 1997; 51:548–553.

58. Kremer JM. Effects of modulation of inflammatory and immune parameters in patients with rheumatic and inflammatory disease receiving dietary supplementation of n-3 and n-6 fatty acids. Lipids 1996; 31:S243–S247.

59. De Caterina R, Endres S, Kristensen SD, Schmidt EB. N-3 fatty acids and renal diseases. Am J Kidney Dis 1994; 24:394–415.

60. Ross E. The role of marine fish oils in the treatment of ulcerative colitis. Nutr Rev 1993; 51:47–49.

61. Stenson WF, Cort D, Rodgers J, Burakoff R, DeSchryver-Kecskemeti K, Gramlich TL, Beeken W. Dietary supplementation with fish oil in ulcerative colitis. Ann Intern Med 1992; 116:609–614.

62. Muggli R. Physiological requirements of vitamin E as a function of the amount and type of polyunsaturated fatty acid. World Rev Nutr Diet 1994; 75:166–168.

63. Bang HO, Dyerberg J, Brøndum-Nielsen A. Plasma lipid and lipoprotein pattern in Greenland west-coat Eskimos. Lancet 1971; 1:1143–1146.

64. Lox CD. The effects of dietary marine oils (omega-3 fatty acids) on coagulation profiles in men. Gen Pharmacol 1990; 21:241–246.

65. Food and Drug Administration. Substances affirmed as generally recognized as safe: menhaden oil. Federal Register 1997; 62:30,751–30,757.

66. Vessby B, Karlsrom B, Boberg M, Lithell H, Berne C. Polyunsaturated fatty acids may impair blood glucose control in type 2 diabetic patients. Diabet Med 1992; 9:126–133.

67. Axelrod L, Camuso J, Williams E, Kleinman K, Briones E, Schoenfeld D. Effects of a small quantity of omega-3 fatty acids on cardiovascular risk factors in NIDDM. A randomized, prospective, double-blind, controlled study. Diabetes Care 1994; 17:37–44.

14 Optimizing Nutrition for Exercise and Sport

Brian Leutholtz and Richard B. Kreider

1. INTRODUCTION

The primary factors that affect exercise performance capacity include an individual's genetic endowment, the quality of training, and the effectiveness of coaching (*see* Fig. 1). Beyond these factors, nutrition plays a critical role in optimizing performance capacity. In order for an athlete to perform well, their training and diet must be optimal. If an athlete does not train enough or has an inadequate diet, their performance may be decreased *(1)*. On the other hand, if an athlete trains too much without a sufficient diet, they may be susceptible to become overtrained (*see* Fig. 2).

Because optimizing training and dietary practices are critical to peak performance, athletes have searched for various ways to improve exercise performance capacity through the use of ergogenic aids. An ergogenic aid is any training technique, mechanical device, nutritional practice, pharmacological method, or psychological technique that can improve exercise performance capacity or enhance training adaptations *(2)*. This includes aids that improve the preparation to performance, the efficiency of physiological and psychological responses to exercise, and/or recovery from exercise. Research has demonstrated that various ergogenic aids can help an athlete optimize performance capacity. This chapter overviews the role that nutrition has on enhancing exercise and sport performance, describes nutritional guidelines that athletes should employ to optimize training adaptations, and evaluates the ergogenic value of various nutrients that have been proposed to improve exercise capacity.

2. ENERGY DEMANDS FOR ACTIVE INDIVIDUALS

The first nutritional principle to optimize performance of athletes is to make sure that they consume enough calories to offset energy demands so as to

From: *Nutritional Health: Strategies for Disease Prevention*
Edited by: T. Wilson and N. J. Temple © Humana Press Inc., Totowa, NJ

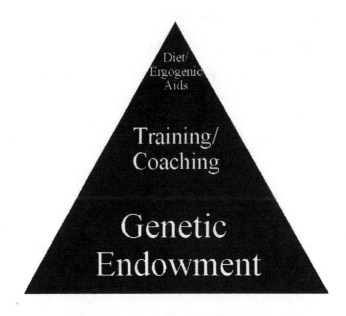

Fig. 1. Factors affecting peak performance.

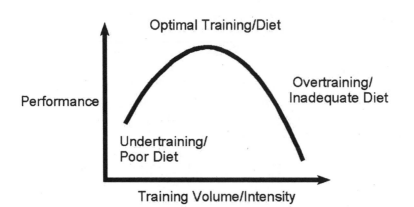

Fig. 2. Training stimulus.

maintain energy balance. Daily caloric intake for untrained individuals typically ranges between 1900–3000 kcal/d (i.e., 27–43 kcal/kg/d for a 70 kg person) *(2–5)*. Obviously, exercise training increases energy expenditure. The longer and more intense an athlete exercises, the greater the energy expenditure. Energy expenditure estimates for athletes have ranged from 3500 kcal/d (50 kcal/kg/d) for individuals training 30–60 min/d up to 12,000 kcal/d (i.e., 170 kcal/kg/d) for cyclists competing in the Tour de France bicycle race (cycling 4–6 h/d) *(3,4)*. For most high school and college athletes training 2–2.5 h/d, energy expenditure estimates range between 60–80 kcal/kg/d *(4)*. However, athletes often do not consume enough calories to offset energy demands *(3)*. This may result in a chronic deficit in energy intake and has been implicated as one potential causative factor in overtraining *(3,6)*. Athletes particularly susceptible to maintaining negative energy intakes during training include runners, cyclists, swimmers, triathletes, gymnasts, skaters, dancers, wrestlers, and boxers *(1–3)*. Additionally, female athletes have been reported to have a high incidence of eating disorders. Consequently, the sports medicine professional should ensure that athletes are well fed and consume enough calories to offset the increased energy demands of training.

3. GENERAL MACRONUTRIENT GUIDELINES FOR ATHLETES

The second principle in supporting the nutritional needs of athletes is to ensure that athletes consume the proper amounts of carbohydrate, fat, and protein in their diet. Table 1 summarizes macronutrient guidelines for athletes. The following discussion provides additional insight on how to structure the diet of athletes in order to optimize performance.

3.1. Carbohydrate

Carbohydrate serves as the primary fuel for high intensity intermittent or prolonged exercise. Carbohydrate is stored in the muscle (about 15 g/kg) and liver (about 80–100 g) *(6)*. Intense exercise depletes muscle and liver glycogen stores. The stores are replenished from dietary carbohydrate. Unfortunately, when significant amounts of carbohydrate are depleted, it may be difficult to fully replenish carbohydrate levels within one day. Consequently, when athletes train once or twice per day over a period of days, carbohydrate levels may gradually decline leading to fatigue, poor performance, and/or overtraining *(3,6)*.

Research has indicated that athletes should ingest between 8–10 g/kg/d of carbohydrate during intense periods of training in order to help maintain carbohydrate stores *(3,6)*. In order to do so, it is recommended that athletes eat frequently (e.g., 4–6 meals/d) and ingest high-calorie carbohydrate foods and/or concentrated carbohydrate drinks. Preferably, the majority of dietary carbohydrate should come from complex carbohydrates with a low to moderate

Table 1
Dietary Macronutrient Guidelines for Athletes

Nutrient	Proposed ergogenic value	Summary of research findings
Carbohydrate	Primary fuel used for anaerobic and high intensity aerobic exercise. Increasing dietary availability proposed to increase glycogen content and increase exercise capacity.	Athletes engaged in heavy training need to consume a diet high in carbohydrate (55–65% of caloric intake). Ingesting 8–10 g/kg/d of carbohydrate during heavy training has been suggested as one strategy to reduce the incidence of overtraining (1,2,3,6).
Protein	Increasing dietary availability of protein has been suggested to be a means of maintaining nitrogen balance and enhancing gains in muscle mass.	Protein balance studies indicate that athletes involved in heavy training need to ingest 1.3–1.7 g/kg/d of protein in order to maintain nitrogen balance (about 1.5 times the RDA for protein). Although most athletes consume enough protein in their diet, some athletes are susceptible to protein malnutrition (dancers, gymnasts, runners, swimmers, etc.). Studies indicate that supplementing the diet with protein above that necessary to maintain protein balance does not increase strength or muscle mass (7,8).
Fat	Primary fuel for moderate- to low-intensity exercise. Some have proposed that increasing fat and/or derivatives of fat may enhance endurance exercise performance. Others suggest that increasing fat content in the diet may help moderate insulin levels leading to a better degree helping to promote fat loss.	It is generally recommended that athletes consume less than 1 g/kg/d of fat in their diet (@ <30% of calories) (3). Studies indicate that individuals who successfully maintain weight loss consume less than 40 g/d of fat (9). Studies generally do not indicate the fat/fat derivative supplements enhance exercise performance. However, supplements that increase fat use during exercise may enhance time to exhaustion.

glycemic index (e.g., grains, starches, fruit, etc.). Although this sounds relatively simple, intense training often suppresses appetite and/or alters hunger patterns *(3)*. Some athletes do not like to exercise within several hours after eating because of sensations of fullness and/or a predisposition to cause gastrointestinal distress. Furthermore, travel and training schedules may limit food availability and/or the access to the types of food athletes are accustomed to eating. This means that care should be taken to coordinate mealtimes with training and make sure athletes have sufficient availability to nutrient-dense foods throughout the day for snacking between meals (e.g., drinks, fruit, carbohydrate/protein bars, etc.).

Research has also demonstrated that the timing and composition of meals consumed may play a role in maintaining carbohydrate stores during training *(7)*. In this regard, it takes about 4 h for carbohydrate to be digested and begin to be stored as muscle and liver glycogen. Consequently, pre-exercise meals should be consumed about 4–6 h before exercise. This means that if an athlete trains in the afternoon, breakfast is the most important meal to top off muscle and liver glycogen levels. Research has also indicated that ingesting a light carbohydrate and protein snack 30–60 min prior to exercise (e.g., 50 g of carbohydrate and 5–10 g of protein) serves to increase carbohydrate availability toward the end of an intense exercise bout *(7)*. This also serves to increase availability of amino acids and decrease exercise-induced catabolism of protein *(7)*.

When exercise lasts more than 1 h, athletes should ingest glucose/electrolyte solution (GES) sports drinks in order to maintain blood glucose levels and help prevent dehydration. Following intense exercise, athletes should consume carbohydrate and protein (e.g., 1 g/kg of carbohydrate and 0.5 g/kg of protein) within 30 min after exercise, as well as consume a high carbohydrate meal within 2 h following exercise. This nutritional strategy has been found to accelerate glycogen resynthesis, as well as promote a more anabolic hormonal profile that may hasten recovery. Finally, for 2–3 d prior to competition, athletes should taper training by 30–50% and consume 200–300 g/d of extra carbohydrate in their diet. This carbohydrate-loading technique has been shown to supersaturate carbohydrate stores prior to competition and improve endurance exercise capacity. Thus, the type of meal and timing of eating are important factors in maintaining carbohydrate availability during training.

3.2. Protein

Historically, there has been considerable debate regarding protein needs of athletes *(7)*. Initially, it was recommended that athletes do not need to ingest more than the RDA for protein (i.e., 0.8–1.0 g/kg/d for children, adolescents, and adults). However, research over the last decade has indicated that athletes engaged in intense training need to ingest about one and a half to two times the RDA of protein (1.3–1.7 g/kg/d) in order to maintain protein balance. If an insufficient amount of protein is obtained from the diet, an athlete will maintain a negative nitrogen balance which can increase protein catabolism and slow recovery. Over time, this may lead to muscle wasting and training intolerance *(1,3,7)*.

Although most athletes ingest this amount of protein in their normal diet, there are some athletes who are susceptible to protein malnutrition due to greater protein degradation, weight restrictions, and/or an inability to ingest enough calories to offset energy expenditure (e.g., runners, cyclists, swimmers, triathletes, gymnasts, dancers, skaters, wrestlers, boxers, etc.). Therefore, care should be taken to ensure that these types of athletes consume a sufficient amount of protein in order to maintain nitrogen balance (e.g., 1.5 g/kg/d). Research has also indicated that ingesting more protein than necessary to maintain nitrogen balance does not promote greater gains in strength or muscle mass *(7,8)*.

3.3. Fat

The dietary fat intake recommendations for athletes are similar to those for non-athletes in order to promote health. Generally, it is recommended that athletes consume less than 30% of their daily caloric intake as fat. For athletes attempting to decrease body fat, it is also recommended that they consume 0.5–1 g/kg/d of fat. This is because weight loss studies indicate that people who are most successful in losing weight and maintaining the weight loss are those who ingest less than 40 g/d of fat in their diet *(9)*. Strategies to help athletes manage dietary fat intake include teaching them which foods contain fat so that they can make better food choices and learn to how to count fat grams.

4. PROPOSED NUTRITIONAL ERGOGENIC AIDS

Nutritional ergogenic aids are the most common type of ergogenic aids used by athletes. They include alterations in the composition of the diet, timing of eating, and/or supplementation of various macro- and micronutrients that may enhance performance. Nutritional strategies that improve the preparation for exercise, the efficiency of exercise, performance capacity, and/or enhance the recovery from exercise may be viewed as ergogenic. Consequently, the final nutritional strategy for enhancing training and/or performance capacity in athletes is the appropriate use of effective and safe nutritional ergogenic aids. Although research has demonstrated that some nutritional strategies and nutrients may affect exercise training and/or performance capacity, the majority of nutritional ergogenic aids marketed to athletes do not affect performance. The following section reviews macro- and micronutrients that have been proposed to improve exercise capacity.

4.1. Carbohydrate and Carbohydrate By-Products

As stated previously, dietary carbohydrate availability can significantly affect muscle and liver carbohydrate stores and performance capacity. For this reason, in addition to the dietary guidelines described, a significant amount of research has been conducted to determine ways to optimize carbohydrate availability during exercise and/or spare muscle glycogen use during exercise. Generally, increasing availability of any form of carbohydrate has the potential to improve exercise capacity by serving as an exogenous fuel source. Table 2 describes the proposed ergogenic value and summary of research findings for several forms of carbohydrate and carbohydrate by-products that have been proposed to enhance exercise performance. Of the products reviewed, glucose electrolyte solution (GES) sport drinks possess the greatest potential to improve exercise capacity. Although some clinical and/or exercise benefits have been reported from dihydroxyacetone phosphate (DHAP), fructose 1,6-diphosphate (FDP), polylactate, pyruvate, and ribose supplementation, it is our view that additional research is necessary to determine the efficacy of these nutrients before they are recommended for athletes.

4.2. Lipids and Lipid By-Products

Because fat can serve as a primary fuel source during low to moderate intensity exercise and most people have a considerable amount of fat stored as potential energy, researchers have also investigated the effects of lipids and lipid byproducts on exercise capacity and training. The basic rationale is that if fat oxidation can be increased during exercise, then carbohydrate stores can be spared, and exercise capacity can be improved. Additionally, if a greater amount of fat can be burned during exercise, this may help in weight management. Table 3 presents the proposed ergogenic value and summary of research findings for selected lipids and lipid by-products that have been proposed to affect exercise performance. Of the nutrients presented, glycerol supplementation used as a means to hyperhydrate athletes susceptible to dehydration appears to possess the most ergogenic potential. Although research to date is promising, more studies are needed in humans to determine whether conjugated linoleic acids (CLA) supplementation affects body composition during training and/or may possess a health benefit. Based on current data, there appears to be a limited ergogenic value of L-carnitine and medium-chain triglyceride (MCT) supplementation. Finally, although there may be some health benefits from diets high in omega 3-fatty acids, there is no evidence that omega 3-fatty acid supplementation with these lipids affects exercise performance.

4.3. Protein and Amino Acids

Amino acids are the foundation of protein in the body and are essential for the synthesis of tissue, specific proteins, hormones, enzymes, and neurotransmitters (7). Amino acids are also involved in the synthesis of energy through gluconeogenesis and regulation of numerous metabolic pathways. Consequently, it has been suggested that athletes may require additional protein in their diet in order to

Table 2
Proposed Nutritional Ergogenic Aids
for Athletes—Carbohydrate and Carbohydrate By-Products

Nutrient	Proposed ergogenic value	Summary of research findings
Glucose/electrolyte solution (GES) sport drinks	Ingesting sport drinks during exercise (e.g., 6–8 oz of 6–8% carbohydrate solution every 5–15 min) during prolonged exercise has been proposed to help maintain blood glucose availability to the muscle and extend time to exhaustion in moderately intense exercise bouts (i.e., 70% of VO_2 max) lasting 3–4 h.	Numerous studies indicate that ingesting GES drinks during exercise maintains blood glucose levels, helps promote fluid retention, and decreases dehydration (12). Recommended for exercise bouts lasting more than 60 min, particularly if exercising in hot/humid environments. Ingesting high concentrated drinks (>15%) may slow gastric emptying.
Fructose 1,6-Diphosphate (FDP)	FDP serves as an intermediate step in glycolysis after the energy requiring steps of converting glucose to glucose-6-phosphate. Theorized to increase blood ATP and 2,3-diphosphoglycerate levels, enhance dissociation of oxygen from hemoglobin, and serve as an efficient source of carbohydrate to enhance exercise capacity.	Studies indicate that FDP supplementation (0.25 g/kg) can serve as an effective fuel source during exercise (11). Some studies indicate that exercise capacity may be improved in patient's with peripheral vascular disease. However, recent studies in healthy subjects indicate that FDP supplementation has no advantage of over other forms of carbohydrate.
Dihydroxyacetone phosphate (DHAP)	Supplementation with DHAP has been suggested to enhance glycolytic and oxidative metabolism. Additionally, DHAP and pyruvate supplementation have been suggested to promote fat loss and extend endurance exercise capacity by serving as a fuel during exercise.	Few well-controlled studies have evaluated the ergogenic value of DHAP. Some studies reported that DHAP supplementation (16–75 g/d) improved maximal VO_2 and promoted fat loss in obese individuals on hypocaloric diets (10). However, more research is needed before definitive conclusions can be made.

Polylactate (PL)	PL is a semisoluble amino acid/lactate salt that has been theorized to be easily converted to pyruvate for entrance into the tricarboxylic acid cycle (TCA) and thereby enhance carbohydrate availability during endurance exercise.	Few studies have evaluated the ergogenic value of PL. One study reported that in comparison to a placebo and maltodextrin, PL supplementation during exercise (7% GES solution) promoted higher pH and bicarbonate levels with no differences in performance (13). Conversely, another study reported that addition of PL to a glucose polymer drink did not affect physiological responses to exercise or performance (14).
Pyruvate	Supplementation of pyruvate with DHAP has been suggested to promote fat loss and extend endurance exercise capacity by serving as a fuel during exercise.	Studies indicate that calcium pyruvate (6–25 g/d) with or without DHAP (16–75 g/d) supplementation promoted significantly more fat loss in obese individuals on hypocaloric diets (15,16). However, there is little data to support that the dosages currently marketed to promote fat loss (0.5–2/d) affects body composition or exercise responses.
Ribose	Ribose is a naturally occurring five-carbon sugar (pentose) that is primarily found in the body as constituents of riboflavin (vitamin B_2), nucleic acids, nucleotides, and nucleosides. Supplementation has been theorized to increase ATP availability and recovery.	Some medical studies indicate that ribose supplementation (10–60 g/d) can increase ATP availability in certain patient populations, blunt ischemia threshold in heart patients, and enhance predictive value of thallium exercise tests (17–19). Whether ribose supplementation affects exercise capacity in trained athletes is unknown.

215

Table 3
Proposed Nutritional Ergogenic Aids—Lipids and Lipid By-Products

Nutrient	Proposed ergogenic value	Summary of research findings
Conjugated linoleic acids (CLA)	CLA are essential fatty acids found primarily in fat from whole dairy products. Animal studies indicate that adding CLA to dietary feed decreases body fat, increases bone mass, has anticarcinogenic properties, enhances immunity, and inhibits atherosclerotic progression. Consequently, CLA supplementation in humans has been suggested to help manage body composition, delay loss of bone, and provide health benefits.	Animal studies provide a strong theoretical rationale as to the potential ergogenic and health benefit of CLA supplementation (20). However, few clinical trials have been conducted. Of the studies available, CLA supplementation does not appear to promote fat loss in humans (21). However, there is some evidence that CLA may affect bone mass and immune status (22). Additional research is necessary in humans.
Glycerol	Glycerol has been reported to promote fluid retention by decreasing urine formation. Glycerol added to water may be beneficial to hyperhydrate athletes prior to exercise in an effort to prevent dehydration during exercise.	Studies indicate that glycerol feedings (1 g/kg with water) can promote fluid retention (23,24). This should help athletes susceptible to dehydration perform better during exercise in the heat. However, the ergogenic effect of glycerol hyperhydration is unclear.
L-Carnitine	Carnitine serves as a transporter of fatty acids from the cytosol into the mitochondria and helps modulate the metabolism of coenzymeA (CoA). Studies indicate that fatty acid oxidation is regulated in part by the ability to shuttle fatty acids into the mitochondria for entrance into the TCA cycle. Consequently, L-carnitine supplementation has been theorized as a means of enhancing fat oxidation and sparing muscle glycogen during exercise as well as promoting fat loss.	Numerous studies have evaluated the potential ergogenic value of L-carnitine supplementation in patient and athletic populations. Although some well-controlled studies indicate that L-carnitine supplementation (0.5–2 g/d) may increase fat oxidation and improve cardiovascular efficiency during exercise, most studies indicate that L-carnitine does not affect energy metabolism, exercise capacity, or body composition (25).

216

| Medium-chain triglycerides | Medium-chain triglycerides (MTC) diffused directly into the mitochondria for entrance into beta-oxidation. Theoretically, MCT feedings should serve as an efficient fuel source for exercise possibly serving to enhance endurance capacity. | Most studies indicate that MCT supplementation does not affect low to moderate-intensity endurance exercise (26). However, recent research suggests that MCT supplementation with carbohydrate may spare muscle glyogen utilization and increase time to exhaustion during intense cycling time trial performance (27). |
| Omega-3 fatty acids | Omega 3FA have been reported to serve as antioxidants, enhance immunity, and to decrease risk of cardiovascular disease. Some have suggested that omega 3FA supplementation in athletes would decrease muscle damage and help maintain immune function. | Several studies have evaluated the potential ergogenic value of omega 3FA supplementation. Although there is evidence that omega 3FA supplementation (1–3 g/d) may affect lipid oxidation and immune responses, most studies indicate no ergogenic benefit on aerobic or anaerobic power (28). |

217

Table 4
Proposed Nutritional Ergogenic Aids—Protein and Amino Acids

Nutrient	Proposed ergogenic value	Summary of research findings
Arginine, ornithine, lysine	Clinical studies indicate that supplementation of these amino acids may stimulate growth hormone release serving to preserve muscle mass during bed rest. Additionally, some studies indicate that arginine supplementation improves immune status. Consequently, some have suggested that supplementation of these amino acids during training may increase muscle mass and strength gains.	Recent studies indicate that supplementation with arginine, ornithine, or lysine (10–25 g/d), either separately or in combination, does not enhance the effect of exercise stimulation on either hGH or various measures of muscular strength or power in experienced weightlifters (7,8).
Aspartate, asparagine	These amino acids serve as precursors to oxaloacetate in the TCA cycle. Supplementation has been theorized to spare muscle glycogen use and enhance endurance performance capacity.	Some well-controlled studies support the ergogenic value of aspartate and arginine supplementation on sparing muscle glycogen use and improving exercise capacity. However, other studies have reported limited effects. Additional research is necessary (7,8,29).
Branched-chain amino acids (leucine, isoleucine, valine)	Exercise-induced decreases in BCAA levels has been suggested to contribute to central fatigue as well as muscle catabolism. Supplementation of BCAA with sports drinks may increase BCAA availability and decrease the ratio of free tryptophan/BCAA. Theoretically, this may minimize serotonin production in the brain and delay central fatigue.	A number of studies have reported that BCAA supplementation can affect physiological and psychological responses to exercise. However, it is unclear the degree to which these potentially beneficial effects may affect performance. Initial research is promising but more studies are needed, particularly during training (7,30).
Creatine	The availability of phosphocreatine (PC) stores in the muscle significantly affects the amount of energy generated during brief periods of high intensity exercise. Creatine supplementation has been hypothesized to increase muscle creatine content, help maintain ATP levels during exercise, and accelerate the rate of resynthesis of ATP during and following high intensity, short duration exercises.	The majority of research studies indicate that short-term creatine supplementation (20 g/d for 5 d) significantly increases muscle creatine and PC content, enhances energy availability during exercise, and improves high intensity, repetitive exercise performance (31). Long-term creatine supplementation has been reported to improve strength and muscle mass gains during training (31).

Glutamine	Glutamine has been reported to affect protein synthesis possibly by increasing cell volume and osmotic pressure. Glutamine availability also directly affects lymphocytic function. Collectively, glutamine supplementation may promote muscle growth and prevent immunosuppression during training.	Exercise decreases serum glutamine levels. This reduction has been suggested to contribute to exercise-induced immunosuppression. Glutamine supplementation has been reported to increase serum levels and there is some evidence that glutamine supplementation can improve postexercise immune profiles. However, although there is strong scientific rationale, no long-term studies have evaluated the effects of glutamine supplementation on training adaptations or body composition (7).
Beta-hydroxy-beta-methylbutyrate (HMB)	Leucine and metabolites of leucine such as α-ketoisocaproate (KIC) have been reported to inhibit protein degradation. The anticatabolic effects have been suggested to be regulated by the leucine metabolite β-HMB. Adding β-HMB to dietary feed improved carcass quality in sows and steers. It has been hypothesized that supplementing the diet with leucine and/or β-HMB may inhibit protein degradation during resistance-training.	Leucine infusion has been reported to decrease protein degradation in humans suggesting that leucine may serve as a regulator of protein metabolism (32). Supplementing the diet with 1.5–3 g/d of calcium β-HMB has been reported to enhance training induced changes in FFM and strength in untrained subjects initiating training. The effects of calcium β-HMB supplementation during resistance-training in well trained athletes are less clear (33). Greater benefits appear to occur during heavy training.
Tryptophan	Blood levels of the amino acid tryptophan increase during prolonged exercise as fatty acids are mobilized for fat oxidation. Increases in brain concentrations of tryptophan have been reported to contribute to fatigue as well as increase endogenous opioid production. Tryptophan supplementation has been theorized to help athletes tolerate pain and enhance endurance exercise capacity.	Most studies indicate that increases in tryptophan in the blood and brain contributes to central fatigue (30). Although an initial study suggested that L-tryptophan supplementation improved endurance exercise performance while exercising at 80% of maximal exercise capacity (34), other studies indicated that L-tryptophan had no effect or promoted an ergolytic effect on performance (35).

enhance muscle and tissue growth, the synthesis of hormones and enzymes necessary for energy metabolism, or serve as a potential energy substrate during exercise.

Table 4 (pp. 218 and 219) describes the potential ergogenic value of amino acids that have been purported to affect exercise capacity and/or promote training adaptations. Of the amino acids reviewed, creatine appears to be one of most effective and safe nutritional supplements to enhance anaerobic exercise capacity, strength, and gains in muscle mass during training *(27)*. Studies have indicated that aspartate, branched-chain amino acids (leucine, isoleucine, and valine), glutamine, and β-hydroxy β-methylbutyrate (HMB) may affect exercise capacity, enhance recovery, and/or promote greater training adaptations. However, not all studies report ergogenic value and additional research is needed. Although there may be some clinical applications, there appears to be little ergogenic value of arginine, ornithine, lysine, and tryptophan supplementation for athletes.

4.4. Vitamins

Vitamins are essential organic compounds that serve to regulate metabolic processes, energy synthesis, neurological processes, and prevent destruction of cells. There are two types of vitamins: fat soluble and water soluble. The fat-soluble vitamins include vitamins A, D, E, and K. The body stores fat-soluble vitamins and therefore excessive intake may result in toxicity. B vitamins and vitamin C are water soluble. Excessive intake of these is eliminated in the urine.

Table 5 describes recommended daily allowance (RDA), proposed ergogenic benefit, and summary of research findings for fat and water soluble vitamins. Although research has demonstrated that specific vitamin supplements may pose some health benefit (e.g., vitamin E, niacin, folate, vitamin C, etc.), few have been reported to directly provide ergogenic value for athletes. However, some vitamins may help athletes tolerate training to a better degree by reducing oxidative damage (vitamins E and C) and/or help to maintain a healthy immune system during heavy training (vitamin C). Theoretically, this may help athletes tolerate heavy training leading to improved performance. The remaining vitamins reviewed appear to have little ergogenic value for athletes who consume a normal, nutrient-dense diet. Since analyses of athlete's diets have found deficiencies in caloric and vitamin intake, some sport nutritionists recommend that athletes consume a low-dose one-a-day multivitamin and/or a vitamin-enriched postworkout carbohydrate/protein supplement during periods of heavy training.

4.5. Minerals

Minerals are essential inorganic elements necessary for a host of metabolic processes. Minerals serve as structure for tissue, important components of enzymes and hormones, and regulators of metabolic and neural control. Some minerals have been found to be deficient in athletes or become deficient in

Table 5
Proposed Nutritional Ergogenic Aids – Vitamins

Nutrient	Proposed ergogenic value	Summary of research findings
Vitamin A	Constituent of rhodopsin (visual pigment) and is involved in night vision. Some suggest that vitamin A supplementation may improve sport vision.	No studies have shown that vitamin A supplementation improves exercise performance *(36)*.
Thiamin (B_1)	Part of the coenzyme (thiamin pyrophosphate), which is needed to convert pyruvate to acetyl CoA for entrance into the Krebs cycle. Supplementation is theorized to improve anaerobic threshold and CO_2 transport. Deficiencies may decrease efficiency of energy systems.	Dietary availability of thiamin does not appear to affect exercise capacity when athletes have a normal intake *(38–40)*.
Riboflavin (B_2)	Constituent of flavin nucleotide coenzymes involved in energy metabolism. Theorized to enhance energy availability during oxidative metabolism.	Dietary availability of riboflavin does not appear to affect exercise capacity when athletes have a normal intake *(39,40)*.
Niacin (B_3)	Constituent of coenzymes involved in energy metabolism. Theorized to blunt increases in fatty acids during exercise, reduce cholesterol, enhance thermoregulation, and improve energy availability during oxidative metabolism.	Studies indicate that niacin supplementation can help decrease blood lipid levels in patients with elevated cholesterol. Niacin supplementation during exercise has been reported to decrease exercise capacity by blunting the mobilization of fatty acids *(41)*.
Pyridoxine (B_6)	Pyridoxine has been marketed as a supplement that will improve muscle mass, strength and aerobic power in the lactic acid and oxygen systems. It also may have a calming effect that has been linked to an improved mental strength.	In well-nourished athletes, pyridoxine failed to improve aerobic capacity, or lactic acid accumulation *(39,40)*. However, when combined with vitamins B_1 and B_{12} it may increase serotonin levels and be beneficial in sports like pistol shooting and archery.

(continued)

Table 5 *(continued)*
Proposed Nutritional Ergogenic Aids – Vitamins

Nutrient	Proposed ergogenic value	Summary of research findings
Cyanocobalamin (B_{12})	Cyanocobalamin is a coenzyme involved in the production of DNA and serotonin. DNA is important in protein and red blood cell synthesis. Theoretically it would increase muscle mass, the oxygen-carrying capacity of blood and decrease anxiety.	In well-nourished athletes, no ergogenic effect has been reported. However, when combined with vitamins B_1 and B_6, cyanocobalamin has been shown to improve performance in pistol shooting. This may be due to increased levels of serotonin, a neurotransmitter in the brain, which may reduce anxiety *(42)*.
Folacin	Folic acid functions as a coenzyme in the formation of DNA and red blood cells. An increase in red blood cells could improve oxygen delivery to the muscles during exercise.	In well-nourished and folate deficient athletes, folic acid did not improve exercise performance *(42)*.
Pantothenic acids	Pantothenic acid acts as a coenzyme for acetyl coenzyme A (acetyl CoA). This may benefit aerobic or oxygen energy systems.	Research has reported no improvements in aerobic performance with acetyl CoA supplementation. However, one study reported a decrease in lactic acid accumulation, without an improvement in performance *(36)*.
β-Carotene	Serves as an antioxidant. Theorized to help minimize exercise-induced lipid perioxidation and muscle damage.	Research indicates that β-carotene supplementation with or without other antioxidants can help decrease exercise-induced perioxidation. Over time, this may help athletes tolerate training. However, it is unclear whether antioxidant supplementation affects exercise performance *(43)*.

Table 5 *(continued)*
Proposed Nutritional Ergogenic Aids – Vitamins

Nutrient	Proposed ergogenic value	Summary of research findings
Vitamin C	Vitamin C is used in a number of different metabolic processes in the body. It is involved in the synthesis of epinephrine, iron absorption, and is an antioxidant. Theoretically, it could benefit exercise performance by improving metabolism during exercise. There is also evidence that vitamin C may enhance immunity.	In well-nourished athletes, vitamin C supplementation does not appear to improve physical performance. However, there is some evidence that vitamin C supplementation following intense exercise may decrease the incidence of upper respiratory tract infections *(44)*.
Vitamin E	As an antioxidant, vitamin E could help prevent the formation of free radicals during intense exercise and prevent the destruction of red blood cells, improving or maintaining oxygen delivery to the muscles during exercise. Some evidence suggests that it may reduce risk to heart disease or decrease incidence of recurring heart attack.	Current research has reported no ergogenic effect at sea level. However, at high altitudes, vitamin E may improve exercise performance *(36,37)*. Additional research is necessary to determine whether long-term supplementation may help athletes tolerate training to a better degree.
Vitamin K	Important in blood clotting. There is also some evidence that vitamin K may affect bone metabolism in post-menopausal women.	Vitamin K supplementation (10 mg/d) in elite female athletes has been reported to increase calcium-binding capacity of osteocalcin and promoted a 15–20% increase in bone formation markers and a 20–25% decrease in bone resorption markers suggesting an improved balance between bone formation and resorption *(38)*.

Table 6
Proposed Nutritional Ergogenic Aids – Minerals

Nutrient	Proposed ergogenic value	Summary of research findings
Boron	Boron has been marketed to athletes as a dietary supplement that may promote muscle growth during resistance training. The rationale was primarily based on an initial report that boron supplementation (3 mg/d) significantly increased β-estradiol and testosterone levels in post-menopausal women consuming a diet low in boron.	Studies which have investigated the effects of 7 wk of boron supplementation (2.5 mg/d) during resistance training on testosterone levels, body composition, and strength have reported no ergogenic value. There is no evidence at this time that boron supplementation during resistance training promotes muscle growth.
Calcium	Involved in bone and tooth formation, blood clotting, and nerve transmission. Diet should contain sufficient amounts especially in growing children/adolescents, female athletes, and post-menopausal women. Vitamin D needed to assist absorption.	Calcium supplementation may be beneficial in populations susceptible to osteoperosis. Calcium supplementation provides no ergogenic effect on exercise performance.
Chromium	Chromium, commonly sold as chromium picolinate has been marketed with claims that the supplement will increase lean body mass and decrease body fat levels.	Animal research indicates that chromium supplementation increases lean body mass and reduces body fat. Early research on humans reported similar results. However, more recent, well-controlled studies reported that chromium supplementation does not improve lean body mass or reduce body fat.
Iron	Iron supplements are used to increase aerobic performance in sports that use the oxygen system. Iron is a component of hemoglobin in the red blood cell, which is a carrier of oxygen.	Iron supplements do not appear to improve aerobic performance, unless there is iron-deficiency anemia.

Table 6 *(continued)*
Proposed Nutritional Ergogenic Aids – Minerals

Nutrient	Proposed ergogenic value	Summary of research findings
Phosphate	Phosphate has been studied for its ability to improve all three energy systems, primarily the oxygen system or aerobic capacity.	Recent well-controlled research studies reported that phosphate supplementation (4 g/d for 3 d) improved the oxygen energy system in endurance tasks. More research is needed to determine the mechanism for improvement.
Magnesium	Activates enzymes involved in protein synthesis. Involved in ATP reactions. Serum levels decrease with exercise. Some suggest that magnesium supplementation may improve energy metabolism/ATP availability.	Well-controlled research indicates that magnesium supplementation does not effect endurance exercise performance in athletes.
Selenium	Selenium has been marketed as a supplement to increase aerobic exercise performance. Working closely with vitamin E and glutathione peroxidase (an antioxidant), selenium may destroy destructive free radical production of lipids during aerobic exercise.	Although selenium may reduce lipid peroxidation during aerobic exercise, improvements in aerobic capacity have not been demonstrated.
Vanadium	Vanadium may be involved in reactions in the body that produce insulin-like effects on protein and glucose metabolism. Owing to the anabolic nature of insulin, this has brought attention to vanadium as a supplement to increase muscle mass, enhance strength and power.	Limited research has shown that noninsulin-dependent diabetics may improve their glucose control, however there is no scientific proof that vanadyl sulfate has any effect on muscle mass, strength or power.

response to training and/or prolonged exercise. When mineral status is inadequate, exercise capacity may be reduced. Dietary supplementation of minerals in deficient athletes has generally been found to improve exercise capacity. Additionally, supplementation of specific minerals in nondeficient athletes has also been reported to affect exercise capacity.

Table 6 (pp. 224 and 225) describes minerals that have been purported to affect exercise capacity in athletes. Of the minerals reviewed, several appear to possess health and/or ergogenic value for athletes under certain conditions. For example, calcium supplementation in athletes susceptible to premature osteoporosis may help maintain bone mass. Iron supplementation in athletes prone to iron deficiency and/or anemia has been reported to improve exercise capacity. Sodium phosphate loading has been reported to increase maximal oxygen uptake, anaerobic threshold, and improve endurance exercise capacity by 8–10%. Increasing dietary availability of salt (sodium chloride) during the initial days of exercise training in the heat has been reported to help maintain fluid balance and prevent dehydration. Finally, zinc supplementation during training has been reported to decrease exercise-induced changes in immune function. Consequently, somewhat in contrast to vitamins, there appear to be several minerals that may enhance exercise capacity and/or training adaptations for athletes under certain conditions. However, although ergogenic value has been purported for the remaining minerals, there is little evidence that boron, chromium, magnesium, or vanadium affect exercise capacity or training adaptations in healthy individuals eating a normal diet.

4.6. Water

The most important nutritional ergogenic aid for athletes is water. Exercise performance can be significantly impaired when 2% or more of body weight is lost through sweat. For example, when a 70-kg athlete loses more than 1.4 kg of body weight during exercise (2%), performance capacity is often significantly decreased. Further, weight loss of more than 4% of body weight during exercise may lead to heat illness, heat exhaustion, heat stroke, and possibly death. For this reason, it is critical that athletes consume a sufficient amount of water and/or GES sports drinks during exercise.

The normal sweat rate of athletes ranges from 0.5–2.0 L/h depending on temperature, humidity, exercise intensity, and their sweat response to exercise. Therefore to maintain fluid balance and prevent dehydration, athletes need to consume 0.5–2 L/h of fluid in order to offset weight loss. This requires frequent ingestion of 6–8 oz of cold water or a GES sports drink every 5–15 min during exercise. Athletes should not depend on thirst to prompt them to drink because people do not typically get thirsty until they have lost a significant amount of fluid through sweat. Additionally, athletes should weigh themselves prior to and following exercise training to ensure that they maintain proper hydration.

Table 7
Proposed Nutritional Ergogenic Aids – Others

Nutrient	Proposed ergogenic value	Summary of research findings
Alcohol	Alcohol has been studied for its use as a psychological stress reducer in precision sports such as riflery, archery and dart throwing. It also has been investigated as an energy source.	Some limited research does support an ergogenic effect in precision sports like riflery when about one drink of alcohol is consumed (a blood alcohol of 0.02), 30–60 min prior to competition. However, its use is illegal in these sports and not recommended. Using alcohol in other high anxiety sports such as figure skating, fencing, and gymnastics may result in sanctions and is unethical.
Alkaline salts (bicarbonate)	Sodium bicarbonate has been researched for its effect on improving power in sports that are of a short duration and use the lactic acid energy system.	An average dose of about 300 mg/kg of body weight taken 1–2 h before exercise has delayed fatigue. However, many athletes report gastrointestinal distress, nausea, bloating, and stomach cramps.
Caffeine	Caffeine has been studied for its ability to stimulate power in the energy systems and mental strength. Caffeine stimulates the central nervous system, increasing arousal. It also stimulates the release of epinephrine which may improve cardiovascular function. Lastly, it may increase free fatty acid use during aerobic exercise and facilitate calcium release from the sarcoplasmic reticulum for stronger muscle contractions in anaerobic events.	Many research studies have concluded that caffeine may improve performance in many of the energy systems. However, doses greater that about 5 cups of coffee may exceed legal limits.
Choline	Choline has been studied for its ability to improve oxygen utilization in aerobic events by maintaining or improving acetylcholine levels for enhanced function of the neuro-muscular system.	The research has reported conclusively that choline supplementations increase blood choline levels, however, and improvement in performance remains equivocal and therefore more research is needed. Daily doses average 1.5–2.0 g.
Coenzyme Q10	Coenzyme Q10 is found in the mitochondria and is involved in oxygen transport and ATP production. It is also an antioxidant that may help destroy free radicals during intense aerobic exercise.	Coenzyme Q10 has been found to improve heart function, aerobic capacity and exercise performance in patients with heart disease, but not in healthy athletes.
Ephedrine, ephedra (Ma Huang)	Ephedrine is a sympathomimetic that may enhance muscle contractility, improve blood flow out of the heart, open bronchial airways and increase blood sugar. It could improve both aerobic and anaerobic types of exercise.	Current research does not seem to support any improvement in exercise capacity. Side effects such as nervousness, headaches, stomach upset, irregular heart beats and seizures may result.
Inosine	Ergogenic claims for inosine range from, improving ATP production, increasing aerobic capacity, reducing lactic acid and improving the use of blood sugar during exercise.	Most studies investigating inosine have been well controlled and designed. The results concluded that inosine had no ergogenic value and may even impair performance.

227

Table 8
Proposed Nutritional Ergogenic Aids – Plant Extracts

Nutrient	Proposed ergogenic value	Summary of research findings
Bee pollen	The multiple nutrients in bee pollen have been promoted for their ability as a good energy source for recovery following intense training.	Well-controlled research studies have reported no ergogenic effect on any of the three energy systems, (i.e., ATP-PC, lactic acid, and oxygen systems) (69).
Echinacea	An herb that is purported to enhance immune function and decrease the severity, duration, and incidence of colds and infections. Proposed to help athletes decrease the risk of upper respiratory tract infections during heavy training.	Medical studies generally support the premise that echinacea may reduce the incidence, severity, and duration of colds and infections. No studies have evaluated whether using echinacea during heavy training would decrease colds and infections (70,71).
Gamma oryzanol (ferulic acid)	Phytosterols theorized to enhance anabolic hormonal responses to training.	Research data are limited. One study reported that 9 wk of supplementation (0.5 g/d) did not affect strength, body composition, or anabolic hormones (72,73).
Ginkgo biloba (GB)	A plant extract purported to enhance memory and improve mental concentration and performance. Theorized to help athletes mental alertness and concentration during competition.	Supplementation of GB has been shown to improve symptoms associated with cognitive deficits in patient populations. There is also some evidence that exercise capacity was improved in peripheral vascular diseased patients administered 120 mg/d for 24 wk (74,75). No studies have evaluated whether GB affects performance capacity in healthy athletes.
Ginseng	By activating the hypothalamic-pituitary-adrenal cortex axis, ginseng may improve the three energy systems, namely ATP-PC, lactic acid and oxygen systems. Improved nitrogen balance and increased stamina also have been proposed.	Well-controlled research does not support any ergogenic effect for ginseng (76).

228

Octacosanol	A long-chain alcohol purported to lower blood lipids and serve as a fuel substrate to enhance exercise performance.	Octacosanol has been reported to lower blood lipid profiles. However, no studies support the purported ergogenic value in athletes (77).
Smilax officianalis (SO)	A compound that contains steroidal saponins purported to enhance immunity as well as provide an androgenic effect on muscle growth.	Some data supports the potential immune enhancing effects of SO (78). There are no data to support the claimed androgenic effect (79).
St. Johns Wort (SJW)	Herbal product purported to serve as a naturally occurring alternative to antidepressants. SJW has been marketed to athletes as a supplement to promote a calming/relaxation effect.	No studies have been conducted to evaluate the potential ergogenic value of SJW supplementation in athletes (80).
Wheat germ oil (WGO)	WGO contains linoleic fatty acids, vitamin E, and octacosanol. Consequently, WGO has been theorized to improve endurance, stamina and vigor, specifically enhanced glycogen metabolism and increased oxygen uptake.	A review of approx 35 studies does not support the use of wheat germ oil as an ergogenic aid (81).
Yohimbine (yohimbe)	Yohimbe has been studied for its ability to increase testosterone levels and improve muscle mass and strength. It also may lead to increased levels of norepinephrine a stimulate used for weight loss.	Well-controlled research studies have failed to report increases in muscle mass, testosterone levels or reductions in body fat when ingesting 15–20 mg/d (82).

Every 1 kg of weight lost during exercise is equivalent to 1 L of fluid (about five cups) the athlete should have consumed during exercise. Athletes should train themselves to tolerate drinking greater amounts of water during training and make sure that they consume more fluid in hotter/humid environments. Preventing dehydration during exercise is one of the most effective ways to maintain exercise capacity. Finally, inappropriate and excessive weight loss techniques (e.g., cutting weight in saunas, wearing rubber suits, severe dieting, vomiting, using diuretics, and so on) are extremely dangerous and should be prohibited.

4.6. Other Nutritional Ergogenic Aids

Tables 7 (p. 227) and 8 (pp. 228 and 229) present other nutrition-related compounds that have been purported to possess ergogenic value for athletes. Of the nutrients described, sodium bicarbonate, caffeine, and echinacea appear to have the greatest potential to affect exercise performance and/or training adaptations. Sodium bicarbonate loading (0.3 g/kg of baking soda) prior to exercise has been consistently reported to enhance high-intensity exercise lasting 1–3 min in duration (e.g., a 400–800-m run). Although some athletes may experience gastrointestinal distress, bicarbonate loading appears to be a highly effective ergogenic aid for athletes as long as they can tolerate the supplementation protocol.

Caffeine is a naturally occurring stimulant found in many foods consumed in the normal diet (e.g., coffee, tea, chocolate). Caffeine ingestion (6–9 mg/kg) prior to exercise has been reported to increase fat oxidation, spare muscle glycogen use, and enhance endurance exercise performance. The ergogenic effects of caffeine appear to be more pronounced in nonhabitual caffeine users and habitual users who abstain from consuming caffeine for about a week prior to competition. Although some athletic governing bodies have banned excessive intake of caffeine as an ergogenic aid, studies show that even when taken within the limits allowed by athletic governing bodies, caffeine may provide ergogenic benefit. One word of caution, however, is that caffeine serves as a mild diuretic. Therefore, caffeine intake prior to exercise may hasten dehydration.

Echinacea is an herb that has been reported to enhance immune function and decrease the severity, duration, and incidence of colds and upper respiratory tract infections. Because intense training may compromise immune function in athletes, some have suggested that echinacea supplementation during heavy training may decrease the incidence of colds and infections. Although there are data to support its immunoenhancing effects, we are aware of no studies that have determined whether use of echinacea specifically in athletes would help maintain immune function during intense training. Herbal effects are further discussed in Chapter 15 by Craig. Likewise, little data support the potential ergogenic value of alcohol, choline, coenzyme Q10, ephedrine/ma huang, inosine, bee pollen, gamma oryzanol, ginkgo biloba, ginseng, octacosanol, smilax officinalis, St. John's Wort, wheat germ oil, or yohimbine.

5. SUMMARY

Dietary and nutritional practices of athletes can significantly affect exercise performance capacity. In order to optimize performance, athletes should (1) eat enough calories to offset energy expenditure (typically 60–80 kcal/kg/d); (2) consume the proper amount of carbohydrate (8–10 g/kg/d), protein (1.5 g/kg/d) and fat (0.5–1 g/kg/d); (3) ingest meals and snacks at appropriate time intervals prior to, during, and/or following exercise in order to provide energy as well as to promote recovery following exercise; and (4) only consider using nutritional supplements that have been found to be an effective and safe means for improving performance capacity. For strength and power athletes, research has indicated that creatine and sodium bicarbonate supplementation possess the greatest ergogenic value. For endurance athletes, research suggests that carbohydrate loading, GES sports drinks, sodium phosphate loading, and caffeine are among the most advantageous ergogenic aids. In addition, several other nutrients have been reported to affect exercise metabolism, improve exercise performance, enhance recovery, and/or help maintain health status under specific conditions (e.g., glycerol, branced-chain amino acids, glutamine, homatropine methylbromide, vitamin E, vitamin C, iron, zinc, and echinacea). However, additional research is needed to determine the potential ergogenic value of these nutrients in various athletic populations.

REFERENCES

1. Kreider RB, Fry AC and O'Toole ML (eds.). Overtraining in Sport. Human Kinetics Publishers, Champaign, IL, 1998.
2. Williams MH. Nutrition for Health, Fitness and Sport. WCB/McGraw-Hill, Dubuque, IA, 1999.
3. Berning JR. Energy intake, diet, and muscle wasting. In: Kreider RB, Fry AC, O'Toole ML eds., Overtraining in Sport. Human Kinetics Publishers, Champaign, IL, 1998, pp. 275–288.
4. American College of Sports Medicine. Encyclopedia of Sports Sciences and Medicine. Macmillan, New York, pp. 1128–1129.
5. Food and Nutrition Board. National Research Council: Recommended Dietary Allowances, revised. National Academy of Sciences. Washington, DC, 1989.
6. Sherman WM, Jacobs KA, and Leenders N. Carbohydrate metabolism during endurance exercise. In: Kreider RB, Fry AC and O'Toole, ML eds. Overtraining in Sport. Human Kinetics Publishers, Champaign, IL, 1998, pp. 289–308.
7. Kreider RB. Dietary supplements and the promotion of muscle growth. Sports Med 1999; 27:97–110.
8. Williams MH. Facts and fallacies of purported ergogenic amino acid supplements. Clin Sports Med 1999; 18:633–649.
9. Miller WC, Koceja DM, Hamilton EJ. A meta-analysis of the past 25 years of weight loss research using diet, exercise or diet plus exercise intervention. Int J Obes Relat Metab Disord 1997; 21:941–947.

10. Stanko RT, Robertson RJ, Galbreath RW, Reilly JJ Jr., Greenawalt KD, Goss FF. Enhanced leg exercise endurance with high-carbohydrate diet and dihydroxyacetone and pyruvate. J Appl Physiol 1990; 69:1651–1656.

11. Myers J, Atwood JE, Forbes S, Sullivan M, Sandhu S, Walsch D, Froelicher V. Effect of fructose 1,6-diphosphate infusion on the hormonal response to exercise. Med Sci Sports Exerc 1990; 22:102–105.

12. Convertino VA, Armstrong LE, Coyle EF, Mack GW, Sawka MN, Senay LC Jr, Sherman WM. American College of Sports Medicine position stand. Exercise and fluid replacement. Med Sci Sports Exerc 1996; 28:i–vii.

13. Fahey TD, Larson JD, Brooks GA, Colvin W, Henderson S, Lary D. The effects of ingesting polylactate or glucose polymer drinks during prolonged exercise. Int J Sport Nutr 1991; 1:49–56.

14. Swensen T, Crater G, Bassett DR Jr., Howley ET. Adding polylactate to a glucose polymer solution does not improve endurance. Int J Sports Med 1994; 15:430–434.

15. Kalman D, Colker CM, Wilets I, Roufs JB, Antonio J. The effects of pyruvate supplementation on body composition in overweight individuals. Nutrition 1999; 15:337–340.

16. Stanko RT, Arch JE. Inhibition of regain in body weight and fat with addition of 3-carbon compounds to the diet with hyperenergetic refeeding after weight reduction. Int J Obes Relat Metab Disord 1996; 20:925–930.

17. Gross M, Kormann B, Zollner N. Ribose administration during exercise: effects on substrates and products of energy metabolism in healthy subjects and a patient with myoadenylate deaminase deficiency. Klin Wochenschr 1991; 26; 69:151–155.

18. Hegewald MG, Palac RT, Angello DA, Perlmutter NS, Wilson RA. Ribose infusion accelerates thallium redistribution with early imaging compared with late 24-hour imaging without ribose. J Am Coll Cardiol 1991; 18:1671–1681.

19. Wagner DR, Gresser U, Zollner N. Effects of oral ribose on muscle metabolism during bicycle ergometer exeircse in AMPD-deficient patients. Ann Nutr Metab 1992; 35:297–302.

20. Park Y, Albright KJ, Sorkson JM, Liu W, Cook ME, Pariza MW. Changes in body composition in mice during feeding and withdrawal of conjugated linoleic acids. Lipids 1999; 34:243–248.

21. Ferreira M, Kreider R, Wilson M, Almada A. Effects of conjugated linoleic acid supplementation during resistance training on body composition and strength. J Str Cond Res 1997; 11:280.

22. Kreider, R, Ferreira M, Wilson M, Almada A. Effects of conjugated linoleic acid (CLA) supplementation during resistance-training on bone mineral content, bone mineral density, and markers of immune stress. FASEB J 1998; 12:A244.

23. Monter P, Zou Y, Robergs RA, Murata G, Stark D, Quinn C, Wood S, Lium D, Greene ER. Glycerol hyperhydration alters cardiovascular and renal function. J Exerc Physiol 1999; Online 2(1): available: http://www.css.edu/users/tboone2/asep/jan12c.htm

24. Wagner DR. Hyperhydrating with glycerol: implications for athletic performance. J Am Diet Assoc. 1999; 99:207–212.

25. Heinonen OJ. Carnitine and physical exercise. Sports Med 1996; 22:109–132.

26. Hawley JA, Brouns F, Jeukendrup A. Strategies to enhance fat utilization during exercise. Sports Med 1998; 25:241–257.

27. Van Zyl CG, Lambet EV, Hawley JA, Noakes TD, Dennis SC. Effects of medium-chain triglyceride ingestion on fuel metabolism and cycling performance. J Appl Physiol 1996; 80:2217–2225.

28. Raastad T, Hostmark AT, Stromme SB. Omega-3 fatty acid supplementation does not improve maximal aerobic power, anaerobic threshold and running performance in well-trained soccer players. Scand J Med Sci Sports 1997; 1:25–31.

29. Lancha AH Jr, Recco MB, Abdalla DS, Curi R. Effect of aspartate, asparagine, and carnitine supplementation in the diet on metabolism of skeletal muscle during a moderate exercise. Physiol Behav 1995; 57:36–71.

30. Kreider RB. Central fatigue hypothesis and overtraining, In: Kreider RB, Fry AC and O'Toole, ML eds. Overtraining in Sport. Human Kinetics Publishers, Champaign, IL, 1998; pp. 309–331.

31. Williams MH, Kreider RB, Branch JD. Creatine: The Power Supplement. Human Kinetics Publishers, Champaign, IL, 1999.

32. Nissen S, Sharp R, Ray M, Rathmacher JA, Rice D, Fuller JC Jr, et al. Effect of leucine metbolite b-hydroxy b-methylbutyrate on muscle metabolism during resistance-exercise training. J Appl Physiol 1996; 81:2095–2104.

33. Kreider RB, Ferrera M, Wison M, Almada AL. Effects of calcium β-hydroxy β-methylbutyrate (HMB) supplementation during resistance-training on markers of catabolism, body composition and strength. Int J Sports Med 1999; 22:1–7.

34. Segura R, Ventura JL. Effect of L-tryptophan supplementation on exercise performance. Int J Sports Med 1988; 9:301–305.

35. Stensrud T, Ingjer F, Holm H, Stromme SB. L-tryptophan supplementation does not improve running performance. Int J Sports Med 1992; 13:481–485.

36. Williams MH. Vitamin supplementation and athletic performance. Int J Vitam Nutr Res Suppl 1989; 30:163–191.

37. Tiidus PM, Houston ME. Vitamin E status and response to exercise training. Sports Med 1995; 20:12–23.

38. Craciun AM, Wolf J, Knapen MH, Brouns F, Vermeer C. Improved bone metabolism in female elite athletes after vitamin K supplementation. Int J Sports Med 1998; 19:479–484.

39. van der Beek E, et al. Thiamin, riboflavin, and vitamins B-6 and C: impact of combined restricted intake on functional performance in man. Am J Clin Nutr 1988; 48:1451–62.

40. Fogelholm M, Ruokonen I, Laakso JT, Vuorimaa T, Himberg JJ. Lack of association between indices of vitamin B1, B2, and B6 status and exercise-induced blood lactate in young adults. Int J Sport Nutr 1993; 3:165–176.

41. Murray R, Bartoli WP, Eddy DE, Horn MK. Physiological and performance responses to nicotinic-acid ingestion during exercise. Med Sci Sports Exerc 1995: 27:1057–62.

42. Herbert V, Dos KC. Folic acid and vitamin B_{12}. In: Shils M, Olson J, Shike M, eds. Modern Nutrition in Health and Disease. Lea & Febiger, Philadelphia, 1994, pp. 1430–1435.

43. Goldfarb AH. Nutritional antioxidants as therapeutic and preventive modalities in exercise-induced muscle damage. Can J Appl Physiol 1999; 24:249–266.

44. Gerster H. The role of vitamin C in athletic performance. J. Am. Coll. Nutr. 1989; 8:636–643.

45. Hemila H. Vitamin C and common cold incidence: a review of studies with subjects under heavy physical stress. Int J Sports Med 1996; 17:379–383.

46. Ferrando AA, Green NR. The effect of boron supplementation on lean body mass, plasma testosterone levels, and strength in male bodybuilders. Int J Sports Nutr 1993; 5:S29–S38.

47. Green NR, Ferrando AA. Plasma boron and the effects of boron supplementation in males. Environ. Health Perspect. 1994; 102, S7:73–77.

48. Singh MA. Combined exercise and dietary intervention to optimize body composition in aging. Ann NY Acad Sci 1998; 20:378–393.

49. Lefavi RG, Anderson RA, Keith RE, Wilson GD, McMillan JL, and Stone MH. Efficacy of chromium supplementation in athletes: emphasis on anabolism. Int J Sport Nutr 1992; 2:111–112.

50. Anderson RA. Effects of chromium on body composition and weight loss. Nutr Rev 1998; 56:266–270.

51. Weaver CM, Rajaram S. Exercise and iron status. J Nutr 1992; 122:782–787.

52. Weller E, Bachert P, Meinck HH, Friedmann B, Bartsch P, Mairbaurl H. Lack of effect of oral Mg-supplementation on Mg in serum, blood cells, and calf muscle. Med Sci Sports Exer 1998; 30:1584–1591.

53. Kreider RB. Phosphorus in exercise and sport, In: Driskell, J.A. and Wolinsky, I., eds., Macroelements, Water, and Electrolytes CRC Press, Boca Raton, FL, 1995, pp. 29–46.

54. Yu-Yahiro JA. Electrolytes and their relationship to normal and abnormal muscle function. Orthop Nurs 1994; 13(5):38–40.
55. Tessier F, Margaritis I, Richard M, Moynot C, Marconnet P. Selenium and training effects on the glutathione system and aerobic performance. Med Sci Sports Exer 1995; 27:390–396.
56. Latzka WA, Montain, SJ. Water and electrolyte requirements for exercise. Clin. Sports Med 1999; 18:513–524.
57. Fawcett J, Farquhar S, Walker R, Thou T, Lowe G, Goulding A. The effect of oral vanadyl sulfate on body composition and performance in weight-training athletes. Int. J. Sport Nutr. 1996; 6:382–90.
58. Singh A, Failla ML, Deuster PA. Exercise-induced changes in immune function: effects of zinc supplementation. J Appl Physiol 1994; 76:2298–2303.
59. American College of Sports Medicine. Position statement on the use of alcohol in sports. Med Sci Sports Exer 1982; 14(6), ix–x.
60. Williams MH. Physical activity, fitness, and substance misuse and abuse, In: Bouchard C, Shepard R, Stephens T, eds. Physical Activity, Fitness and Health. Human Kinetics Publishers, Champaign, IL, 1994.
61. Horswill CA. Effects of bicarbonate, citrate, and phosphate loading on performance. Int J Sport Nutr 1995; 5:S111–S118.
62. Linderman JK, Gosselink KL. The effects of sodium bicarbonate ingestion on exercise performance. Sports Med, 1994; 18:75–80.
63. Graham TE, Spriet LL. Caffeine and exercise performance. Sports Sci Exch 1996; 9:1–5.
64. Kanter MM, Williams MH. Antioxidants, carnitine and choline as putative ergogenic aids. Int. J Sport Nutr, 1995; 5:S120–S131.
65. Laaksonen R, Fogelholm M, Himberg J, Laakso J, Salorinne Y. Ubiquinone supplementation and exercise capacity in trained young and older men. Eur J Appl Physiol, 1995; 72:95–100.
66. Malm C, Svensson M, Sjoberg B, Ekblom B, Sjodin B. Supplementation with Ubiquinone-10 causes cellular damage during intense exercise. Acta Physiol Scand, 1996; 157:511–512.
67. Fitch K. The use of anti-asthmatic drugs: Do they affect sports performance? Sports Med, 1986; 3:136–150.
68. Williams MH, Kreider RB, Hunter DW, Somma CT, Shall LM, Woodhouse ML, Rokitski L. Effect of inosine supplementation on 3-mile treadmill run performance and VO$_2$ peak. Med. Sci Sports Exer, 1990; 22:517–522.
69. Woodhouse ML, Williams MH, Jackson CW. The effects of varying doses of orally ingested bee pollen extract upon selected performance variables. Ath Training, 1987; 22:26–28.
70. Barrett B, Kiefer D, Rabago D. Assessing the risks and benefits of herbal medicine: an overview of scientific evidence. Altern Ther Health Med, 1999; 5(4):40–49.
71. Brinkeborn RM, Shah DV, Degenring FH. Echinaforce and other echinacea fresh plant preparations in the treatment of the common cold. A randomized, placebo controlled, double-blind clinical trial. Phytomedicine, 1999; 6(1):1–6.
72. Wheeler KB, Garleb KA. Gamma oryzanol-plant sterol supplementation: metabolic, endocrine, and physiologic effects. Int J Sport Nutr, 1991; 1:17017–7.
73. Fry AC, Bonner E, Lewis DL, Johnson RL, Stone MH, Kraemer WJ. (1997) The effects of gamma-oryzanol supplementation during resistance exercise training. Int J Sport Nutr 7, 318–329.
74. Soholm B. (1998) Clinical improvement of memory and other cognitive functions by Ginkgo biloba: review of relevant literature. Adv Ther 15, 54–65.
75. Blume J, Kieser M, Holscher U. (1996) Placebo-controlled double-blind study of the effectiveness of Ginkgo biloba special extract Egb 761 in trained patients with intermittent claudication. Vasa 25(3), 265–274.
76. Bahrke MS, Morgan WP. Evaluation of the ergogenic properties of ginseng. Sports Med 1994; 18:229–248.

77. Stusser R, Batista J, Padron R, Sosa F, Pereztol O. Long-term therapy with policosanol improves treadmill exercise-ECG testing performance of coronary heart disease patients. Int J Clin Pharmacol Ther 1998; 36:469–473.

78. Bernardo RR, Pinto AV, Parente JP. Steroidal saponins from Smilax officinalis. Phytochemistry. 1996; 43:465–459.

79. Grunewald KK, Bailey, RS. Commercially marketed supplements for bodybuilding athletes. Sports Med 1993; 15:90–103.

80. Deltito J, Beyer D. The scientific, quasi-scientific and popular literature on the use of St. John's Wort in the treatment of depression. J Affect Disord 1998; 51:345–351.

81. Cureton T. The Physiological Effects of Wheat Germ Oil on Humans in Exercise. CC Thomas, Springfield, IL, 1972.

82. Riley AJ. Yohimbine in the treatment of erectile disorder. Bri J Clin Pract 1994; 48:133–136.

15 Health Promoting Herbs as Useful Adjuncts to Prevent Chronic Diseases

Winston J. Craig

1. INTRODUCTION

Plants have played a significant role in maintaining the health and improving the quality of human life for thousands of years. The majority of the earth's inhabitants rely on traditional medicine for their primary health-care needs, and a major part of this therapy involves the use of plants, plant extracts, or their active principles. For centuries, American Indians have utilized a number of native herbs for medicinal purposes. During the past decade, many more Americans have turned to herbal remedies for the treatment of a variety of medical conditions including coughs and colds, insomnia, digestive problems, headache, premenstrual syndrome, prostate problems, anxiety, and depression. The increasing use of herbs in the United States has been fueled by the high cost of drugs, the fear of side effects experienced with conventional drugs, and the desire to take more personal responsibility for one's health in a way that is perceived as more natural.

Some of the more popular herbs in use today include echinacea, ginkgo, garlic, ginseng, goldenseal, saw palmetto, St. John's Wort, chamomile, cranberry, aloe vera, kava, valerian, milk thistle, and feverfew. Recently, research has validated the usefulness of echinacea for stimulating the immune function; saw palmetto berries and stinging nettle for the treatment of benign prostate hypertrophy; hops, passionflower, and valerian for the treatment of insomnia; St. John's Wort for anxiety and depression; chamomile for its anti-inflammatory effects; cranberry for urinary tract infections; aloe vera for healing burns and wounds; kava for anxiety disorders; milk thistle to protect and restore liver function; and feverfew for the relief of migraine headaches *(1)*.

From: *Nutritional Health: Strategies for Disease Prevention*
Edited by: T. Wilson and N. J. Temple © Humana Press Inc., Totowa, NJ

2. UNIQUE HERBAL FLAVORS AND USES

Herbs and spices can be defined as fragrant, aromatic, or pungent edible plant substances (bark, buds, bulbs, flowers, leaves, fruit, seeds, rhizomes, and roots) that contribute flavor to food and beverages. Herbal teas have become very popular as an alternative to caffeinated beverages. Dried herbs usually smell and taste somewhat differently from their fresh counterparts. The drying process usually causes a loss or change in the volatile oil of the plant material. Hence, the nonvolatile components become concentrated, resulting in the domination of bitter elements. Furthermore, the flavor of most dried herbs diminish with time.

Culinary herbs and spices have been used since antiquity to flavor and preserve food. The ability of herbs and spices to delay food spoilage is due in large part to their rich content of antioxidants. The unique flavors associated with different herbs are provided by the aromatic ingredients of their essential oils and oleoresins (mixtures of terpenes such as thymol, menthol, carvone, cineole, etc.), whereas their pungency is due to their alkaloids (such as piperine in black pepper and capsaicin in red pepper). In addition, some herbs such as saffron, paprika, and turmeric are used to add color to food.

With the current emphasis on eating more healthful diets that are low in fat and salt, people are turning to various herbs and spices to flavor their food. This trend is in line with the recommendations of various government health agencies and professional health organizations. The culinary herbal seasonings that can be safely used to enhance the flavor of vegetables, soups, stews, and pasta dishes include basil, caraway, cilantro, coriander, cumin, dill, fennel, ginger, marjoram, oregano, parsley, pepper, rosemary, sage, and thyme. Sometimes these herbs are blended together, as in Italian seasoning, to produce a richer, more pleasing aroma and flavor to the food.

During the past two centuries, immigrants to the United States brought with them their own culture and ethnic dishes resulting in the highlighting of new flavors. The present popularity of Italian, Mexican, Indian, and other ethnic dishes has resulted in an increased use of herbal seasonings. For example, oregano is essential in the preparation of Italian and Spanish food and is commonly used to flavor pizza. Chili pepper is commonly used in many Italian, Mexican, and Indian dishes. Italians use sweet basil for flavoring beans and many of their tomato dishes. Thyme has a prominent place in French cuisine, and rosemary is a common ingredient in Italian and French dishes. For centuries, garlic has been used in Mediterranean, Indian, and Oriental dishes. Many Americans are now using garlic in a variety of dips, vegetable dishes, soups, and some baked goods. Similarly, onions or dehydrated onion can be used to enhance the flavor of most vegetables, salads, soups, gravies, and many entrees.

A number of the culinary herbs contain physiologically active compounds that make them useful in treating certain disorders, or generally to promote health.

In this fashion, the herb can provide a typical druglike action. For example, fennel and various mints have been successfully used to treat coughs and colds; ginger is effective as an antiemetic for preventing nausea and vomiting associated with motion sickness as well as for morning sickness; licorice root can help heal stomach and duodenal ulcers; and peppermint is used in the treatment of irritable bowel syndrome *(1,2)*. These physiological effects of herbs are parallel to those observed with some conventional medicines, but without the undesirable side effects.

Many commonly consumed plant foods, such as broccoli, carrots, citrus, grapes, soy, and tomatoes, contain physiologically active phytochemicals or phytonutrients that promote health and protect against chronic diseases *(3,4)*. This has given rise to the term "functional foods" to designate those foods that provide health benefits beyond basic nutrition *(5)*. However, the distinction between a basic nutrient and a phytochemical is increasingly blurred. This situation is highlighted when substances such as soluble fiber and linolenic acid provide a variety of health-promoting properties (*see* Table 1), in addition to their traditional roles in normal digestion and metabolism. This has led some people to look on food not only as a source of nutrients but also as medicine.

3. HERBS FOR CARDIOVASCULAR PROBLEMS

A plant-based diet, rich in whole grains, fruits, vegetables, and legumes, modest in nuts, and low in saturated fat, along with a regular aerobic exercise program, is recommended for anyone with an elevated risk of cardiovascular disease. In addition, there are herbs that appear to provide help for persons with hyperlipidemia, an abnormal tendency to form blood clots, impaired blood flow, or other cardiovascular problems.

Garlic (*Allium sativum* L.) has been used therapeutically for many centuries. The compound producing much of the activity of garlic is allicin, which is released when intact cells of a clove are cut or crushed. Allicin inhibits the growth of a wide variety of bacteria, molds, yeasts (including *Candida*), and viruses. The regular use of garlic can also be useful in lowering the risk of heart attacks and strokes, as it lowers both total and low-density lipoprotein (LDL) cholesterol levels and triglyceride levels, without affecting high-density lipoprotein (HDL) cholesterol levels *(6,7)*. On average, consuming one-half to one clove of garlic per day for 3–6 mo reduces hypercholesterolemia by about 10% of its initial value *(7)*. Garlic also increases fibrinolytic activity and inhibits platelet aggregation due in part to the presence of ajoenes, allyl methyl trisulfide, vinyldithins, and other sulfur compounds produced from the breakdown of allicin *(6,8,9)*. Different forms of garlic exhibit various levels of activity. The odor-modified garlic extract (Kyolic) has been found to be just as effective as fresh garlic for lowering blood cholesterol levels *(10)*. The use of enteric-coated garlic pills, which dis-

Table 1
Commonly Used Health-Promoting Herbs,
Their Functions and Phytochemical Content

Physiological function	Herb with desired function	Active phytochemicals
Lowers total and LDL cholesterol	Garlic	Disulfides
	Psyllium	Soluble fiber
	Flaxseed	Soluble fiber, phytosterols
	Fenugreek	Soluble fiber, saponins
	Gugulipid	Guggulsterones
	Lemon grass oil	Terpenoids
Inhibits LDL oxidation	Green tea	Catechins
	Black tea	Theaflavins
	Licorice root	Glabridin
	Grape seed	Proanthocyanidins
	Pine bark	Pycnogenols
Inhibits blood clots	Garlic	Ajoenes, vinyldithiins, diallyl trisulfide
	Onions	Alpha-sulfinyl disulfides
	Flaxseed	Linolenic acid
	Ginger	Diterpene dialdehydes
	Asian ginseng	
	Hawthorn	Proanthocyanidins
	Evening primrose oil	Linolenic acid
Improves circulation or vascular function/ arterial compliance	Ginkgo biloba	Flavonoids, terpenoids
	Hawthorn	Flavonoids
	Horse chestnut	Escin
	Red clover	Isoflavones
Improves glycemic control or insulin utilization	Bitter melon	Steroids, polypeptide
	Fenugreek	Soluble fiber
	Gurmar	
	Flaxseed	Soluble fiber
	Psyllium	Soluble fiber
	Asian ginseng	
	Cinnamon	
Enhances immune function	Echinacea	Isobutylamides, flavonoids
	Garlic	
	Cat's claw	Flavonoids, terpenoids
	Licorice root	Glycyrrhizin, chalcones
	Astragalus	Saponins
	Black currant seed	

Table 1 *(continued)*

Physiological function	Herb with desired function	Active phytochemicals
Cancer chemopreventive activity	Garlic	Sulfides, disulfides, and trisulfides
	Onions, chives, leeks	Disulfides and trisulfides,
	Labiatae herbs (mint family)	Terpenoids, flavonoids, ursolic acid
	Umbelliferous herbs (carrot family)	Coumarins, phthalides, terpenoids, polyacetylenes
	Licorice root	Glycyrrhizin, chalcones
	Green tea	Catechins
	Flax	Lignans
	Ginger	Curcuminoids, gingerols, diarylheptanoids
	Turmeric	Curcuminoids
	Asian ginseng	Ginsenosides

solve in the intestinal tract, are another way to cut down on odor problems while still enjoying the benefits of garlic. However, a steam-distilled garlic oil preparation was recently found to be inactive when fed for 3 mo to hypercholesterolemic patients *(11)*. The results of a meta-analysis suggest that garlic may also be useful for patients with mild hypertension *(12)*.

Onions (*Allium cepa* L.) contain many compounds that are identical or similar to those found in garlic. However, garlic is considered more potent because it contains about three times the level of sulfur compounds found in onions. Onions are considered anticlotting agents because they possess substances with fibrinolytic activity and can suppress platelet aggregation *(6,8,13)*. A whole family of sulfinyl disulfides isolated from onions have been shown to strongly inhibit platelet aggregation *(13)*. However, onion consumption has not been linked to modifications of the plasma lipid profile.

Diets rich in soluble fiber are also known to influence the lipid profile. Psyllium (*Plantago psyllium*), the major component of Metamucil, is a rich source of soluble fiber in the diet and hypercholesterolemic patients have experienced decreases in total and LDL cholesterol levels of about 10–15 mg/dL (0.26–0.4 mmol/L), respectively *(14)*. In a meta-analysis of 12 studies hypercholesterolemic adults experienced decreases in total cholesterol and LDL cholesterol levels of 0.31 and 0.35 mmol/L (5% and 9%), respectively, without changes in HDL cholesterol levels after consumption of a psyllium-enriched cereal for an average of 42 d *(15)*. The regular use of ground flaxseed (*Linum usitatissimum*) can also lower both total cholesterol and LDL cholesterol levels about 10% as well as producing a substantial decrease in platelet aggregation, without altering HDL cholesterol and triglyceride levels *(16,17)*. Flax has a very low saturated fat content, and a high content of polyunsaturated fat and phytosterols, in addition to its soluble fiber content.

Other herbal products have also been shown to exert effects on cardiovascular risk factors. Blood cholesterol levels may be reduced by fenugreek (*Trigonella foenum-graecum*) *(18)*, gugulipid *(19)*, the oils of lemon grass (*Cymbopogon citratus*) *(20)*, and evening primrose (*Oenothera biennis*) *(21)*, and by the terpenoids found in *Labiatae* (mint family) and *Umbellifereae* (parsley family) herbs *(22)*. Asian ginseng (*Panax ginseng*) is reported to inhibit platelet aggregation and increase blood clotting times *(23)*. Many herbs also contain a variety of antioxidant phenolic compounds such as caffeic acid, ferulic acid, and ellagic acid which can inhibit atherosclerosis *(24)*.

Flavonoids are plant pigments responsible for the colors of flowers, fruits, and some leaves *(25)*. Flavonoids have extensive biological properties that promote human health and help reduce the risk of disease. Suggested activities include the extension of the activity of vitamin C, acting as antioxidants, protection of LDL cholesterol from oxidation, inhibition of platelet aggregation, as well as anti-inflammatory and antitumor activity *(26,27)*. In the Zutphen study, it was shown that flavonoid intake from fruit, vegetables, and herbs was inversely associated with heart disease mortality, and incidence of heart attack and stroke over a 5-yr and 15-yr period, respectively. Those in the highest tertile of flavonoid intake had a 68% lower risk of mortality from heart disease (after adjustment for potential confounders) compared with those in the lowest tertile of flavonoid intake *(28)*. Similarly, those in the highest quartile of flavonoid intake had a 73% lower risk of stroke compared with those in the lowest quartile of flavonoid consumption *(29)*. In a prospective study of postmenopausal women in Iowa, total flavonoid intake was associated with a 38% decreased risk of coronary heart disease (CHD) mortality (for the highest pentile of flavonoid intake vs the lowest) but no association was observed between flavonoid intake and stroke mortality *(30)*. Among the commonly consumed herbs, there are a number that contain substantial levels of flavonoids. These include chamomile, dandelion, ginkgo, green and black tea, hawthorn, licorice, passionflower, milk thistle, onions, rosemary, sage, and thyme *(25)*.

Anthocyanins are the water-soluble pigments responsible for the red, pink, mauve, purple, blue, and violet color of most flowers and fruits. They are useful for the treatment of vascular disorders and symptoms associated with capillary and venous fragility *(25)*. Grape seeds (*Vitis vinifera* L.) are a good source of proanthocyanidins, polyphenolics that provide protection against LDL oxidation and show good promise for the treatment of vascular disorders such as inadequate circulation *(25,31)*. Similar compounds are found in the bark of the French maritime pine, *Pinus maritima*, and are marketed as pycnogenol. An extract of horse chestnut seeds contains escin, a triterpene glycoside, that is also useful for chronic venous insufficiency *(32)*.

Ginkgo biloba and hawthorn appear to exert their cardiovascular effects by acting as vasodilators. *Ginkgo biloba* leaf extract appears to be somewhat effective, especially in geriatric patients, against conditions such as memory loss, dizziness, depression, confusion, and other ailments. These conditions often respond to the vasodilation and improved cerebral blood flow induced by the Ginkgo extract which contains flavone glycosides and diterpenoids (ginkgolides) *(1,33,34)*. The leaves, fruits, and flowers of hawthorn (*Crataegus* spp.) can improve blood flow and have been suggested to improve the pumping capacity of the heart. Hawthorn probably causes dilation of the smooth muscles of the coronary vessels, thereby increasing blood flow and reducing the tendency for angina, *(1)*, Proanthocyanidins, the active principles in the flower heads of hawthorn (*Crataegus oxyacantha*), can inhibit platelet aggregation *(35)*.

LDL oxidation is believed to play a key role in atherosclerosis (*see* Chapter 8 by Woodside and Young). Plants contain a variety of antioxidants that can offer defense against LDL oxidation. LDL cholesterol isolated from 10 normolipidemic subjects, who consumed licorice root extract for 2 wk, was more resistant to oxidation than LDL isolated before the licorice was consumed. When a licorice extract (free of glycyrrhizinic acid) or glabridin, a flavonoid found in licorice, was fed to apo-E–deficient mice, they also experienced a reduced susceptibility of their LDL cholesterol to oxidation and a reduction in the extent of atherosclerotic lesions compared with the control mice *(36)*. The use of licorice had no effect on either the total or LDL cholesterol levels, and blood coagulation was unaffected. Because glabridin was found to be less active than the whole licorice extract, it is thought that licorice contains a number of other antioxidants, including licochalcones and other polyphenols.

LDL oxidation is also inhibited by tea flavonoids—the catechins from green tea or the theaflavins (catechin dimers) from black tea *(37)*. Of the catechins, epigallocatechin gallate appears to provide the most protection, whereas the theaflavins exert stronger inhibitory effects than the catechins. Several epidemiological studies have suggested that drinking either green or black tea may lower blood cholesterol and blood pressure levels and provide a degree of protection against cardiovascular disease. The protective effect of tea may result from the ability of the catechins and similar compounds to reduce intestinal cholesterol absorption, as well as to lower blood coagulability and inhibit proliferation of human aortic smooth muscle cells *(38)*.

4. BLOOD SUGAR MODIFICATION

Diabetes is a disease characterized by elevated blood sugar levels. A more general discussion is provided in Chapter 12 by Franz. The unregulated blood sugar may result from either a lack of insulin or a reduction in its effectiveness. Careful dietary habits and regular exercise are essential components in the management of type II diabetes (non-insulin-dependent diabetes mellitus). In addition, there are a few herbs that may be therapeutically useful. These herbs may lower blood glucose levels or improve the body's ability to release and use insulin.

Bitter melon or balsam pear (*Momordica charantia*) is a green, cucumber-shaped tropical fruit with a bitter taste and gourdlike bumps that is eaten unripe like a vegetable. It is used traditionally throughout India, Sri Lanka, Africa, and the West Indies as a diabetic remedy and is available in the United States in Asian food stores. Clinical trials have established that the use of the bitter melon extract can effectively lower blood sugar levels and improve glucose tolerance in persons with type II diabetes (39). Bitter melon contains a mixture of steroidal glycosides that have a potent hypoglycemic effect and a polypeptide that mimics insulin activity (40).

The consumption of fenugreek seeds (*Trigonella foenum-graecum*) can also lower blood sugar levels in diabetics. Research in India found that glucose tolerance improved, urinary glucose excretion decreased 70%, and insulin responses were reduced in diabetics after defatted fenugreek was used for 10 d (18). Total serum cholesterol, LDL cholesterol, and triglyceride levels, but not HDL cholesterol, all significantly decreased by about 20% when fenugreek was added to the diet. These changes in blood lipids are advantageous for a diabetic who has hyperlipidemia. Fenugreek, which belongs to the legume family, contains a high level of viscous gum (soluble fiber). A daily use of 25–100 mg of fenugreek seeds could serve as an effective supportive therapy in the management of diabetes.

Gurmar (*Gymnema sylvestre*), a native plant of the forests of India, has been effectively used in the management of diabetes mellitus (types I and II). The leaves of this climbing vine contain certain components that block the sensation of sweetness when applied to the tongue. An extract of the leaves of *Gymnema* reduces insulin requirements (or oral hypoglycemic drug dosage), improves fasting blood glucose levels, and improves blood glucose control by enhancing the action of insulin and possibly by rejuvenating the dysfunctional beta cells of the pancreas (41,42). It may also produce lower levels of blood cholesterol and triglycerides. These effects are seen in diabetics only, and not in healthy volunteers.

Flaxseed, ginseng, psyllium, cinnamon, and other herbs may also provide benefits to diabetics. Because flaxseed (*Linum usitatissimum*) is very rich in soluble fiber it is also a candidate for the management of abnormal glucose levels. Subjects consuming bread containing 25% flax seed meal showed an almost 30% improvement in a glucose tolerance test compared with those who ate plain bread (17). For centuries, ginseng has been used to treat diabetes by practitioners of traditional Chinese medicine. In a double-blind, placebo-controlled study, patients with type II diabetes who took 200 mg of ginseng daily for 8 wk experienced improved fasting blood glucose levels and improved glycated hemoglobin levels *(43)*. Men with type II diabetes who took 5 g of psyllium (*Plantago psyllium*) twice a day for 8 wk experienced an 11% drop in daily blood glucose levels in addition to a 13 % drop in LDL cholesterol levels *(44)*. An extract from cinnamon has been found to potentiate insulin activity *(45)*. It has been suggested that compounds in cinnamon may find use in adult-onset diabetes. Preliminary studies have reported antihyperglycemic activity or improved glucose tolerance from a number of other herbs including garlic, onions, bay leaves, cloves, coriander, cumin, cloves, juniper berries, prickly pear cactus, turmeric, and ivy gourd leaves *(46,47)*. Further research is needed to validate these findings and discover if there is any clinical significance to the hypoglycemic effects of these herbs.

5. HELP FOR THE IMMUNE SYSTEM

Echinacea, licorice, cat's claw, and garlic are some of the herbal products that may help enhance the immune system *(1,25)*. In the early 1900s, *Echinacea* (purple coneflower) was the major plant-based antimicrobial medicine in use. With the development of sulfa drugs, the use of *Echinacea* rapidly declined. *Echinacea* is known to promote the activity of lymphocytes, increase phagocytosis, and induce interferon production *(1)*. *Echinacea* appears to be useful in moderating the symptoms of the common cold, flu, and sore throat. However, not all studies have shown that *Echinacea* extracts significantly decrease the incidence, duration, or severity of colds and respiratory infections *(48)*. The immuno-enhancing activity of *Echinacea* is believed to be provided by certain polysaccharides and isobutylamides *(25)*.

Glycyrrhizin, a sweet tasting triterpenoid saponin in licorice root (*Glycyrrhiza glabra* L.), and its aglycone (glycyrrhetinic acid) have been reported to augment interferon activity and natural killer cell activity *(49)*. The chalcones in licorice also possess antiviral activity against the human immunodeficiency virus (HIV), and glycyrrhizin possesses noticeable anti-inflammatory and antiallergic properties *(50)*.

For over 2000 yr, the Peruvian Indians have used for medicinal purposes two species of cat's claw, *Uncaria guianesis* and *U. tomentosa*. Today, preparations of the bark from the root and stalk of these plants are attracting much attention in the West because of their immunostimulant properties and their potential to help fight AIDS and leukemia *(51,52)*. Extracts of cat's claw are reported to stimulate T-cells, macrophages, and other components of the immune system. Extracts are also reported to have antimutagenic and anti-inflammatory properties *(51,52)*. Recently, blackcurrant seed oil, an oil rich in linolenic acid, has a moderate immune-enhancing effect because of its effect on prostaglandin metabolism *(53)*.

Garlic preparations have also been reported to stimulate the immune system of patients with AIDS *(54)*. Garlic can increase the number of helper cells and killer cell activity as well as improving AIDS-related conditions such as diarrhea and fungal and viral infections *(55)*. Validation of the immunostimulant activities of garlic may be of particular importance for the treatment of AIDS in developing countries, where a lack of hard currency may limit access to Western drugs and medicine.

6. HERBS WITH CANCER CHEMOPREVENTIVE ACTIVITY

A number of commonly used herbs have been identified as possessing cancer-protective properties. These include members of the *Allium* sp. (garlic, onions, chives, leeks), members of the mint family (basil, mints, oregano, rosemary, sage, sweet savory, thyme), turmeric, ginger, licorice root, green tea, flax, and members of the *Umbelliferae* (carrot) family, such as anise, caraway, celery, chervil, cilantro, coriander, cumin, dill, fennel, and parsley *(56)*.

Unique cancer chemoprotective phytochemicals have been identified in all of these herbs. In addition, many herbs contain a variety of phytosterols, terpenoids, flavonoids, saponins, and carotenoids, which also have cancer chemoprotective activity *(57)*. These beneficial substances act as antioxidants, immune system stimulants, inhibit the formation of DNA adducts from carcinogens, inhibit hormonal actions and metabolic pathways associated with the development of cancer, or induce protective phase I or II detoxification enzymes such as glutathione-*S*-transferase *(57–62)*.

Examples of phytochemicals that stimulate glutathione-*S*-transferase activity include the phthalides in the umbelliferous herbs, the sulfides in garlic and onions, curcumin in turmeric and ginger, and terpenoids such as limonene, geraniol, cineole, alpha-pinene, and carvone found in commonly used culinary herbs *(57,58,61)*. Rosemary and sage contain the antioxidant diterpenoids (rosmanol, carnosol, rosmarinic acid, carnosic acid, epirosmanol, and isorosmanol) and ursolic acid, a triterpenoid with antitumor activity *(59)*.

Garlic (*Allium sativum*) has been shown to reduce the development of bladder, skin, stomach, and colon cancer *(10,63)*. In a review of case-control and cohort studies of all types of cancer, 27 out of 34 studies revealed an inverse association between cancer and the consumption of allium vegetables *(64)*. A prospective study in Iowa revealed that risk of colon cancer was 32% less in those in the highest quartile of garlic consumption compared with those in the lowest quartile *(65)*. Garlic can inhibit the formation of nitrosamines, which are potent carcinogens, and also inhibit the formation of DNA adducts *(66)*. The rich content of sulfides, disulfides and trisulfides in garlic also helps to explain its cancer chemopreventive properties. In China, those in the highest quartile of intake of garlic, onions, and other allium herbs have a risk of stomach cancer that is 40% less than those in the lowest quartile *(67)*. Case-control studies in Greece have also shown a high consumption of garlic, onion, and other allium herbs to be protective against stomach cancer *(57)*. Finally, a Dutch study revealed that cancer in the noncardia section of the stomach for those consuming the highest level of onions (at least half an onion a day) was about 50% lower than that in persons consuming no onions *(68)*.

Flaxseed, turmeric, and ginger have all been suggested to prevent cancer proliferation. Flaxseed *(Linum usitatissimum)* contains a rich supply of lignans. Metabolites of these lignans act as phytoestrogens by binding to estrogen receptors and inhibiting the growth of estrogen-stimulated breast cancer *(69)*. Turmeric *(Curcuma longa)* contains phenolic compounds that inhibit cancer development as well as having antimutagenic activity. Turmeric has been shown to suppress the development of stomach, breast, lung and skin tumors *(70)*. Its activity is largely a result of its content of the antioxidant curcumin. Ginger also contains curcumin in addition to a dozen powerful antioxidant phenolic compounds, known as gingerols and diarylheptanoids *(60)*.

Carotenoid pigments are also effective antioxidants that quench free radicals, provide protection against oxidative damage to cells, and stimulate immune function. Persons with high levels of serum carotenoids typically have a reduced risk of cancer *(71)*. Carotenoids are the pigments found in rose hips, paprika, and the green, leafy herbs. However, studies using β-carotene supplements have not provided the expected health benefits, and in some cases have produced adverse effects such as an increased risk of lung cancer and overall mortality in smokers *(72,73)*. These findings suggest that although the consumption of carotenoid-rich fruits and vegetables promote health, caution should be exercised in the use of β-carotene supplements.

Polyphenolics in green tea *(Camellia sinensis)* are known to possess antimutagenic and anticancer activity. Some evidence suggests a protective effect of tea against cancer of the stomach and colon *(37)*. Tumor incidence and average tumor yield in rats with chemically induced colon carcinogenesis was significantly reduced when the rats received (-)-epigallocatechin gallate, a major polyphenolic constituent of green tea *(74)*. Extracts of both black and green tea have significantly inhibited leukemia and liver tumor cells *(75)*. Extracts of gotu kolu *(Centella asiatica)* were recently shown to be very effective in killing cultured tumor cells. Centella appears to have selective toxicity against tumor cells, as it lacked toxicity towards human lymphocytes. In follow-up studies, Centella extract more than doubled the life span of mice with tumors, and showed a remarkable lack of toxicity even at high doses *(76)*. Centella is also therapeutic for the treatment of ulcers, wounds, and eczema.

Recent Korean studies suggest that ginseng *(Panax ginseng)* may also lower the risk of cancer in humans *(77)*. Ginseng extract and powder has been found to be more effective than fresh sliced ginseng, the juice, or a ginseng tea, in reducing the risk of cancer *(78)*. In a case-control study, the incidence of human cancer was seen to steadily decrease with duration of ginseng use and total lifetime use of ginseng. Those who had taken ginseng for 1 yr had 36% less risk of cancer than nonusers, whereas those who used ginseng for 5 yr or more had 69% less risk *(79)*. Ginseng seems to be most protective against cancer of the ovaries, larynx, pancreas, esophagus, and stomach but less effective against breast, cervical, bladder, and thyroid cancer. The protective properties of ginseng root are believed to be partly due to its content of ginsenosides, a family of triterpene saponins *(25)*.

7. CONCERNS WITH HERBAL USAGE

Health practitioners, when taking clinical histories, often fail to ask patients, about their use of herbal products. In addition, patients may not volunteer this information because they do not realize its importance. Furthermore, patients may not wish to frustrate the health practitioner by telling them they are self-medicating with botanical materials or herbal supplements. Because herbs can often enhance or negate the effect of a conventional drug, it is important for physicians to know which herbs their patients take, how much, and how often. There are a number of possible drug–herb interactions to be considered *(80)*. For example, nonsteroidal anti-inflammatory drugs may negate the usefulness of feverfew in the treatment of migraine headaches; ginkgo, garlic, ginger, and ginseng should not be used concomitantly with warfarin, as they may alter bleeding time; immunostimulants such as *Echinacea* should not be given with immunosuppressants such as corticosteroids; evening primrose oil should not be used with an anticonvulsant, as it may lower the seizure threshold; excessive sedation may result when kava and barbiturates are used together; and licorice may offset the effect of spironolactone.

Another problem with the use of herbs or herbal extracts is the fact that the contents of many are not standardized so that the dose of a particular active ingredient is unknown *(1)*. The phytochemical content of an herb can vary from plant to plant based on where the herb was grown, the light conditions, and the maturity of the plant when harvested. The level of phytochemicals can vary greatly even between cultivars of the same species. Furthermore, different parts of an herb usually contain different amounts of the active ingredient *(26,81)*. Methods of preparation of the herbal extract also influence the activity of the final product for the consumer. The level of ginsenosides has been found to vary as much as 60-fold among 10 common brands of ginseng on the market *(82)*. Occasionally, there are also some reports of adulteration of herbal products. For example, *Echinacea* is sometimes adulterated with the inactive root of wild quinine, *Parthenium integrifolium*, for reasons of cost.

8. CONCLUSION

A variety of commonly used herbs containing different phytochemicals have the potential for use in the treatment of chronic diseases. Some of these herbs provide assistance in the treatment of hypercholesterolemia, some provide protection against cancer, some help with blood sugar control, and others are known to stimulate the immune system. Furthermore, a diet in which culinary herbs are generously used to flavor the food will provide a variety of active phytochemicals that promote health and protect against chronic diseases. Herbs have been described as both a friend of physicians and the praise of cooks *(83)*. Although the discriminate use of some herbal products is safe and some therapeutic benefits may be derived from their proper usage, the indiscriminate or excessive use of herbs can be unsafe *(1)*.

REFERENCES

1. Tyler V. Herbs of Choice. The Therapeutic Use of Phytomedicinals. Haworth Press, New York, 1994.
2. Dew MJ, Evans BK, Rhodes J. Peppermint oil for the irritable bowel syndrome: a multicentre trial. Br J Clin Pract 1984; 38:394–398.
3. Beecher GR. Phytonutrients' role in metabolism: effects of resistance to degenerative processes. Nutr Rev 1999; 57: S3–S6.
4. Craig WJ. Phytochemicals: guardians of our health. J Am Diet Assoc 1997; 97:S199–S204.
5. Thomson C, Bloch AS, Hasler CM. Position of the American Dietetic Association: functional foods. J Am Diet Assoc 1999; 99:1278–1285.
6. Kleijnen J, Knipschild P, ter Riet GT. Garlic, onions and cardiovascular risk factors. A review of the evidence from human experiments with emphasis on commercially available preparations. Br J Clin Pharmacol 1989; 28:535–544.
7. Warshafsky S, Kramer RS, Sivak SL. Effect of garlic on total serum cholesterol: a meta-analysis. Ann Intern Med 1993; 119:599–605.
8. Kendler B.S. Garlic (*Allium sativum*) and onion (*Allium cepa*): a review of their relationship to cardiovascular disease. Prev Med 1987; 16:670–685.
9. Nishimura H, Ariga T. Vinyldithiins in garlic and Japanese domestic allium (*A. Victorialis*), In: Huang MT, Osawa T, Ho CT, Rosen, RT, eds. Food Phytochemicals for Cancer Prevention I. Fruits and Vegetables. American Chemical Society, Washington DC, 1994, pp. 128–143.
10. Dauusch JG, Nixon DW. Garlic: a review of its relationship to malignant disease. Prev Med 1990; 19:346–361.
11. Berthold HK, Sudhop T, von Bergmann K. Effect of a garlic oil preparation on serum lipoproteins and cholesterol metabolism: a randomized controlled trial. JAMA 1998; 279:1900–1902.
12. Silagy CA, Neil HA. A meta-analysis of the effect of garlic on blood pressure. J Hypertens 1994; 12:463–468.
13. Kawakishi S, Morimitsu Y. Sulfur chemistry of onions and inhibitory factors of the arachidonic acid cascade, In: Huang MT, Osawa T, Ho CT, Rosen RT, eds. Food Phytochemicals for Cancer Prevention I. Fruits and Vegetables. American Chemical Society, Washington DC, 1994, pp. 120–127.
14. Sprecher DL, Harris BV, Goldberg AC, Anderson EC, Bayuk LM, Russell BS, et al. Efficacy of psyllium in reducing serum cholesterol levels in hypercholesterolemic patients on high- or low-fat diets. Ann Intern Med 1993; 119:545–554.
15. Olson BH, Anderson SM, Becker MP, Anderson JW, Hunninghake DB, Jenkins DJA, et al. Psyllium-enriched cereals lower blood total cholesterol and LDL cholesterol, but not HDL cholesterol, in hypercholesterolemic adults: results of a meta-analysis. J Nutr 1997; 127:1973–1980.
16. Bierenbaum ML, Reichstein R, Walkins T. Reducing atherogenic risk in hyperlipemic humans with flax seed supplementation: a preliminary report. J Am Coll Nutr. 1993; 12:501–504.

17. Cunnane SC, Ganguli S, Menard C, Liede AC, Hamadeh MJ, Chen ZY, Wolever TM, Jenkins DJ. High alpha-linolenic acid flaxseed *(Linum usitatissimum):* some nutritional properties in humans. Br J Nutr 1993; 69:443–453.

18. Sharma RD, Raghuram TC. Hypoglycaemic effect of fenugreek seeds in non-insulin dependant diabetic subjects. Nutr Res 1990; 10:731–739.

19. Nityanand S, Srivastava JS, Asthana OP. Clinical trials with gugulipid, a new hypocholesterolemic agent. J Assoc Physicians India 1989; 37:323–328.

20. Elson CE, Underbakke GL, Hanson P, Shrago E, Wainberg RH, Qureshi AA. Impact of lemongrass oil, an essential oil, on serum cholesterol. Lipids 1989; 24:677–679.

21. Sugano M, Ide T, Ishada T, Yoshida K. Hypocholesterolemic effect of gamma-linolenic acid as evening primrose oil in rats. Ann Nutr Metab 1986; 30:289–299.

22. Case GL, He L, Mo H, Elson CE. Induction of geranyl pyrophosphate pyrophosphatase activity by cholesterol-suppressive isoprenoids. Lipids 1995; 30:357–359.

23. Park HJ, Rhee MH, Park KM, Nam KY, Park KH. Effect of non-saponin fraction from *Panax ginseng* on cGMP and thromboxane A2 in human platelet aggregation. J Ethnopharmacol 1995; 49:157–162.

24. Decker EA. The role of phenolics, conjugated linoleic acid, carnosine, and pyrroloquinoline quinone as nonessential dietary antioxidants. Nutr Rev 1995; 53:49–58.

25. Bruneton J. *Pharmacognosy, Phytochemistry, Medicinal Plants.* C.K. Lavoisier Publishers, Paris, 1995.

26. Manach C, Regerat F, Texier O, Agullo G, Demigne C, Remesy C. Bioavailability, metabolism and physiological impact of 4-oxo-flavonoids. Nutr Res 1996; 16:517–544.

27. Cook NC, Samman S. Flavonoids–chemistry, metabolism, cardioprotective effects, and dietary sources. J Nutr Biochem 1996; 7:66–76.

28. Hertog MGL, Feskens EJM, Hollman PC, Katan MB, Kromhout D. Dietary antioxidant flavonoids and risk of coronary heart disease. Lancet 1993; 342:1007–1011.

29. Keli SO, Hertog MG, Feskins EJ, Kromhout D. Dietary flavonoids, antioxidant vitamins, and incidence of stroke: the Zutphen study. Arch Intern Med 1996; 156:637–642.

30. Yochum L, Kushi LH, Meyer K, Folsom AR. Dietary flavonoid intake and risk of cardiovascular disease in postmenopausal women. Am J Epidemiol 1999; 149:943–949.

31. Nuttall SL, Kendall MJ, Bombardelli E, Morazzoni P. An evaluation of the antioxidant activity of a standardized grape seed extract, Leucoselect. J Clin Pharm Ther 1998; 23:385–389.

32. Pittler MH, Ernst E. Horse-chestnut seed extract for chronic venous insufficiency. A criteria-based systematic review. Arch Dermatol 1998; 134:1356–1360.

33. Kleijnen J, Knipschild P. Gingko biloba for cerebral insufficiency. Br J Clin Pharmacol 1992; 34:352–358.

34. Curtis-Prior P, Vere D, Fray P. Therapeutic value of Ginkgo biloba in reducing symptoms of decline in mental function. J Pharm Pharmacol 1999; 51:535–541.

35. Vibes J, Lasserre B, Gleye J, Declume C. Inhibition of thromboxane A2 biosynthesis in vitro by the main components of *Crataegus oxyacantha* (Hawthorn) flower heads. Prostaglandins Leukotrienes Essential Fatty Acids 1994; 50:173–175.

36. Fuhrman B, Buch S, Vaya J, Belinky PA, Coleman R, Hayek T, Aviram M. Licorice extract and its major polyphenol glabridin protect low-density lipoprotein against lipid peroxidation: in vitro and ex vivo studies in humans and in atherosclerotic aoplipoprotein E-deficient mice. Am J Clin Nutr 1997; 66:267–275.

37. Ishikawa T, Suzukawa M, Ito T, Yoshida H, Ayaori M, Nishiwaki M, et al. Effect of tea flavonoid supplementation on the susceptibility of low-density lipoprotein to oxidative modification. Am J Clin Nutr 1997; 66:261–266.

38. Dreosti IE. Bioactive ingredients: antioxidants and polyphenols in tea. Nutr Rev 1996; 54(11):S51–S58.

39. Srivastava Y, Venkatakrishna-Bhatt H, Verma Y, Venkaiah, K, Raval BH. Antidiabetic and adaptogenic properties of *Momardica charantia* extract: an experimental and clinical evaluation. Phytother Res 1993; 7:285–289.
40. Marles RJ, Farnsworth NR. Antidiabetic drugs and their active constituents. Phytomedicine 1995; 2:137–189.
41. Shanmugasundaram ERB, Rajeswari G, Baskaran K, Rajesh Kumar BR, Shanmugasundaram KR, Arhmath BK. Use of *Gymnema sylvestre* leaf extract in the control of blood glucose in insulin-dependant diabetes mellitus. J Ethnopharmacol 1990; 30:281–294.
42. Baskaran, K., Kizar Ahamath B, Shanmugasundaram KR, Shanmugasundaram ER. Antidiabetic effect of a leaf extract from *Gymnema sylvestre* in non-insulin dependent diabetes mellitus patients. J Ethnopharmacol 1990; 30:295–305.
43. Sotaniemi EA, Haapakoski E, Rautio A. Ginseng therapy in non-insulin-dependent diabetic patients. Diabetes Care 1995; 118:1373–1375.
44. Anderson JW, Allgood LD, Turner J, Oeltgen PR, Daggy, BP. Effects of psyllium on glucose and serum lipid responses in men with type 2 diabetes and hypercholesterolemia. Am J Clin Nutr 1999; 70:466–473.
45. Imparl-Radosevich J, Deas S, Polansky MM, Baedke DA, Ingebritsen TS, Anderson RA, Graves DJ. Regulation of PTP-1 and insulin receptor kinase by fractions from cinnamon: implications for cinnamon regulation of insulin signalling. Horm Res 1998; 50:177–182.
46. Broadhurst CL. Keeping diabetes in check. Herbs Health 1997; 1 (4):30–33.
47. Khan A, Bryden NA, Polansky MM, Anderson RA. Insulin potentiating factor and chromium content of selected foods and spices. Biol Trace Elem Res 1990; 24:183–188.
48. Grimm W, Muller HH. A randomized controlled trial of the effect of fluid extract of Echinacea purpurea on the incidence and severity of colds and respiratory infections. Am J Med 1999; 106:138–143.
49. Abe N, Ebina T, Ishida N. Interferon induction by glycyrrhizin and glycyrrhetinic acid in mice. Microb Immunol 1982; 26:535–539.
50. Shibata S. Antitumor-promoting and anti-inflammatory activities of licorice principles and their modified compounds, In: Huang MT, Osawa T, Ho CT, Rosen RT, eds. Food Phytochemicals for Cancer Prevention II. Teas, Spices and Herbs. American Chemical Society, Washington DC, 1994, pp. 308–321.
51. Rizzi R, Re F, Bianchi A, De Feo V, de Simone F, Bianchi L, Stivala LA. Mutagenic and antimutagenic activities of *Uncaria tomentosa* and its extracts. J Ethnopharmacol 1993; 38:63–77.
52. Aquino R., De Feo V, De Simone F, Pizza C, Cirino G. Plant metabolites. New compounds and anti-inflammatory activity of *Uncaria tomentosa*. J Nat Prod 1991; 54:453–459.
53. Wu D, Meydani M, Leka LS, Nightingale Z, Handelman GJ, Blumberg JB, Meydani SN. Effect of dietary supplementation with black currant seed oil on the immune response of healthy elderly subjects. Am J Clin Nutr 1999; 70:536–543.
54. Burger RA, Warren RP, Lawson LD, Hughes BG. Enhancement of in vitro human immune function by *Allium sativum* L (garlic) fractions. Int J Pharmacogn 1993; 31:169–174.
55. Abdullah TH, Kirkpatrick DV, Carter J. Enhancement of natural killer cell activity in AIDS with garlic. Deutsch Zeishrift Oncol 1989; 21:52–53.
56. Caragay AB. Cancer-preventative foods and ingredients. Food Tech 1992; 46(4):65–68.
57. Huang MT, Ferraro T, Ho CT. Cancer chemoprevention by phytochemicals in fruits and vegetables. An overview. In: Huang MT, Osawa T, Ho CT, Rosen RT, eds. Food Phytochemicals for Cancer Prevention I. Fruits and Vegetables. American Chemical Society, Washington DC, 1994, pp. 2–16.
58. Bisset NG, ed. Herbal Drugs and Phytopharmaceuticals. A Handbook for Practice on a Scientific Basis. Medpharm Scientific Publishers, Stuttgart, 1994.

59. Ho CT, Ferraro T, Chen Q, Rosen RT, Huang MT. Phytochemicals in teas and rosemary and their cancer-preventive properties, In: Huang MT, Osawa T, Ho CT, Rosen RT, eds. Food Phytochemicals for Cancer Prevention II. Teas, Spices and Herbs. American Chemical Society, Washington DC, 1994, pp. 2–19.
60. Kikuzaki H, Nakatani N. Antioxidant effects of some ginger constituents. J Food Sci 1993; 58:1407–1410.
61. Nakatani N. Chemistry of antioxidants from *Labiatae* herbs, In: Huang MT, Osawa T, Ho CT, Rosen RT, eds. Food Phytochemicals for Cancer Prevention II. Teas, Spices and Herbs. American Chemical Society, Washington DC, 1994, pp. 144–153.
62. Steinmetz KA, Potter JD. Vegetables, fruit, and cancer, II. Mechanisms. Cancer Causes Control 1991; 2:427–442.
63. Lau BHS, Tadi PP, Tosk JM. *Allium sativum* (garlic) and cancer prevention. Nutr Res 1990; 10:937–948.
64. Steinmetz KA, Potter JD. Vegetables, fruit, and cancer prevention: a review. J Am Diet Assoc 1996; 96:1027–1039.
65. Steinmetz KA, Kushi LH, Bostick RM, Folsom AR, Potter JD. Vegetable, fruit, and colon cancer in the Iowa women's health study. Am J Epidemiol 1994; 139:1–15.
66. Milner JA. Garlic: its anticarcinogenic and antitumorigenic properties. Nutr Rev 1996; 54(11):S82–S86.
67. You WC, Blot WJ, Chang YS, Ershow A, Yang ZT, An Q, et al. Allium vegetables and reduced risk of stomach cancer J Natl Cancer Inst 1989; 81:162–164.
68. Dorant E, van den Brandt PA, Goldbohm RA, Sturmans F. Consumption of onions and a reduced risk of stomach carcinoma. Gastroenterology 1996; 110:12–20.
69. Serraino M, Thompson LU. The effect of flaxseed supplementation on the initiation and promotional stages of mammary tumorigenesis. Nutr Cancer 1992; 17:153–159.
70. Nagabhushan M, Bhide SV. Curcumin as an inhibitor of cancer. J Am Coll Nutr 1992; 11:192–198.
71. Van Poppel G, Goldbohm RA. Epidemiologic evidence for beta-carotene and cancer prevention. Am J Clin Nutr 1995; 62:1393S–1402S.
72. Lee I, Cook NR, Manson JE, Buring JE, Hennekens CH. Beta-carotene supplementation and incidence of cancer and cardiovascular disease: the Women's health study. J Natl Cancer Inst 1999; 91:2102–2106.
73. Albanes D. Beta-carotene and lung cancer: a case study. Am J Clin Nutr 1999; 91:2102–2106.
74. D-Limonene, an anticarcinogenic terpene. Nutr Rev 1988; 46:363–365.
75. Lea MA, Xiao Q, Sadhukhan AK, Cottle S, Wang ZY, Yang CS. Inhibitory effects of tea extracts and (-)-epigallocatechin gallate on DNA synthesis and proliferation of hepatoma and erythroleukemia cells. Cancer Lett 1993: 68:231–236.
76. Babu TD, Kuttan G, Padikkala J. Cytotoxic and anti-tumor properties of certain taxa of Umbelliferae with special reference to *Centella asiatica* urban. J Ethnopharmacol 1995; 48:53–57.
77. Yun TK. Experimental and epidemiological evidence of the cancer-preventive effects of *Panax ginseng* CA Meyer. Nutr Rev 1996; 54(11):S71–S81.
78. Yun TK, Choi SY. A case-control study of ginseng intake and cancer. Int J Epidemiol 1990; 19:871–876.
79. Yun TK, Choi SY. Preventive effect of ginseng intake against various human cancers: a case-control study on 1987 pairs. Cancer Epidemiol Biomarkers Prev 1995; 4:401–408.
80. Miller LG. Herbal medicinals. Selected clinical considerations focusing on known or potential drug-herb interactions. Arch Intern Med 1998; 158:2200–2211.
81. Bravo L. Polyphenols: chemistry, dietary sources, metabolism, and nutritional significance. Nutr Rev 1998; 56:317–333.
82. Ansley D, ed. Ginseng. Much ado about nothing? Consumer Reports 1995; 60:699.
83. Farrell KT. Spices, Condiments and Seasonings. AVI Publishing, Westport, CT, 1985, p. 17.

16 Fetal Nutrition and Cardiovascular Disease in Adult Life

David J. P. Barker and Keith M. Godfrey

1. THE CORONARY HEART DISEASE EPIDEMIC

At the start of the twentieth century, the incidence of coronary heart disease (CHD) rose steeply; it rapidly became the most common cause of death in Western countries. Its incidence is now rising in other parts of the world to which Western influences are extending, such as India, China, Eastern Europe, and Russia. As such rapid increases in incidence over a relatively short time cannot be the result of changes in gene frequency, attention has been directed at the environment, particularly the lifestyles of men and women in industrialized countries.

Given that the other major heart disorder in adult life, chronic rheumatic heart disease, was already known to be caused by events in childhood, it may seem surprising that adults rather than children were the early focus of research into CHD. Perhaps discovery of the powerful effects of cigarette smoking on lung cancer directed attention in this way. Whatever the reason, 40 yr of research into adult lifestyle have met with limited success in explaining the origins of CHD: obesity and cigarette smoking have been implicated, and evidence on dietary fat has accumulated to the point where a public health policy of reduced intake is prudent, although unproven: preliminary evidence points to a role for psychosocial stress. Much, however, remains unexplained.

Unfortunately, formulation of public health policies to prevent CHD, policies based on the best available advice, has simultaneously created a scientific orthodoxy. This states that the disease results from the 'unhealthy' lifestyles of westernized adults together with a contribution from genetic inheritance. Such a view of CHD, however, leaves its changing incidence and geography largely unexplained, and offers little insight into why, within westernized communities, one person develops the disease but another does not. The effectiveness of preventative measures based on this view of the disease is being questioned.

From: *Nutritional Health: Strategies for Disease Prevention*
Edited by: T. Wilson and N. J. Temple © Humana Press Inc., Totowa, NJ

In many Western countries the steep rise of CHD has been followed by a fall; in the United States this has been of the order of 45% over 25 yr *(1)*. No parallel changes in adult lifestyle seem to explain it. In Britain, there were large changes in lifestyle during World War II, especially in diet. Government food policy led to major and widespread changes in diet, so that fat and sugar consumption fell sharply and fiber consumption rose. Death rates from CHD in middle-aged men and women, however, continued to rise throughout the war and the period of postwar rationing *(2)*.

The geography of CHD in Britain is paradoxical. Rates are twice as high in the poorer areas of the country, and in lower-income groups. The steep rise of the disease in Britain and other Western countries was associated with rising prosperity, so why should its rates be lowest in the most prosperous places, such as London and the home counties, and in the highest-income groups? Biochemical and physiological measurements in adult life, including serum cholesterol and blood pressure, have been shown to be linked to CHD *(3)*. Yet, even when combined with these biological risk factors, adult lifestyle has limited ability to predict CHD *(4)*. Rose *(5)* has pointed out that, for a man falling into the lowest risk groups for cigarette smoking, serum cholesterol concentration, blood pressure, and preexisting symptoms of CHD, the most common cause of death is still CHD.

It is, perhaps, surprising that it was geographical studies of death rates among babies in Britain during the early 1900s that gave the early clue that explanations for these paradoxes may come from events *in utero (6)*. The usual certified cause of death in newborn babies at that time was low birthweight. Death rates in the newborn differed considerably between one part of the country and another, being highest in some of the northern industrial towns and the poorer rural areas in the north and west. This geographical pattern in death rates was shown to closely resemble today's large variations in death rates from CHD, variations that form one aspect of the continuing North/South divide in health in Britain. One possible conclusion suggested by this observation was that low rates of growth before birth are in some way linked to the development of CHD in adult life. The suggestions that events in childhood influence the pathogenesis of CHD was not new. A focus on intrauterine life, however, offered a new point of departure for research.

2. LOW BIRTHWEIGHT AND CHD

The early epidemiological studies that pointed to the possible importance of programing in CHD were based on the simple strategy of examining men and women in middle and late life whose body measurements at birth were recorded. Among nearly 16,000 men and women born in Hertfordshire, UK, during 1911–1930, death rates from CHD fell twofold between those at the lower and upper ends of the birthweight distribution (*see* Table 1) *(7)*. A study in Sheffield, where detailed obstetric records are available from the early years of the last

Table 1
Death Rates from CHD Among 15,726 Men and Women According to Birthweight

Birthweight lb (kg)	Standardized mortality ratio	No. of deaths
≤5.5 (2.50)	100	57
–6.5 (2.95)	81	137
–7.5 (3.41)	80	298
–8.5 (3.86)	74	289
–9.5 (4.31)	55	103
–9.5 (4.31)	65	57
All	74	941

century, showed that it is people who were small at birth because they failed to grow, rather than being born prematurely, who are at increased risk of the disease *(8)*. In both the Hertfordshire and Sheffield studies, low birthweight was also associated with an increased risk of stroke *(9)*. The association between low birthweight and CHD has been confirmed in studies in Uppsala, Sweden *(10)*, Helsinki, Finland *(11)*, Caerphilly, Wales, *(12)* and the United States, where among 80,000 women in the Nurses Study, there was a similar twofold fall in the relative risk of nonfatal CHD across the range of birthweight *(13)*. An association between low birthweight and prevalent CHD has also been shown in South India *(14)*. Among men and women aged 45 yr and over the prevalences of the disease fell from 15% in those who weighed 5.5 lb (2.5 kg) or less at birth to 4% in those who weighed 7 lb (3.2 kg) or more.

In studies exploring these associations, the trends in CHD with birthweight were found to be paralleled by similar trends in two of its major risk factors— hypertension and non-insulin-dependent diabetes mellitus *(15,16)*. Table 2 illustrates the size of these trends, the prevalence of non-insulin dependent diabetes and impaired glucose tolerance falling threefold between men who weighed 5.5 lb at birth and those who weighed 9.5 lb. This association has been confirmed in men and women in studies in the UK *(17)*, three in the United States *(18–20)* and one in Sweden *(21)*. Thirty-eight studies on populations totaling one quarter of a million people confirm that low birthweight is associated with raised blood pressure through childhood and into adult life *(22,23)*.

One response to such findings has been to argue that people who were exposed to an adverse environment *in utero* and failed to grow continue to be exposed to an adverse environment in childhood and adult life. It is this later adverse environment, the argument goes, that produces the effects attributed to programing *in utero*. This argument has been addressed in recent publications and there is little evidence to support it *(21)*. Instead, associations between birthweight and later disease are found in each social group, and are independent of influences such as smoking and obesity in adult life. Findings in children also help to resolve

Table 2
Prevalence of Non-Insulin Dependent Diabetes
and Impaired Glucose Tolerance in Men Aged 59–70 yr

Birthweight lb (kg)	No. of men	% With impaired glucose tolerance or diabetes	Odds ratio adjusted for BMI (95% confidence interval)	
≤5.5 (2.50)	20	40	6.6	(1.5–28)
–6.5 (2.95)	47	34	4.8	(1.3–17)
–7.5 (3.41)	104	31	4.6	(1.4–16)
–8.5 (3.86)	117	22	2.6	(0.8–8.9)
–9.5 (4.31)	54	13	1.4	(0.3–5.6)
>9.5 (4.31)	28	14	1.0	
All	370	25		

these difficulties. Studies in several countries have shown that children who were small at birth have raised blood pressure and evidence of impaired ability to respond to an oral glucose challenge (17). These findings are further evidence that the associations in adults do not reflect unknown confounding variables linked to lifestyle. Because many of the studies were done in countries where child mortality is low, they also argue against suggestions that associations with birth size reflect bias due to differential survival or migration (19). Adult lifestyle does, however, add to intrauterine effects. The highest prevalences of non-insulin-dependent diabetes and impaired glucose tolerance, for example, are seen in people who were small at birth but obese as adults (15,21). Around the world, the communities with high prevalences of diabetes generally conform to this pattern, they include Ethiopian Jews air-lifted to Israel, and Indian people who migrated to the UK, among whom fetal growth was generally poor but obesity common in adult life (24).

3. FETAL NUTRITION

In common with other living creatures, human beings are "plastic" in their early life, and are shaped by the environment. Although the growth of a fetus is influenced by its genes, studies in humans and animals suggest that it is usually limited by the environment, in particular the nutrients and oxygen it receives from the mother (25,26). There are many possible evolutionary advantages in the body remaining plastic during development, rather than having its development driven only by genetic instructions acquired at conception (27). A recent study of babies born after ovum donation illustrates how birth size is essentially controlled by the mother's body and the nutritional environment it affords (28). The birthweights of the babies were strongly related to the weight of the recipient mother, heavier mothers having larger babies. Birthweights were, however, unrelated to the weights of the women who donated the eggs.

4. FETAL ADAPTATIONS TO UNDERNUTRITION

Studies in animals show that the fetus may respond to undernutrition in a number of ways *(16)*. It can redistribute its cardiac output to protect key organs, the brain in particular *(29)*; it can alter its metabolism, for example, by switching from glucose to amino-acid oxidation; and it can change the production of, or tissue sensitivity to, hormones regulating growth, in which insulin has a central role *(30)*. Slowing of growth is also adaptive because it reduces the requirements for the substrate. Unlike physiological adaptations in adult life, adaptations during development tend to have lasting effects on the structure and function of the body. Experiments show that even minor modifications to the diets of pregnant animals may be followed by life long changes in the offspring in ways that can be related to human disease, for example, raised blood pressure and altered glucose metabolism *(31,32)*. A wide range of organs and systems can be permanently changed or "programmed" by experimental manipulation of the intrauterine environment. This suggests that programing may reflect a general principle in developmental biology *(33)*. Men and women who were *in utero* at the time of the Dutch famine were only around 200 g lighter at birth than those *in utero* before or after the famine. Nevertheless, they have reduced glucose tolerance and evidence of insulin resistance *(34)*. A conclusion from this is that fetuses can adapt to undernutrition and continue to grow, although at the price of an increased risk of disease in postreproductive life.

Birthweight serves as a marker of fetal nutrition and growth, but it is an imperfect one. The same birthweight may be the outcome of many different paths of growth *(35)*. Where more detailed measurements of body size at birth are available, they may give insights into adaptations that the fetus has made. Babies that are thin (as defined by a low ponderal index, birthweight/length^3) though within the normal range of birthweight, tend to be insulin resistant as children and adults and are therefore liable to develop non-insulin-dependent diabetes *(36)*. This has been confirmed in studies in Sweden *(21)*. It suggests that the thin baby responded to undernutrition through endocrine and metabolic changes. Babies that are short in relation to their head circumference, and have a reduced abdominal circumference, tend to have persisting abnormalities of vascular structure, including reduced elasticity, and of liver function, including elevated serum low-density lipoprotein (LDL) cholesterol and plasma fibrinogen concentrations *(37–39)*. They have increased death rates from CHD *(40)*. Replication of these observations has been limited, however, because few data sets include abdominal circumference at birth. Babies that have small abdominal circumference in relation to their head circumference may result from "brain-sparing" circulatory adaptations by which cardiac output is diverted to the brain at the expense of the trunk. These adaptations increase the load on the heart, and there is preliminary evidence suggesting that persisting left ventricular hypertrophy, a known risk factor for CHD, may be a consequence of this *(41)*.

Two other patterns of body proportions at birth have been linked with adult disease. Studies in South India have shown that babies who are short and fat tend to become insulin deficient and have high rates of non-insulin-dependent diabetes *(42)*. This is consistent with findings in the Pima Indians and with the U-shaped association between abdominal circumference at birth and death from CHD *(19,40)*. Babies that are short and fat are thought to be the result of maternal hyperglycemia. Babies whose placentas are disproportionately large in relation to their own size tend to have raised blood pressure and increased death rates for CHD *(9,43)*. Although such associations have been replicated, they are not consistently found. Animal studies offer a possible explanation for this. In sheep the placenta enlarges in response to moderate undernutrition in midpregnancy. This is thought to be an adaptive response to extract more nutrients from the mother. It is not, however, a consistent response but occurs only in ewes that were well-nourished before pregnancy *(44)*.

5. MATERNAL INFLUENCES ON FETAL GROWTH

Size at birth reflects the product of the fetus's trajectory of growth, set at an early stage in development, and the maternoplacental capacity to supply sufficient nutrients to maintain that trajectory. It has been thought that in Western populations regulatory mechanisms in the maternal and placental systems act to ensure that human fetal growth and development is little influenced by normal variations in maternal nutrient intake, and that there is a simple relationship between a woman's body composition and the growth of her fetus. Recent experimental studies in animals and our own observations in humans challenge these concepts *(45)*. These studies suggest that a mother's own fetal growth and her dietary intakes and body composition can exert major effects on the balance between the fetal demand for nutrients and the maternoplacental capacity to meet that demand. Failure of the maternoplacental supply line to satisfy fetal nutrient requirements results in a range of fetal adaptations and developmental changes. Although these may be beneficial for short-term survival, they may lead to permanent alterations in the body's structure and metabolism, and thereby to cardiovascular and metabolic disease in adult life *(45)*. Figure 1 shows a conceptual framework illustrating this hypothesis.

Quite apart from any long-term effects on health in adult life, specific issues that have not been adequately addressed in previous studies of maternal nutrition include (1) effects on the trajectory of fetal growth, (2) intergenerational effects, (3) paradoxical effects on placental growth, and (4) effects on fetal proportions and specific tissues. The effects of the mother's body composition and dietary balance also need to be addressed and are discussed next.

5.1. The Fetal Growth Trajectory

A rapid trajectory of growth increases the fetus's demand for nutrients. This reflects effects on both maintenance requirements, which are greater in fetuses that have achieved a larger size as a result of a faster growth trajectory, and on

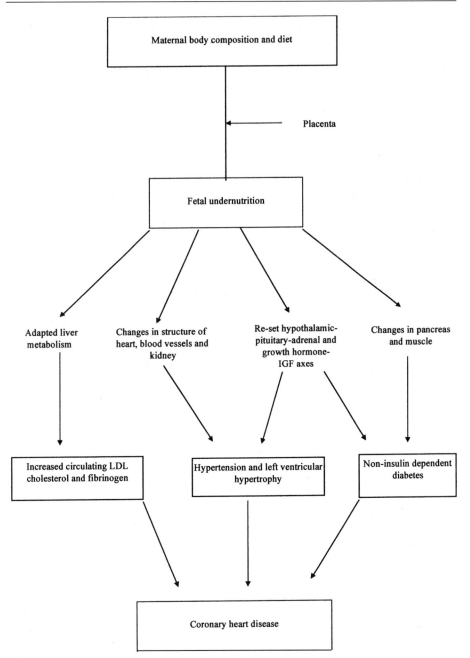

Fig. 1. A framework of possible mechanisms linking fetal undernutrition and coronary heart disease.

requirements for future growth. In absolute terms, the fetal demand for nutrients is small until late in pregnancy. Experimental studies of pregnant ewes have shown that, though a fast growth trajectory is generally associated with larger fetal size and improved neonatal survival, it does render the fetus more vulnerable to a reduced maternoplacental supply of nutrients in late gestation. Thus, maternal undernutrition during the last trimester adversely affected the development of rapidly growing fetuses with high requirements while having little effect on those growing more slowly *(46)*. Rapidly growing fetuses were found to make a series of adaptations in order to survive, including fetal wasting and placental oxidation of fetal amino acids to maintain lactate output to the fetus *(46)*.

The trajectory of fetal growth is thought to be set at an early stage in development. Experiments in animals have shown that periconceptional alterations in maternal diet and plasma progesterone concentrations can alter gene expression in the pre-implantation embryo to change the fetal growth trajectory *(47,48)*. Environmental effects have been demonstrated on both embryonic growth rates and on cell allocation in the preimplantation embryo. Maternal progesterone treatment can, for example, permanently alter the trajectory of fetal growth by changing the allocation of cells between the inner cell mass that develops into the fetus and the outer trophectoderm that becomes the placenta *(47,48)*. The trajectory of fetal growth is thought to increase with improvements in periconceptional nutrition, and is faster in male fetuses *(49)*. One possibility is that the greater vulnerability of such fetuses on a fast growth trajectory could contribute to the rise in CHD with Westernization and the higher death rates in men.

5.2. Intergenerational Effects

Experimental studies in animals have shown that undernutrition over many generations can have cumulative effects on reproductive performance. Thus, feeding rats a protein deficient diet over 12 generations resulted in progressively greater fetal growth retardation over the generations; following refeeding with a normal diet it then took three generations to normalize growth and development *(50)*.

Strong evidence for major intergenerational effects in humans has come from studies showing that a woman's birthweight influences the birthweight of her offspring *(51,52)*. We have, moreover, found that whereas low birthweight mothers tend to have thin infants with a low ponderal index (birthweight/birth length^3), the father's birthweight is unrelated to ponderal index at birth *(see* Fig. 2); crown–heel length at birth is, however, more strongly related to the father's birthweight than to the mother's *(53)*. The effect of *maternal* birthweight on thinness at birth is consistent with the hypothesis that the maternoplacental supply line may be unable to satisfy fetal nutrient demand in low-birthweight mothers. Potential mechanisms underlying this effect include alterations in the uterine or systemic vasculature, programed changes in maternal metabolic status, and impaired placentation. The strong effect of *paternal* birthweight on crown–heel length may reflect paternal imprinting of genes important for skeletal growth, such as those regulating the concentrations of insulin-like growth factors *(54)*.

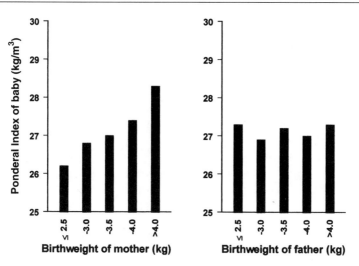

Fig. 2. Ponderal index at birth of 492 term babies according to the birthweight of their mothers and fathers.

5.3. Placental Size and Transfer Capabilities

Although the size of the placenta gives only an indirect measure of its capacity to transfer nutrients to the fetus, it is nonetheless strongly associated with fetal size at birth. Experiments in sheep have shown that maternal nutrition in early pregnancy can exert major effects on the growth of the placenta, and thereby alter fetal development *(55,56)*. The effects produced depend on the nutritional status of the ewe in the periconceptional period. In ewes poorly nourished around the time of conception, high nutrient intakes in early pregnancy increase the size of the placenta. Conversely, in ewes well nourished around conception, high intakes in early pregnancy result in small placental size *(55)*. Although this suppression appears paradoxical, in sheep farming it is common practice for ewes to be put on rich pasture prior to mating and then on poor pasture for a period in early pregnancy *(57)*.

As part of a study designed to evaluate whether the normal variations in maternal diet found in Western communities could influence fetal growth and development, we have found evidence of a similar suppressive effect of high dietary intakes in early pregnancy on placental growth *(58)*. Thus, among 538 women who delivered at term, those with high dietary intakes in early pregnancy, especially of carbohydrate, had smaller placentas, particularly if combined with low intakes of dairy protein in late pregnancy *(see* Table 3) *(58)*. These effects were independent of the mother's body size, social class, and smoking, and resulted in alterations in the ratio of placental weight to birthweight (placental ratio).

Effects on placental growth may be of long-term importance as a follow-up study of men born early in the 20th century in Sheffield found a U-shaped relation

Table 3
Mean Placental Weight(g) Adjusted for Baby's Sex and Duration
of Gestation According to Mother's Daily Intakes of Carbohydrates
in Early Pregnancy and Dairy Protein in Late Pregnancy[a]

Dairy protein intake in late pregnancy (g/d)	Carbohydrate intake in early pregnancy (g/d)			
	≤265	–340	>340	All
≤18.5	539 (72)	507 (49)	494 (54)	516 (175)
–26.5	556 (73)	546 (63)	509 (48)	540 (184)
>26.5	582 (36)	533 (60)	536 (83)	544 (179)
All	554 (181)	531 (172)	517 (185)	534 (538)

[a]Figures in parentheses are numbers of subjects.

between the placental ratio and later CHD *(9)*. Although babies with a disproportionately small placenta may suffer as a consequence of an impaired placental supply capacity, those with a disproportionately large placenta may experience fetal catabolism and wasting to supply amino acids for placental consumption *(16,59)*. Consequent fetal adaptations may underlie the increased adult CHD death rates in those with both low and high placental ratios.

5.4. Effects on Specific Fetal Tissues

Experimental studies in animals have shown that dietary manipulations during early development can have tissue-specific effects, resulting in alterations in an animal's proportions. For example, in pigs fed differing diets in the first year of life, those fed a protein-deficient diet had a disproportionately large head, ears, and genitalia compared with those fed an energy-deficient diet *(25)*. Recent experiments in guinea pigs have shown that maternal undernutrition in pregnancy resulted in offspring that not only had altered body proportions at birth, but also showed profound elevation of serum cholesterol concentrations when fed a high-cholesterol diet in the postweaning period *(60)*.

In humans, few studies have examined the possibility of maternal nutrition during pregnancy having tissue-specific effects on the fetus, leading to greater alterations in neonatal proportions than in birthweight. Any such effects may be of importance as adult CHD and non-insulin-dependent diabetes are more strongly associated with altered birth proportions than with birthweight *(11,21)*. We have found that women with low dairy protein intakes in late pregnancy tend to have babies that are thinner at birth *(53)*; maternal dairy protein intakes were not however related to birthweight *(58)*.

6. PRIMARY PREVENTION OF CHD

The thesis which is developing from these findings is that the primary prevention of CHD depends on (1) prevention of imbalances in fetal growth, and between pre- and postnatal growth, and (2) prevention of imbalances in nutrient supply to the fetus. We suggest that the epidemics of CHD that regularly accompany the transition from chronic malnutrition to adequate nutrition are the result of these imbalances.

6.1. Imbalances in Growth

As already described, babies that are thin or short in relation to their head circumference, or short and fat, or have disproportionately large placentas, are at increased risk of cardiovascular disease (CVD) or non-insulin-dependent diabetes. As yet, we do not understand the maternal antecedents of these patterns of imbalanced fetal growth, though we have some insights. A recent study in Finland illustrates the consequences of imbalance between pre- and postnatal growth. Table 4 is taken from a study of 3641 men born in Helsinki. The highest death rates from CHD were among men who were thin at birth but whose weight had "caught-up" by the age of 7 yr so that they had an above-average body mass index (BMI) thereafter *(61)*. Catch-up growth could be associated with adverse outcomes in adult life through altered body composition. Babies who are thin at birth have a lower muscle mass *(62)*. It is possible that if they develop a high body mass in childhood, they have a disproportionately high fat mass. Another possibility is that accelerated postnatal weight gain is intrinsically damaging. In rats, the combination of prenatal undernutrition and retarded fetal growth and good postnatal nutrition with accelerated growth leads to striking reductions in life span *(63)*. Why catch-up growth is detrimental is not known, but one speculation is that fetal growth restriction leads to reduced cell numbers and subsequent catch-up growth is achieved by overgrowth of a limited cell mass *(64)*. A third possible link between catch-up growth and later disease is that it reflects persisting changes in hormonal secretion, including insulin, insulin-like growth factor-1, and growth hormone, which are established in utero in response to undernutrition, and influence both childhood growth and later disease *(16)*.

Whatever underlies the association between death from CHD and accelerated weight gain in early childhood it illustrates an imbalance between pre- and postnatal growth. The effects of adult obesity provide a further illustration. Obesity has a greater effect on impaired glucose tolerance in people who had low birthweight *(15,21)*. Similarly, the Dutch famine had its greatest effect on glucose tolerance in men and women who were overweight as adults *(34)*.

6.2. Imbalances in Nutrient Supply to the Fetus

Indications that the *balance* of macronutrients in the mother's diet can have important short- and long-term effects on the offspring has come from a series

Table 4
Hazard Ratios for Death from CHD According to Ponderal Index at Birth
and Body Mass Index at Age 11 yr, Adjusted for Length of Gestation[a]

Ponderal index (kg/m^3) at birth	Body mass index (kg/m^2) at age 11 yr			
	≤15.5	–16.5	–17.5	>17.5
= 25	2.7 (21)	3.3 (26)	3.7 (19)	5.3 (14)
–27	1.5 (14)	3.2 (40)	4.0 (35)	2.7 (14)
–29	2.2 (17)	1.6 (18)	1.8 (19)	3.2 (21)
> 29	1.0 (4)	1.7 (11)	1.5 (12)	1.9 (12)

[a]Figures in parentheses are numbers of deaths. BMI cutpoints are approximately quartiles.

of experimental studies in pregnant rats. These have found that maternal diets with a low ratio of protein to carbohydrate and fat alter fetal and placental growth and result in lifelong elevation of blood pressure in the offspring (31). A follow-up study of 40-yr-old men and women in Aberdeen, UK, suggested that alterations in the maternal macronutrient balance during pregnancy could have similar adverse effects on the offspring (65); the relations with maternal diet were, however, complex and studies to replicate them are in progress. Among women with low intakes of animal protein, a higher carbohydrate intake was associated with a higher adult blood pressure in the offspring; among those with high animal protein intakes, a lower carbohydrate intake was associated with higher blood pressure. These increases in blood pressure were associated with decreased placental size (65). Support for the thesis that alterations in fetal and placental development may result from a low ratio of animal protein to carbohydrate comes from observational studies of maternal nutrition in pregnancy (58). Support for adverse effects of a high ratio of animal protein to carbohydrate comes from a review of 16 trials of protein supplementation showing that supplements with a high protein density were consistently associated with lower birthweight (66).

Evidence that maternal body composition has important effects on the offspring has come from studies showing that extremes of maternal body composition in pregnancy are associated with adverse long-term outcomes in the offspring. Follow-up of a group of Jamaican children showed that those whose mothers had thin skinfold thicknesses in pregnancy and a low pregnancy weight gain had higher blood pressure at the age of 11 yr (67). A subsequent study of 11-yr-old children in Birmingham, UK, found similar associations (68). Studies in India have found that a low maternal weight in pregnancy is associated with an increased risk of CHD in the offspring in adult life (14). Among men and women exposed to the Dutch famine in utero those whose mothers had low

Table 5
Standardized Mortality Ratios for CHD in Finnish Men According
to Ponderal Index at Birth and Mother's BMI in Late Pregnancy[a]

	BMI of mother (kg/m^2) of baby (kg/m^3)					
Ponderal index	≤ 24	–26	–28	–30	> 30	All
–25	56 (6)	134 (20)	158 (17)	131 (7)	171 (7)	124 (57)
–27	88 (12)	87 (21)	123 (26)	104 (11)	131 (11)	104 (81)
–29	46 (5)	76 (17)	55 (13)	98 (12)	116 (16)	76 (63)
>29	38 (2)	61 (7)	45 (7)	68 (6)	72 (9)	58 (31)
All	62 (25)	89 (65)	89 (63)	97 (36)	111 (43)	89 (232)

[a]Figures in parentheses are numbers of deaths.

weight in pregnancy had the most impaired glucose tolerance (34). At the other extreme of maternal body fatness, evidence for long-term effects of maternal *obesity* has come from follow-up of a group of men born in Finland early in the 20th century (11). Markedly raised CHD rates were found in men whose mothers had a high body mass index in pregnancy (*see* Table 5). This effect was independent of an association between thinness at birth and increased rates of adult CHD. Modeling the data to derive contour lines of similar CHD death rates indicated that increasing maternal BMI had little effect on the offspring's death rates in tall women, but strong effects in short women (11,45). One interpretation of these findings is that greater maternal body fatness may increase fetal growth and hence the fetal demand for nutrients; short women may not be able to meet this increased demand as a result of a constrained nutrient supply capacity determined during their own intrauterine development (11).

Studies in South India and among the Pima Indians in Arizona suggest that non-insulin dependent diabetes may originate through maternal obesity and consequent hyperglycemia, which results in babies that are short and fat at birth (19,42). As adults, they tend to be insulin deficient. An interpretation of this is that high circulating glucose concentrations impair development of the pancreatic beta cells *in utero*, as has been shown experimentally in animals.

7. FUTURE RESEARCH

The complexities of fetal growth and development are such that currently available data form only a limited basis for changing dietary recommendations to pregnant women. Previous studies of maternal nutrition have adopted too simplistic an approach to assessing the true impact of nutrition on fetal development. They have failed to address the possibility of long-term effects on the health of the offspring in adult life

In order to reduce chronic disease in later life, we now need to understand how the human fetus is nourished, and how undernutrition programs its metabolism.

Fetal development is, of course, governed by complex, nonlinear systems. Components of these systems interact, and the systems will have generic properties that do not depend on the details of their components *(69)*. We cannot, therefore, solve our problems by reductionist science alone. We need to combine it with further clinical and epidemiological research.

REFERENCES

1. Pisa Z, Uemura K. Trends of mortality from ischaemic heart disease and other cardiovascular diseases in 27 countries, 1968–1977. World Health Stat Q 1982; 35:11–47.
2. Barker DJP, Osmond C. Diet and coronary heart disease in England and Wales during and after the second world war. J Epidemiol Community Health 1986; 40:37–44.
3. Keys A. 1980. Seven Countries. Harvard University Press, Cambridge, MA.
4. Rose G, Marmot MG. Social class and coronary heart disease. Br Heart J 1981; 45:13–19.
5. Rose G. Sick individuals and sick populations. Int J Epidemiol 1985; 14:32–38.
6. Barker DJP, Osmond C. Infant mortality, childhood nutrition and ischaemic heart disease in England and Wales. Lancet 1986; 1:1077–1081.
7. Osmond C, Barker, DJP, Winter, PD, Fall, CHD, Simmonds, SJ. Early growth and death from cardiovascular disease in women. BMJ 1993; 307:1519–1524.
8. Barker DJP, Osmond C, Simmonds SJ, Wield GA. The relation of small head circumference and thinness at birth to death from cardiovascular disease in adult life. BMJ 1993; 306:422–426.
9. Martyn CN, Barker DJP, Osmond C. Mothers' pelvic size, fetal growth, and death from stroke and coronary heart disease in men in the UK. Lancet 1996; 348:1264–1268.
10. Leon DA, Lithell HO, Vagero D, Koupilova I, Mohsen R, Berglund L, et al. Reduced fetal growth rate and increased risk of death from ischaemic heart disease: cohort study of 15,000 Swedish men and women born 1915–29. BMJ 1998; 317:241–245.
11. Forsen T, Eriksson JG, Tuomilehto J, Teramo K, Osmond C, Barker DJP. Mother's weight in pregnancy and coronary heart disease in a cohort of Finnish men: follow up study. BMJ 1997; 315:837–840.
12. Frankel S, Elwood P, Sweetnam P, Yarnell J, Davey Smith G. Birthweight, body- mass index in middle age, and incident coronary heart disease. Lancet 1996; 348:1478–1480.
13. Rich-Edwards JW, Stampfer MJ, Manson JE, Rosner B, Hankinson SE, Colditz GA, et al. Birth weight and risk of cardiovascular disease in a cohort of women followed up since 1976. BMJ 1997; 315:396–400.
14. Stein CE, Fall CHD, Kumaran K, Osmond C, Cox V, Barker DJP. Fetal growth and coronary heart disease in South India. Lancet 1996; 348:1269–1273.
15. Hales CN, Barker DJP, Clark PMS, Cox LJ, Fall C, Osmond C, Winter PD. Fetal and infant growth and impaired glucose tolerance at age 64. BMJ 1991; 303:1019–1022.
16. Barker DJP, Gluckman PD, Godfrey KM, Harding JE, Owens JA, Robinson JS. Fetal nutrition and cardiovascular disease in adult life. Lancet 1993; 341:938–941.
17. Barker DJP. Fetal origins of coronary heart disease. BMJ 1995; 311:171–174.
18. Valdez R, Athens MA, Thompson GH, Bradshaw BS, Stern MP. Birthweight and adult health outcomes in a biethnic population in the USA. Diabetologia 1994; 37:624–631.
19. McCance DR, Pettitt DJ, Hanson RL, Jacobsson LTH, Knowler WC, Bennett PH. Birth weight and non-insulin dependent diabetes: thrifty genotype, thrifty phenotype, or surviving small baby genotype? BMJ 1994; 308:942–945.
20. Curhan GC, Willett WC, Rimm B, Stampfer MJ. Birth weight and adult hypertension and diabetes mellitus in US men. Am J Hypertens 1996; 9:11.
21. Lithell HO, McKeigue PM, Berglund L, Mohsen R, Lithell UB, Leon DA. Relation of size at birth to non-insulin dependent diabetes and insulin concentrations in men aged 50–60 yr. BMJ 1996; 312:406–410.

22. Law CM, Shiell AW. Is blood pressure inversely related to birth weight? The strength of evidence from a systematic review of the literature. J Hypertens 1996; 14:935–941.

23. Nilsson PM, Ostergren PO, Nyberg P, Soderstrom M, Allebeck P. Low birth weight is associated with elevated systolic blood pressure in adolescence: a prospective study of a birth cohort of 149 378 Swedish boys. J Hypertens 1997; 15:1627–1631.

24. Cohen MP, Stern E, Rusecki Y, Zeidler A. High prevalence of diabetes in young adult Ethiopian immigrants to Israel. Diabetes 1988; 37:824–828.

25. McCance RA, Widdowson EM. The determinants of growth and form. Proc R Soc Lond B 1974; 185:1–17.

26. Gluckman PD, Breier BH, Oliver M, Harding J, Bassett N. Fetal growth in late gestation—a constrained pattern of growth. Acta Paediatr Scand Suppl 1990; 367:105–110.

27. Stearns, S. Evolution in health and disease. Oxford University Press, Oxford, UK, 1998.

28. Brooks AA, Johnson MR, Steer PJ, Pawson ME, Abdalla HI. Birth weight: nature or nurture? Early Hum Dev 1995; 42:29–35.

29. Dicke JM. Poor obstetrical outcome. In: Pauerstein CJ, ed. Clinical Obstetrics. John Wiley and Sons, New York, 1987, pp. 421–439.

30. Fowden AL. The role of insulin in prenatal growth. J Dev Physiol 1989; 12:173–182.

31. Langley-Evans SC, Jackson AA. Increased systolic blood pressure in adult rats induced by fetal exposure to maternal low protein diets. Clin Sci 1994; 86:217–222.

32. Desai M, Crowther NJ, Ozanne SE, Lucas A, Hales CN. Adult glucose and lipid metabolism may be programmed during fetal life. Biochem Soc Trans 1995; 23:331–335.

33. Hoet JJ, Hanson MA. Intrauterine nutrition: its importance during critical periods for cardiovascular and endocrine development. J Physiol 1999; 514.3:617–627.

34. Ravelli ACJ, van der Meulen JHP, Michels RPJ, Osmond C, Barker DJP, Hales CN, Bleker OP. Glucose tolerance in adults after prenatal exposure to famine. Lancet 351:173–177.

35. Harding JE, Johnston BM. Nutrition and fetal growth. Reprod Fertil Dev 1995; 7:539–547.

36. Barker DJP, Hales CN, Fall CHD, Osmond C, Phipps K, Clark PMS. Type 2 (non-insulin-dependent) diabetes mellitus, hypertension and hyperlipidaemia (syndrome X): relation to reduced fetal growth. Diabetologia 1993; 36:62–67.

37. Martyn CN, Greenwald SE. Impaired synthesis of elastin in walls of aorta and large conduit arteries during early development as an intiating event in pathogenesis of systemic hypertension. Lancet 1997; 350:953–955.

38. Barker DJP, Meade TW, Fall CHD, Lee A, Osmond C, Phipps K, Stirling Y. Relation of fetal and infant growth to plasma fibrinogen and factor VII concentrations in adult life. BMJ 1992; 304:148–152.

39. Barker DJP, Martyn CN, Osmond C, Hales CN, Fall CHD. Growth in utero and serum cholesterol concentrations in adult life. BMJ 1993; 307:1524–1527.

40. Barker DJP, Martyn CN, Osmond C, Wield GA. Abnormal liver growth in utero and death from coronary heart disease. BMJ 1995; 310:703–704.

41. Vijayakumar M, Fall CHD, Osmond C, Barker DJP. Birth weight, weight at one year, and left ventricular mass in adult life. Br Heart J 1995; 73:363–367.

42. Fall CHD, Stein CE, Kumaran K, Cox V, Osmond C, Barker DJP, Hales CN. Size at birth, maternal weight, and type 2 diabetes in South India. Diabet Med 1998; 15:220–227.

43. Barker DJP, Bull AR, Osmond C, Simmonds SJ. Fetal and placental size and risk of hypertension in adult life. BMJ 1990; 301:259–262.

44. McCrabb GJ, Egan AR, Hosking BJ. Maternal undernutrition during mid-pregnancy in sheep; variable effects on placental growth. J Agric Sci 1992; 118:127–132.

45. Barker DJP. Mothers, Babies and Health in Later Life. Churchill Livingstone, Edinburgh, 1998.

46. Harding JE, Liu L, Evans P, Oliver M, Gluckman P. Intrauterine feeding of the growth-retarded fetus: can we help? Early Hum Dev 1992; 29:193–197.

47. Kleeman DO, Walker SK, Seamark RF. Enhanced fetal growth in sheep administered progesterone during the first three days of pregnancy. J Reprod Fertil 1994; 102:411–417.

48. Walker SK, Hartwich KM, Seamark RF. The production of unusually large offspring following embryo manipulation: concepts and challenges. Theriogenology 1996; 45:111–120.
49. Leese HJ. The energy metabolism of the pre-implantation embryo. In: Heyner S, Wiley L eds. Early Embryo Development and Paracrine Relationships. Alan R. Liss, New York, 1990, pp. 67–78.
50. Stewart RJC, Sheppard H, Preece R, Waterlow JC. The effect of rehabilitation at different stages of development of rats marginally malnourished for ten to twelve generations. Br J Nutr 1980, 43:403–412.
51. Klebanoff MA, Meirik O, Berendes HW. Second-generation consequences of small-for-dates birth. Pediatrics 1989; 84:343–347.
52. Emanuel I, Filakti H, Alberman E, Evans SJW. Intergenerational studies of human birthweight from the 1958 birth cohort. I. Evidence for a multigenerational effect. Br J Obstet Gynaecol 1992; 99:67–74.
53. Godfrey KM, Barker DJP, Robinson S, Osmond C. Maternal birthweight and diet in pregnancy in relation to the infant's thinness at birth. Br J Obstet Gynaecol 1997; 104:663–667.
54. DeChiara T, Efstratiadis A, Robertson EJ. A growth-deficiency phenotype in heterozygous mice carrying an insulin-like growth fctor II gene disrupted by targeting. Nature 1990; 345:78–80.
55. Robinson JS, Owens JA, de Barro T, Lok F, Chidzanja S. Maternal nutrition and fetal growth. In: Ward RHT, Smith SK, Donnai D, eds. Early fetal growth and development. Royal College of Obstetricians and Gynaecologists, London, 1994, pp. 317–334.
56. Robinson JS, Hartwich KM, Walker SK, Erwich JJHM, Owens JA. Early influences on embryonic and placental growth. Acta Paediatr Suppl 1997; 423:159–163.
57. Slen, SB. Wool production and body growth in sheep. In: Cuthbertson D, ed. Nutrition of Animals of Agricultural Importance. Part 2. Assessment of and Factors Affecting the Requirements of Farm Livestock. Pergamon Press, Oxford, 1969, pp. 827–848.
58. Godfrey K, Robinson S, Barker DJP, Osmond C, Cox V. Maternal nutrition in early and late pregnancy in relation to placental and fetal growth. BMJ 1996; 312:410–414.
59. Robinson JS, Chidzanja S, Kind K, Lok F, Owens P, Owens JA. Placental control of fetal growth. Reprod Fertil Dev 1995; 7:333–344.
60. Kind KL, Clifton PM, Katsman AI, Tsiounis M, Robinson JS, Owens JA. Restricted fetal growth and the response to dietary cholesterol in the guinea pig. Am J Physiol 1999; 277:R1675–R1682.
61. Eriksson JG, Forsen T, Tuomilehto J, Winter PD, Osmond C, Barker DJP. Catch-up growth in childhood and death from coronary heart disease: longitudinal study. BMJ 1999; 318:427–431.
62. Robinson SM, Wheeler T, Hayes MC, Barker DJP, Osmond C. Fetal heart rate and intrauterine growth. Br J Obstet Gynaecol 1991; 98:1223–1227.
63. Hales CN, Desai M, Ozanne SE, Crowther NJ. Fishing in the stream of diabetes: from measuring insulin to the control of fetal organogenesis. Biochem Soc Trans 1996; 24:341–350.
64. Pitts GC. Cellular aspects of growth and catch-up growth in the rat: A reevaluation. Growth 1986; 50:419–436.
65. Campbell DM, Hall MH, Barker DJP, Cross J, Shiell AW, Godfrey KM. Diet in pregnancy and the offspring's blood pressure 40 years later. Br J Obstet Gynaecol 1996; 103:273–280.
66. Rush D. Effects of changes in maternal energy and protein intake during pregnancy, with special reference to fetal growth. In: Sharp F, Fraser RB, Milner RDG, eds. Fetal Growth. Royal College of Obstetricians and Gynaecologists, London, 1989, pp. 203–233.
67. Godfrey KM, Forrester T, Barker DJP, Jackson AA, Landman JP, Hall JStE, Cox V, Osmond C. Maternal nutritional status in pregnancy and blood pressure in childhood. Br J Obstet Gynaecol 1994; 101:398–403.
68. Clark PM, Atton C, Law CM, Shiell A, Godfrey K, Barker DJP. Weight gain in pregnancy, triceps skinfold thickness and blood pressure in the offspring. Obstet Gynaecol 1998, 91:103–107.
69. Goldberger AL. Non-linear dynamics for clinicians: chaos theory fractals, and complexity at the bedside. Lancet 1996; 347:1312–1314.

17 Impact of Nutritional Epidemiology

Barrie M. Margetts

1. INTRODUCTION

Nutritional epidemiology is concerned with exploring the relationship between nutrition and health in human populations *(1)*. It has developed out of an epidemiological approach, classically defined as the study of the *distribution* and *determinants* of health-related conditions or events in defined populations, and the application of this study to the control of health problems *(2)*. Distribution refers to analysis of time, place, and classes of persons affected; determinants are all the physiological, biological, social, cultural, and behavioral factors that influence health. Why nutritional epidemiology? Nutritional epidemiology is the only method in nutritional sciences that provides direct information on nutrition and health in human populations consuming usual amounts of foods and nutrients. Whenever information on diet or nutrition is being collected and related to a health problem, there are important methodological issues that need to be considered to minimize the likelihood of obtaining biased, and therefore, unhelpful, information. The underlying objective of all nutritional epidemiological research should be to improve health. Poor quality information does not help achieve this objective.

The impact of nutritional epidemiology is to provide an insight into the nutritional factors that may cause, and prevent, nutrition-related health problems; used properly, it should guide metabolic research that can explore causal mechanisms in more depth. Metabolic studies can highlight the clues that can be further assessed in epidemiological studies to explore whether the proposed mechanism may have some relevance in human health. Much metabolic research is undertaken on the justification of the impact the research will have on human health, but often with little consideration as to how the work fits in with epidemiological research. For example, the effects of specific carcinogens or phytochemicals in the potential food supply are studied in animal models in vivo in doses that are

From: *Nutritional Health: Strategies for Disease Prevention*
Edited by: T. Wilson and N. J. Temple © Humana Press Inc., Totowa, NJ

not relevant to human exposure, or based on assumptions about bioavailability in humans that are not tested or justified. Researchers across the breadth of nutrition have a responsibility to work together to provide information in a coherent manner that can be used to inform those responsible for making decisions about what we should or should not eat or about the risk/harm of foods we are exposed to. Nutritional epidemiology helps provide an evidence-based approach to the solution of important public health problems.

This chapter provides some guidance as to how to design and interpret nutritional epidemiological studies; to help the non-specialist in nutritional epidemiology to make sense of work in this area. It seems almost a rule of nature that "experts" in a field develop language and jargon to describe their field of work in such a way as to exclude others. It is hoped that this chapter can shed some light on the big issues in nutritional epidemiology in a clear and helpful manner, and encourage you to read further *(3,4)*.

2. EXPOSURE, OUTCOME, AND OTHER VARIABLES

Before starting any nutritional epidemiological study, it is essential to be clear about what you want to measure and how accurately you need to measure these factors. The research should begin with a sound review of the relevant literature that identifies the key factors, and likely strength of associations, being investigated. Without this information, it will not be possible to design a sound study. A clear research question (hypothesis) will identify the relevant measures of exposure, outcome, and also other factors or variables that may influence the relationship between exposure and outcome.

2.1. Exposure

Exposure is a generic term to describe factors (variables or measures) to which a person or group of people come into contact with and that may be relevant to their health *(5)*. This could include food and the constituents of foods (nutrients and nonnutrients), smoking, alcohol, air pollution, noise, dietary advice, or health promotion via advertisements or the social environment; in other words, any factor that has an impact on a person or group may be defined as an exposure.

2.2. Outcome

Outcome is another generic term used to describe factors (variables/ measures) that are being studied in relation to the effects of an exposure; often these outcome measures are disease states, but they may also be anthropometric or physiological measures. Depending on the study, these outcome measures may be expressed as continuous or discrete variables. Often an outcome with a continuous distribution will be divided into categories and a measure of effect assessed across these categories. For example, blood pressure may be analyzed as a continuous outcome measure or subjects may be categorized into those with or without hypertension on the basis of whether they fall above or below an agreed cutoff point. Even for nominally discrete outcome measures, such as disease state, it should be recognized that there is not a clear distinction between presence and absence of disease, that diseases progress and at some point in that progression, the disease may become diagnosed.

2.3. Other Variables: Confounding and Effect Modification

A major issue to consider in interpreting epidemiological research is the possibility that variables other than the exposure of interest have influenced the true relationship between exposure and outcome. These other variables need to be measured so that their effects on the exposure–outcome relationship can be properly investigated. It is common practice to adjust the relationship between exposure and outcome for these other variables using regression, or some other, statistical approach. However, this approach may mislead. If a variable that has been adjusted for is in the causal pathway then the adjusted estimate of the effect of the exposure on the outcome will be weakened. If the relationship between exposure and outcome differs at different levels of the other variable, an adjusted effect will mask important biological interaction. It is, therefore, important to consider the way in which the other variables that are being adjusted for may relate to the exposure, the outcome and the relationship between exposure and outcome.

Confounders are associated with both exposure and outcome and distort the relationship under investigation. For a variable to be a confounder:

1. It must be associated with, but not causally dependent on the exposure of interest;
2. It must be a risk factor for outcome, independent of its association with the exposure of interest;
3. The foregoing must apply within the population under study.

A confounder cannot lie in the causal pathway.

Effect modifiers are variables where the effect of the exposure on the outcome operates differently at different levels of the other variable. Such an effect is referred to as an interaction. An effect modifier will lie in the causal pathway that relates the exposure of interest to the outcome.

It is never possible to eliminate the effects of all potential confounders (this is referred to as residual confounding), and it is therefore important to measure known or suspected confounders so that they can be considered in the analysis. Where variables are known to be confounders, the investigator can control for them either in the design (by randomization, restriction (e.g., exclude smokers), or matching) or in the analysis (by stratification and/or multiple regression), provided sufficient valid information is available on the confounding factor. It will not be possible to control the confounder if it has not been measured, or has been measured poorly.

It is not always easy to disentangle the effects of other variables. Always check before statistically adjusting as to whether the other variables are likely to be confounders or effect modifiers. It is optimal to do this before the study starts, so that the study can be designed accordingly, but if this is not possible, it can be done in the analysis. The best approach is to undertake a series of analyses stratified by the variable of interest. Confounding can be adjusted for in an analysis; when there is effect modification, the results for each stratum of the variable should be presented separately and the variable should not be adjusted for. The need for undertaking stratum specific analyses should be considered in the way the study is designed to ensure that there are sufficient subjects in each stratum of analysis. If the sample size is too small, stratum specific estimates of effect may have wide confidence intervals that may suggest no statistically significant effect when in fact there is one.

Diet is a most complex exposure to measure where there may be both confounding and effect modification between aspects of diet, and between sociodemographic factors, and other biological variables such as body mass. One of the major challenges over the next few years will be to understand the effects of dietary patterns where higher consumption of "protective" factors may simply reflect lower consumption of "harmful" factors. For example, in Europe and North America, people who eat more fruits and vegetables tend to eat less meat and animal fat. Is the apparent protective effect of fruit and vegetable intake due to increased intake of substances in these foods, or the lower consumption of other harmful substances in meat and animal fats? How to deal with this? If the exposure of interest is fruit intake, the researchers should stratify subjects by level of meat consumption and assess whether the relationship between fruit and cancer differs at different levels of meat intake. If it does, this would suggest an interaction between meat and fruit, and stratum specific, rather than meat adjusted results should be presented. If the effect of fruit does not interact with the effect of meat, but meat consumers have a higher risk of cancer independently of fruit and they also eat less fruit, then meat will be a confounder and should be adjusted for in the analysis. Gender is often considered to be a confounder, because intake differs by gender, and disease rates are usually higher in men. However, gender may be an effect modifier in some circumstances, for example, where there may be some hormone-related effect with gender acting as a proxy for an underlying etiological difference.

3. MEASUREMENT OF NUTRITIONAL EXPOSURE, OUTCOME, AND OTHER VARIABLES

Whenever information is obtained from any source about exposure, outcome, or other variables of interest, it is important to consider whether the information that is collected measures what is required with an appropriate level of accuracy. In this chapter, the emphasis is placed on measures of nutritional exposure, but it is essential to have some indication of the validity of the measures of outcome (e.g., accuracy and completeness in an unbiased sample) *and* potential confounders and effect modifiers. There is no one right way to make any of these measures, the method used must be appropriate for the study being undertaken. It is important to be able to check the assumptions that the measures used are valid (consider also whether the measures are able to differentiate between subjects above and below cutoff points—sensitivity and specificity) before the study begins because it may not be possible to adjust for measurement error appropriately in the analysis.

3.1. Nutritional Exposure

Nutritional exposure may cover individual foods or dietary patterns as well as the substances added to foods. It may include:

1. The components found in foods (either nutrients or nonnutrients, such as phytochemicals)
2. Substances added to food during the growing, manufacture, and processing of the food (additives, preservatives, pesticides)
3. Chemical alterations that occur during cooking
4. Markers of the dietary intake measured in body tissues or in bodily excretions

In some situations, nutritional exposure is inferred from anthropometric measurements or clinical signs of deficiency. Depending on which of the above measures is the intended exposure, different approaches will be required, and different assumptions need to be made (and checked) about the validity and quality of the measures used to approximate the exposure.

The exposure needs to be measured with sufficient accuracy to enable the primary question of the research to be answered with reasonable confidence.

4. METHODS USED TO MEASURE DIET

The selection of an appropriate method to measure exposure and the correct use of that method must be considered before the study proper begins. Other texts have covered the different approaches that can be used to measure diet (6,7).

Broadly the appropriate methods may be described in terms of:
- The sample:
- Individual
  - Group
  - Population
- Time frame
  - Current or past intake
  - Usual intake
- Critical period (biologically relevant)

- Unit of interest:
  - Food
  - Food patterns
  - Nutrients
  - Nonnutrients (as currently defined)
- Unit of expression:
  - Absolute or relative intake (grams of fat or percent energy from fat)
  - Cumulative exposure over time (e.g., total lifetime calcium intake)
  - The average exposure over time (e.g., amount of fat per day)
  - Peak exposure at a critical time (e.g., folate intake in first trimester of pregnancy)
- Level of accuracy required: study specific based on question being addressed

5. VALIDATION

As mentioned earlier, whenever any information is being collected it is important to asses whether it is *fit for purpose*, i.e., whether the measure used is valid. A measure is valid if it measures what it purports to measure. This implies that there is a true measure of the variable against which the new or alternative measure *(test)* is compared. In most situations it is not possible to have an absolute measure of the true exposure, and the new or test measure of exposure is usually compared with another measure that is considered from previous research to be more accurate (the *reference measure*) than the new measure. A study that compares these measures is a validation study, but should be referred to as a study of the *relative validity* (sometimes called concurrent validity) of the test compared with the reference measure.

If a test measure is compared with a reference measure, it is assumed that the reporting errors in the test measure are not related to the errors in the reference measure. If they are, then the measure of agreement used to express the relationship between test and reference measure will be invalid (usually an overestimate of the true agreement). It is becoming more common to include a third measure, usually a biological measure, in to a study of the validity of a test measure *(8)*. The rationale for this is that the errors associated with measuring a biological sample are likely to be independent from the errors of a measure derived from information supplied by a subject (e.g., the test measure may be a food-frequency questionnaire and the reference measure may be a 4–7-d weighted record.). An important assumption is that the biological measure is a relevant marker of the true exposure and is sensitive to changes in intake across the range of exposure in the population under study.

The correct way to express the results from a validation study depend on how the measures are going to be used in the main study. If absolute intakes are required, then the validation must assess how well the test measure assesses absolute intake. If the purpose is to rank subjects and assess change in risk across levels of exposure (say fourths or fifths), then the validation study must assess the degree of misclassification likely between fourths or fifths of the distribution. Simply expressing the association between a test and reference measure using a correlation coefficient may be misleading, and unhelpful. Ideally, the required level of accuracy of the test measure should be established before the study begins. The measure of validity can then be used in the design, analysis, and interpretation of the main study. Where the measure of validity is assessed during, rather than before, the main study careful thought needs to be given as to how the results will be analyzed and used in the interpretation of the main study.

5.1. Adjustment for Measurement Error

It is not sufficient to state that the measure was validated; the impact of the lack of perfect agreement between the test measure and the true measure (as judged by comparison with a reference measure) must be considered in the analysis and interpretation of the main study. There are now statistical techniques available to adjust for this lack of perfect agreement, and is usually described as adjusting for measurement error (4). Before believing these adjusted results, it is important to judge whether assumptions used in these adjustment models are robust and appropriate for the data being analyzed. Most adjustment approaches assume that the errors are random; in practice this is rarely likely to be the case.

Current guidance would suggest that both adjusted and unadjusted results should be presented to allow the reader to see the impact that adjustment has on the results.

6. UNDER- AND OVERREPORTING

Much has been written about underreporting; some might conclude that it is not possible to assess dietary intake based on self-reported measures because people lie about how much they eat. This may be true where absolute levels of exposure are required, but may not be the case where relative measures (ranking, categorizing) are required. It is not really helpful to make blanket statements about the usefulness of any methods. A more subtle approach is required that takes into account the requirements for the appropriate use of the measure being used. Of particular concern is when people with certain characteristics under or over report their intake differently from the whole sample. For example, overweight subjects underreporting their intake differently from those of average weight, or women with breast cancer over estimating their fat intake compared to women without breast cancer. If it is assumed the error is random, and therefore the estimate of effect is attenuated (reduced), when in fact the errors are nonrandom and differential, then the measure of effect can either be attenuated or exaggerated, leading to the wrong interpretation of the meaning of the results.

It is therefore necessary to assess the likely size and effect of under- or overreporting in the study. This can be done by comparing measured intakes with true intakes or proxy measures. Most work has been done on energy intake, using measures of energy expenditure as a check. If energy intake is less than measured energy expenditure, then it may be concluded that energy intake is underreported if subjects are not losing weight or in an unstable metabolic condition. Black and colleagues *(9)* have shown that underreporting can occur across the whole range of intakes, and that it may be misleading to use an arbitrary cutoff to define underreporting. For epidemiological purposes, energy expenditure can be estimated using a regression equation that only requires information on the age, gender, and weight of the subject *(10)*. This simple measure of basal metabolic rate (BMR) relates well to measured energy expenditure and can be used to compare energy expenditure with a measure of dietary intake. If the estimated energy intake is less than the BMR (or a bit more to allow for some level of activity—often 1.2 × BMR, *see* ref. *9* for more details), it suggests that the estimated energy intake is unrealistically low.

There are several ways that this measure of underreporting should be used in the analysis and interpretation of the study. It is often assumed that all subjects below an agreed level of the energy/BMR (E/BMR) ratio should simply be excluded from the study. However, before doing this, and thereby losing considerable statistical power, it is worth exploring whether the underreporting has led to a biased estimate of effect (altered the relationship between the measured exposure estimate and outcome). Ideally, the relationship between exposure and outcome should be explored separately in people with E/BMR ratios above and below the agreed cutoff. If the relationship found within each stratum of E/BMR is different, then there is a suggestion of bias and the results from the two strata should not be combined because the estimated measure of effect would be incorrect. If, however, the relationship is similar in each stratum, it may suggest that there is no bias and that the estimate of effect would not be distorted by leaving all the subjects in the analysis. It is also worth checking whether the E/BMR ratio is different in different levels of other potentially confounding factors such as age, gender, and body mass index (BMI). If overweight people underestimate their intake more than average-weight people, and if BMI is associated with the exposure–outcome relationship, then it will be important to take account of the differential underreporting of energy intake in overweight subjects.

Intakes of other nutrients or foods may also be under- or overreported. The direction of effect may depend on a host of factors related to the perception of subjects and the methods used. It is often assumed that vegetable and fruit consumption is overestimated and that fat intake is underestimated. However, the analysis of recalled fat intake in women with breast cancer, when compared to actual intake 10 yr before, suggested that women overestimated their past intake *(4)*. The reason put forward was that women who had breast cancer and "knew fat caused breast cancer" overestimated their true past exposure. Apart from a reasonably accurate biological marker of energy expenditure and perhaps protein intake (multiple 24 h urinary nitrogen excretion), there are few measures of true dietary exposure that can be used to check the accuracy of reported intakes.

7. REPRODUCIBILITY

Reproducibility assesses the repeatability of a measure while taking account of the circumstances in which the measures were taken. The repeatability is often referred to as precision or reliability and assesses the consistency with which a method measures exposure. Differences between repeat measures may be due either to:

1. True subject variation for that measure
2. The effect of observer (measurement) error
3. Changes in the circumstances of the application of the method
4. Differences in other characteristics of the subjects

It is difficult to distinguish between the true subject variation; observer effects, and changes in the circumstances under which the repeat measure is obtained. This may be particularly true in repeat measures of diet where learning effects may over estimate the agreement between repeat measures. Although theoretically straight-forward, assessing the reproducibility of a measure is difficult.

8. ENERGY ADJUSTMENT

The concept of energy density and the optimal approach to expressing the levels of intakes, particularly of macronutrients (protein, fat, and carbohydrate), has been debated for many years. The prevailing view suggests that the relevant measure of exposure for macronutrients is the intake relative to energy intake, rather than a simple measure of absolute intake. One reason for expressing macronutrient intake relative to energy intake is that it makes it easier to compare intakes across different levels of energy intake, for example, men and women and different ages. In judging whether it is appropriate to adjust for energy intake, it is important to consider whether it is logical from a biological or mechanistic perspective. Data should be analyzed with and without adjusting for energy to assess the impact that adjusting may have on the interpretation of results. It may be that for some situations the absolute level of intake is a more relevant measure of exposure.

Energy adjustment is most useful when the following conditions hold true (after Flegal, *11*):

- The exposure of interest is not the absolute amount of the nutrient but the amount relative to energy.
- Energy over- or underreporting is proportionally the same for all foods, so that the correct proportion of the nutrient to energy intake is reported.

If these conditions do not apply, energy adjustment may be misleading.

9. BIOLOGICAL SAMPLES

Samples may be taken from a wide range of body tissues and fluids and are potentially useful markers or indicators of exposure and outcome. The use of biological markers of dietary intake is attractive because they appear to be more objective measurements of exposure than measures of intake derived by questioning the subjects themselves. This assumption should always be tested before using biological markers to infer dietary intake. A particular issue to consider is that most markers do not provide a measure of absolute intake, only the relative ranking of intakes. Although the technical errors of measurement of markers may be smaller, the marker may not be a relevant measure of the dietary exposure of interest. For a biological marker to be a useful indicator of exposure, it must be sensitively and specifically related to dietary intake across the range of intakes in the population under study. Ideally, as the level of dietary exposure increases or decreases, so to should the level of the biological marker. That is, there should be a time-related relationship between the marker and the dietary intake of interest. This may be the case, for example, between urinary nitrogen excretion and dietary protein intake, but for most other readily available markers this is not the case. Most markers used at present are concentrations in blood, which may not accurately reflect the intake over the time frame required. There are a complex series of steps involved in the absorption, transport, and distribution of a nutrient found in food and subsequently measured as a biological sample. The circulating level may be dependent on a range of other potentially rate-limiting factors. It may be, therefore, that there is only a weak relationship between dietary intake and a marker because the level measured in blood, for example, is dependent on a transport protein or other coenzymes. Kaaks and others *(12)* have discussed these issues further, as have other texts *(3,4)*.

Although the potential benefits of biomarkers are attractive, they should not be used uncritically. The following should be considered:

- Most markers can generally only be used as indicators of the relative ranking of individual dietary intakes in a group and do not generally provide a measure that is relevant to the absolute dietary intake.
- Most markers are measured as a concentration that may not reflect the amount of the substance available at the site of biological function; blood levels may be regulated by the body and may not truly reflect the availability of the substance; removal or addition of a substance to the measure used in the blood may be limited by the availability of other related limiting substances (e.g., retinol binding protein).
- Correlations between true intake levels and markers tend not be any better than between true intake and more traditional dietary methods (such as recalls and questionnaires). This may be partly explained by the relatively fast turnover rates in many markers and large intraindividual variation in true intake.
- The level of a marker, such as plasma β-carotene may only be partly determined by the dietary intake of carotene. The marker may be a proxy or indicator of a dietary pattern.
- The level of the marker may be affected by other factors, such as smoking, or drugs.

10. TYPES OF EPIDEMIOLOGICAL STUDIES

Broadly, epidemiological studies can be divided into experimental and observational investigations (*see* Table 1). The main study designs are briefly summarized; other texts provide more detail *(3)*. For all studies where data are collected from individuals, some *a priori* information is required about how common the exposure and outcome are likely to be in the study population, and what effect the exposure is expected to have on outcome. Without this information, it will not be possible to ascertain how many subjects to include in a study, or how accurately exposure must be able to be measured. This assumes that in *all* studies before beginning the study, a thorough literature should be conducted to help in the design of the study.

10.1. Ecological Studies

In ecological studies of the association between nutrition and health, population or group indices of dietary intake or nutritional status (exposure) are related to population or group indices of health status (outcome). The unit of analysis is not an individual but a group defined by time (e.g., calendar year, birth cohort), geography (e.g., country, province, or city), or sociodemographic characteristics (e.g., ethnicity, religion, or socioeconomic status). For example, national dietary fat intake for each country in Europe (from FAO food balance sheet data) can be plotted against rates of heart disease for each country. Within a country, national trends for consumption of foods may be plotted against trends for morbidity or mortality. Ecological studies are helpful when within group (country or region) variation in exposure is small compared with between group variation. It is often difficult in ecological studies to control for other potentially confounding factors and to explore interactions. When comparing national levels of exposure and outcome it is important to consider the relevant time frame for comparison; there is likely to be some lag time between exposure and its effect on outcome.

Ecological studies are ideal for exploring newly proposed hypotheses; this serves as a basis for developing more detailed individual level studies in the future. Ecological studies are weak in terms of drawing causal inferences about the effects of factors operating at an individual level. In some situations, individual level data are not available, and an ecological approach is all that is available. Ecological studies may be very useful for monitoring national trends in health indicators and the wider social, cultural, economic, and environmental factors that influence health that cannot be measured at an individual level.

10.2. Cross-Sectional Studies

Cross-sectional studies (sometimes described as prevalence surveys) measure both exposure and outcome in the present and at the same point in time in individuals. Generally, cross-sectional studies sample from the population in such a

Table 1
Summary of Study Designs Used in Nutritional Epidemiological Research

Study design	Study group	
	Populations	Individuals
Experimental	Community trials or community intervention studies	Clinical trials (therapeutic or secondary or tertiary prevention) Field trials (primary prevention) Field intervention studies
Observational	Ecological studies	Cross-sectional (prevalence) studies Case-control (referent) studies Cohort (longitudinal) studies

way as to reflect the population characteristics for both exposure and outcome and thus can be used to describe the prevalence of nutrition problems in a community. If information on population characteristics (e.g., age, gender, income, education) are also collected, they can assess the influence these factors may have on the exposure-outcome relationship. When repeated in the same population, a cross-sectional survey can be used for surveillance and monitoring.

The sampling frame, number of subjects (sample size and power), response rate, and potential information bias may all influence the validity of the prevalence estimates derived. If a particular sector of the sample is excluded (e.g., malnourished children too sick to participate), the prevalence estimate and reported associations may be misleading. The optimal sample size should be calculated before the study starts to ensure that enough subjects are included. Sample size is determined by the prevalence of the measures of interest, differences expected in the estimates of prevalence between groups in the study, the accuracy of the measures, and the required level of statistical power. Failure to detect statistically significant differences between groups may be a function of sample size. If exposure and outcome measures are rare in a general population sample, a very large sample size will be required to estimate the prevalence of these measures with any accuracy.

In a cross-sectional study, the measure of interest is often expressed at a group level such as the average intake or proportion above a cutoff. As long as the distribution of the population can be correctly described to ensure that the measure of central tendency (such as the average) is correct, assuming a sufficiently large sample and that the errors of reporting exposure are random (rather than systematic in some way that may lead to bias), it does not matter if each individual's actual intake is not measured exactly. This means that a 24-h recall could be used, which does not estimate within-person variation. The researcher cannot describe individual intakes using this approach, and the identification of individuals at risk (of being too high or low) cannot be made; what can be said is that a certain proportion of the population may be above or below a cutoff.

The main disadvantage of cross-sectional studies is that it is not possible to disentangle cause from effect because the exposure is not measured before the onset of the outcome. It may be that, for example, the outcome or illness may have altered the dietary patterns, rather than the other way around (e.g., someone starts drinking milk after they get an ulcer to relieve symptoms). Although cross-sectional studies can take into account other potentially confounding factors, causal inferences cannot be drawn from such studies, primarily because the temporal sequence cannot be established.

10.3. Case-Control Studies

In case-control studies (or sometimes termed case-referent studies), patients with a disease (cases) are compared with controls who do not have the disease. Ideally, a population is defined (e.g., the catchment area of a hospital or the walking distance for mothers to bring malnourished children to a clinic) from which all cases of interest are identified over a specified period of time. This population must be sufficiently large to generate a statistically viable number of cases. Controls are then drawn at random from the same population from which the cases are drawn. All noncases could be recruited for comparison, but it is more statistically efficient to take a sample of the population. Controls are often selected at random and matched on certain characteristics that are known to influence outcome, but that of themselves are of no direct interest in the study (e.g., age and gender). Case-control designs are efficient where the outcome (e.g., ovarian or liver cancer) is rare (in an absolute sense) and all available cases can be recruited from the population of interest.

It is important to consider how commonly the exposure of interest (e.g., low meat intake or fat intake) occurs in the population; what determines the required sample size for the whole study is the number in the level of exposure at which it is believed risk of disease (or being a case) will be higher. For example, if the hypothesis was that being a vegetarian was protective against colon cancer, and the number of vegetarians required was, say 200, then the total number of subjects required would not be 400 cases and 400 controls, but 200 times the prevalence of vegetarianism (in the UK about 5%; thus need 20×200 cases and controls or 4000 cases and 4000 controls). If everybody has the same dietary intake, the study cannot help assess the role of variations in diet on disease outcome. The exposure must be able to be measured in the same way in cases and controls to avoid bias.

The dietary exposure of interest is usually some time in the past nearer to the time when diet may have been "causing" the disease to develop. A major potential weakness in case-control studies is differential recall bias between cases and controls, where cases recall past exposure either more or less accurately than controls. Case-control studies do not need to have absolutely accurate measures of exposure, but they must correctly rank the level of exposure in the same way in cases and controls. It is also possible that the disease process may affect the recall of past diet.

10.4. Cohort Studies

Cohort studies (sometimes called prospective studies) measure exposure in the present and outcome is assessed at some point in the future. Unlike cross-sectional surveys, a cohort study can be used to draw causal inferences about the effect of the exposure on outcome, as the exposure is measured before the outcome is known, and therefore not influenced by knowledge of the outcome status. The sample for a cohort study is not always selected to represent the distribution within the whole population. The sample may be weighted to maximize heterogeneity of exposure, or it might be selected to minimize loss to follow-up; both of these factors may be considered to be of more importance than the representativeness of the sample. For both cohort and experimental studies, the primary concern is to select a sample that is not going to be lost in the follow-up period. For example, a number of large cohort studies follow-up health professionals who have to be registered to maintain their practice, and so can be traced through these registers.

Cohort designs can be an efficient way of sampling rare exposures from the population; the benefit here is that it is possible to maximize the range of dietary exposure that can be studied. For example, vegetarians with very different dietary habits from the general population can be recruited and compared with a sample of omnivores to explore the effects of the dietary differences on health outcomes. If one was to take a random sample of the population, only about 5% are vegetarians, and so the sample would need to be very large to recruit sufficient vegetarians to have a statistically viable sample. It is important to consider how many people are required to be followed over what length of time to have sufficient disease endpoints to calculate an estimate of the risk of disease in the vegetarian group compared with the omnivore group.

In a cohort study, the exposure measure is often divided into thirds or fourths of the distribution and the change of risk assessed across these categories (logistic regression). The requirement for the measure of exposure in this type of analysis is that the measured intakes of subjects can accurately rank the true intake of the population (i.e., so that people with a high and low intake can be differentiated). The selection of the cutoff points used to define groups may critically affect the estimate of risk obtained. Some authors prefer to use a regression approach where instead of grouping data, each individual observation contributes to the regression equation (multiple regression); what is then described is the change in outcome per unit change in exposure. Both approaches, logistic and multiple regression, allow for the adjustment of the effects of other factors.

Cohort studies are often very large and may take many years to be conducted, and are usually expensive. As in other study designs, confounding factors need to be considered, as does the accuracy of the measures of exposure used. Measurement error and misclassification may lead to nonstatistically significant associations that may not reflect the true underlying associations.

10.5. Experimental Studies

Experimental studies are the most robust test of a causal hypothesis. An experiment is the only study design where the exposure "treatment" is actually manipulated by the researcher and the effect that manipulation has on outcome can be assessed. The most important aspect of experimental studies is that allocation to different treatment groups is random and not influenced either by the observer or the participant. In other respects, apart from random allocation of treatment, experimental studies may be considered to be similar to cohort studies. Experimental studies sometimes select representative samples of the whole population (community interventions), or sometimes samples of people from selected outcome groups (clinical trials). The primary issues to consider in designing an experiment are: what is the required length of follow-up to ensure that the treatment, if it is going to effect outcome, has time to alter metabolic processes necessary to affect outcome; how to check compliance with treatment regime; how to minimize observer and participant effects; and is the sample size adequate to measure the hypothesized effect with reasonable statistical confidence.

11. DEVELOPING CULTURALLY SENSITIVE AND SPECIFIC MEASURES OF EXPOSURE

Considerable effort has been expended in identifying optimal approaches to measuring dietary exposure in North American and European populations who are literate and numerate. Most approaches that have been developed assume a certain degree of literacy and numeracy. Extrapolating methods from one social group to another within a country is likely to lead to problems; these are magnified many times when extrapolating from one country and culture to another. The following list summarizes a number of key points to consider when developing methods, particularly where the researcher may not be familiar with the local situation. Wherever the research is conducted the best possible approach should be used, and where some compromise must be made, the effects this has on the validity of the study should be considered before the study begins. A poorly conducted study will not help address major public health problems because it will not answer the key questions. Lack of resources, although it is a real constraint for research and development in many parts of the world, should not be used as an excuse for poorly thought-through research. Priority must be given to addressing issues that are of major public health concern. It is also patronizing to suggest that a cheaper, secondhand approach is good enough in poorer countries, in many ways the opposite could be argued. Greatest effort and attention to detail should be directed to places of greatest need and potential impact. An important part of research should be to develop the human resources and skills base in each country in which the work is done.

General issues:
- If things can go wrong they probably will, so assume this as a starting point and avoid making assumptions based on your previous experience.
- When undertaking fieldwork consider the local infrastructure required to do the work.
- Consider the effect your presence will have on local coworkers' responsibilities and consider their needs, just as you would expect to be treated yourselves. Consider what local colleagues will get out of the work you are doing.
- If you use equipment in remote areas, consider what might happen if it goes wrong (and halfway through your study!). Always consider robust simple accurate methods and have a backup strategy.
- Decide what you really need to know and what level of support you require to gather that level of information (i.e., can individuals do what you want, do you have to use observational techniques or other approaches not dependent upon numeracy or literacy).
- Check whether your proposed fieldworkers are acceptable to the local community (in some communities women do not like strangers either watching them cook, or touching their food, but may be quite happy for a locally known person to do this).
- How do you get informed consent from subjects; if the community elders approve, is this adequate?

Specific dietary issues:
- Start the process by talking to the target group (focus group discussion) to identify how they describe foods and their preparation (and names used); this will help clarify whether your concepts are similar to those of the target group.
- Some foods may be taboo at certain times in certain groups of people; check this before you start; check fasting or festival days—in many cultures these occur very often and should be considered as part of a normal or usual diet (i.e., they should not always simply be excluded).
- Do not make assumptions about what appears to be a simple diet; consider the role of rarely eaten but rich sources of nutrients (or foods gathered in the field while working, as well as those cooked at home).
- Consider using complimentary methods such as 24-h recalls and FFQs together in cross-sectional or cohort studies; this combination of approaches may allow an estimate of gram weights of foods as well as an estimate of the frequency of consumption of rarely eaten foods that may be rich in nutrients.
- Assess whether you need to use an observational approach or whether you can rely on self-reported intakes (consider literacy, but also social desirability bias leading to dietary change).
- Where families eat from a communal pot, observational techniques may be required (if the research requires individual level assessment).
- Pretest and pilot different approaches before you start proper; it is likely your preconceived ideas are not appropriate.

- If you want amounts of foods consider all options; portion size estimation and assumptions may not be valid (e.g., in our study in India within-household variation in roti a local type of unleavened bread, size was very small from day to day, but between-household roti size was great; our approach was to weigh a series of rotis in each family before the study and use that as the portion size for that family).
- Where a staple is the main source of energy (or a single food item is the main source of a vitamin or mineral) estimating the correct portion size may be more important for that staple or food item, than where there is a wider variety of foods contributing to the nutrient of interest.
- Consider potential seasonal variation and other sources of foods not immediately obvious (such as food sent by friends or relatives in a city).
- Do you need to consider income elasticity and social issues when planning interventions to change dietary patterns? Consider income that may be sent from abroad and other family responsibilities.
- How to check the validity of the measures obtained?

Physical activity:

- Check concepts of distance and time before asking simple questions about length of time engaged in different activities; proxy measures may be required, and the validity of these measures will need to be checked.

12. SUMMARY OF KEY POINTS TO CONSIDER IN DESIGNING A NUTRITIONAL EPIDEMIOLOGICAL STUDY

Key points are summarized that may help the reader in either designing or critically reading a report of original research in nutritional epidemiology. The following information has been modified after Sempos et al. *(13)*.

- The goal is to assess how dietary exposure relates to health risk; different epidemiological approaches can be used, with strengths and weaknesses that need to be considered.
- The relationship between dietary exposure and health risk is complex; the link between what is eaten, absorbed, and incorporated into cell function, and the effect this has on biological processes that may affect "health" (i.e., the host's ability to maintain optimal function at the cellular, organ and whole body level), the effect may be modulated by other factors that need to be considered at the same time.
- Before using a method, it is essential to check whether it provides a measure that is appropriately accurate; this assumes that a validation study is undertaken before the proper study begins; the development of the method needs to take into account the social and cultural context in which it will be used.
- Covariates (dietary and other factors), related to the exposure of interest, need to be measured with minimal and known error (same issues as applied to measurement error and impact for exposure of interest).
- Check that the nutrient database used is complete for the foods and nutrients you are interested in.

- The method used to assess exposure must reflect the above complexity.
- Exposure can be measured using traditional dietary survey methodology, but may also include measures of nutritional status (biochemical, anthropometric, clinical); biomarkers of intake; biological intermediaries, concentrations of which are influenced by diet.
- All dietary survey methods have flaws; for what ever purpose the dietary data are collected, the measure derived from the method will have some error and will not be a perfect measure of the true required exposure.
- Measures derived from biological samples are likely to have less technical error (no underreporting or information bias) than dietary measures and where it is possible to establish a dose-response relationship with dietary exposure may be the preferred method from which to derive the measure of exposure; it is important to consider whether the biological measure is related to the relevant exposure of interest (in terms of time frame and dose); concentrations in blood may not indicate the true functional dynamic state of the availability of the measure being made.
- Prospective studies must be able to capture changes in dietary patterns over time with sufficient accuracy to determine whether that change is related to the change in outcome; this is related to sample size and the variability of the measure used, and assumes nondifferential errors in reporting exposure.
- It is always good practice to check for differential reporting errors in subjects in the study; this can be done by age, gender, BMI, or energy expenditure.
- Statistical modeling cannot adjust for or eliminate the effects of bias; nor can it eliminate the effects of the complex biological interaction between different aspects of diet (and in some cases it should not be used where dietary patterns interact as discussed in Section 8).
- It may not be appropriate to use the estimates of the errors of dietary measures derived from validation studies to "adjust or correct" the measure of exposure–outcome relationship. The assumption about the direction, specificity and effects of the error need to be carefully considered, before assuming that the effect of the error is to lead to attenuation of effect; it is possible that differential error may lead to an exaggeration of effect.
- Evaluation of causal relationships generally requires the integration of information from the basic, clinical, and population sciences including epidemiology.
- Causal inferences should be drawn with caution and only after considering the possible effects of chance, bias, and confounding, and the effects of study design (particularly in observational studies) and measurement error on the size and direction of measures of effect reported.

ACKNOWLEDGMENTS

The author thanks colleagues Rachel Thompson and Daniel Warm for helpful comments on drafts of this chapter. Any errors or omissions are the sole responsibility of the author.

REFERENCES

1. Byers T. The role of epidemiology in developing nutritional recommendations: past, present and future. Am J Clin Nutr 1999; 69:1340S–1348S.
2. Last JM, ed. A Dictionary of Epidemiology. Third Edition. Oxford University Press, New York, 1995.
3. Margetts BM, Nelson M, eds. Design Concepts in Nutritional Epidemiology. Second Edition. Oxford University Press, Oxford, 1997.
4. Willett W. Nutritional Epidemiology. Second Edition. Oxford University Press, New York, 1998.
5. Armstrong BK, White E, Saracci R. Principles of Exposure Measurement in Epidemiology. Oxford University Press, Oxford, 1992.
6. Cameron ME, van Staveren WA, eds. Manual on Methodology for Food Consumption Studies. Oxford University Press, Oxford, 1988.
7. Margetts BM, Nelson M. Measuring dietary exposure in nutritional epidemiological studies. Nutr Res Rev 1995; 5:165–178.
8. Ocke M, Kaaks R. Biochemical markers as an additional measurement in dietary validity studies: application of the method of triads with examples from the European Prospective Investigation into Cancer and Nutrition. Am J Clin Nutr 1997; 65:1240S–1245S.
9. Black AE, Prentice AM, Goldberg GR, Jebb SA, Bingham SA, Livingstone MBE, et al. Measurements of total energy expenditure provide insights into the validity of dietary measurements of energy intake. J Am Diet Assoc 1993; 93:572–579.
10. Food and Agricultural Organization/World Health Organization/United Nations University. Energy and protein requirements. Report of a joint expert consultation. WHO Technical Report Series WHO no. 724, Geneva.
11. Flegal KM. Evaluating epidemiologic evidence of the effects of food and nutrient exposures. Am J Clin Nutr 1999; 69:1339S–1344S.
12. Kaaks R, Riboli E, Sinha R. Biochemical markers of dietary intake, in Application of biomarkers in Cancer Epidemiology. Toniolo P, et al., eds. IARC Scientific Publications No. 142, International Agency for Research on Cancer, Lyon, France, pp. 103–126.
13. Sempos CT, Liu K, Ernst ND. Food and nutrient exposures: what to consider when evaluating epidemiologic evidence. Am J Clin Nutr 1999; 69: 1330S–1338S.

18 Use of Biotechnology to Improve Food Production and Quality

Donald C. Beitz

1. INTRODUCTION

This chapter describes the use of biotechnology by the food industry to increase the efficiency of production and the quality of foods for use by humans. Selected examples are presented in which new technologies of food production by plants and animals are being used because of economic advantages to producers and because of nutritional benefits to human consumers. Some benefits of biotechnology can be summarized as follows *(1)*:

1. Plant production
   a. Higher yielding varieties and more nutritious foods and feeds
   b. Improved resistance to diseases, pests, and adverse conditions
   c. Decreased need for fertilizers and other chemical treatments
2. Animal production
   a. Improved efficiency of converting feeds into useful animal products
   b. Greater control of diseases
   c. Improved composition of foods derived from animals

The remainder of the chapter amplifies of the benefits of using biotechnology to produce animal feed and human food by plants and animals.

2. USING BIOTECHNOLOGY TO IMPROVE FOOD PRODUCTION BY PLANTS

During the past 50 yr, tremendous success has been achieved in food production by plants through development of production systems and varieties of crops. Major improvements in varieties have been made by traditional breeding practices of identifying and selecting strains of crops that exhibit specific valuable traits such as yield, standability, composition, and

From: *Nutritional Health: Strategies for Disease Prevention*
Edited by: T. Wilson and N. J. Temple © Humana Press Inc., Totowa, NJ

resistance to pests and adverse conditions *(2)*. Biotechnological producers are catalyzing another revolution by allowing specific crops to be identified, selected, and even created that have desired traits. Generally speaking, new crop varieties are created by development of cell cultures of the plant under study, inserting new genes into the plant cells, and promoting the differentiation of plant cells in culture into plantlets that eventually are grown into mature plants.

2.1. Extent of Use of Genetically Modified Crops

Agricultural biotechnology companies such as Monsanto, Dupont, Novartis, and Dow Chemical have invested billions of dollars in development of genetically engineered crops. Monsanto, in 1996, introduced the first genetically modified crop to farmers. This crop, Roundup Ready soybeans, was accepted readily; about 50% of the soybeans grown in the United States in 1999 were Roundup Ready soybeans *(3)*. In the same year, about a third of the corn grown in the United States was insect-resistant (Bt) corn. Other countries readily have used the "new" varieties; for example, 60% of Canada's canola crop in 1999 and about 50% of Argentina's soybeans were genetically engineered.

During 1999, consumer concerns resulted in a backlash against genetically modified crops and foods derived from those crops *(4)*. Scientific, moral, ethical, and emotional objections to and support for biotechnology are being expressed openly and vigorously as regulatory agencies, governments, and consumer groups debate the health, environmental, and commercial risks and benefits of technology.

2.2. Modifying Plants to Improve Nutrition

The health and well-being of humans are entirely dependent on foods derived directly from plants or indirectly when plants are consumed by food animals. Carbohydrates, lipids, and proteins make up the bulk of plants and supply energy for human life. Organic and inorganic micronutrients provide essential roles in life processes. Essential dietary micronutrients include 17 minerals and 13 vitamins *(5)*. Nonessential compounds include a variety of unique organic phytochemicals that are linked to promotion of good health. Modification of the content of macronutrients, micronutrients, and phytochemicals in plant foods is an urgent need worldwide, but especially in developing countries where people exist on a few staple foods that are deficient in essential nutrients *(5)*. Deficiencies of vitamin A, iron, and iodine are especially common. Even in developed countries, where food is abundant and caloric intake is often excessive, deficiencies of micronutrients such as iron are prevalent because of poor eating habits. Hence, genetic modification of nutrient content of plants can have significant impact on nutritional status and human health.

In contrast to the situation with essential nutrients, primary evidence for health-promoting roles of phytochemicals are more difficult to prove and comes from epidemiological studies. In fact, exact identity of many active phytochemicals still needs to be determined. Selected phytochemicals that are considered candidates for genetic modification of plants are *(5)*:

1. Carotenoids such as lycopene in tomatoes and lutein in kale and spinach,
2. Glucosinolates such as glucoraphanin in broccoli and broccoli sprouts,
3. Phytoestrogens such as genistein and diadzein in soybeans, tofu, and other soy products, and
4. Phenolics such as resveratrol in red wine and red grapes.

Traditional breeding programs of plants have emphasized increased yields of foods; little emphasis, however, has been placed on micronutrient content. Variation in micronutrient content is known to exist and can be used by breeders to improve plants foods.

Today, tools of biotechnology allow manipulation of plant food composition. Genes for synthesis of carotenoids, biotin, thiamin, and vitamin E and for iron uptake have become available for transfer between different plants. Genes for other nutrients and phytochemicals are being isolated and studied as tools to improve human nutrition.

2.3. Modification of Some Nonstaple Crops

Research is underway to improve resistance of potatoes to several viral, fungal, and bacterial diseases. Cassava that is resistant to the African cassava mosaic virus has been developed. Palm plants are being engineered to produce improved oils (e.g., more oleic acid) and possibly even biodegradable plastics. Bananas are being engineered for improved viral resistance and edible vaccines (e.g., *Escherichia coli* diarrhea).

2.4. Other Engineered Traits of Economic Importance

Along with diseases, drought, and pests, plant growth is retarded by excesses of specific metals in soils. Recently, scientists have identified metal-resistant genes in plants and other organisms *(6)*. Now, the potential exists for making food-producing plants more tolerant to excess aluminum, mercury, copper, or cadmium in soil by introducing genes for phytochelatins that sequester the metal complexes in cells. This technology could improve the acreage of tillable land available for food production. Such modified plants may have greater use as cost-effective agents of environmental remediation. To perform such remediation, the plants could be harvested and incinerated to clean polluted soils. Soil cleaned of pollutants then might become available for the production of consumable foods.

2.5. *Improved Lipid Composition of Selected Plants*

Vegetable oils comprise as much as 25% of the average caloric intake of humans *(2)*. Biotechnology has made it possible to tailor the composition of plant-derived lipids with respect to food functionality and human dietary needs. Plant breeders have taken advantage of the natural diversity in fatty acids that exist among plant varieties and closely related species to develop plants that produce unique oils. For example, low linolenic acid and high linoleic/low palmitic acid soy oils have been made commercially available by traditional breeding.

Directed genetic modifications of plant lipids depends on availability of genes of interest. Fatty acyl desaturase genes are available for synthesis of both α- and γ-linolenate. A Δ^5-desaturase for synthesis of eicosapentaenate recently has become available *(7)*. Genes for several thioesterases for production of medium-chain fatty acids are now available. Moreover, genes for fatty acid elongases for synthesis of eicosamonoenoate (20:1) and docosamonoenoate (22:1) from oleate are available. Thus, several genes to control chain length and degree of unsaturation are available for use in causing plants to produce unique and novel oils.

Because plant oils may form potentially toxic oxidized products when exposed to oxidative stress, increasing monounsaturated fatty acids at the expense of polyunsaturated fatty acids may be desired for improved heat stability and shelf life. By using antisense technology (oleate desaturase), oleic acid-rich (>80%) canola oil has been produced. Similar antisense technology has been used to produce soy oil with greater than 80% oleate and about 11% saturated fatty acids and to decrease linolenate in soy oil from 8% to 2% *(7)*. Investigators continue to study ways to change fatty acid composition of oils (e.g., increased stearate content) to decrease formation of *trans* fatty acids during hydrogenation. This research is of clinical significance for decreasing the intake of the atherogenic *trans* fatty acids by humans.

Another application is the increased synthesis of the very-long-chain fatty acids with 20 and 22 carbons by plants *(7)*. These acids are important constituents of animal cell membranes, and the 20-carbon acids serve as precursors for the biologically active eicosanoids such as prostaglandins, leukotrienes, and thromboxanes. Intake of these very-long-chain fatty acids, especially crucial for newborn infants, is beneficial for cardiovascular disease, renal function, and retinal and brain development.

Investigations are being made to engineer plant oils to increase their content of α-tocopherol, the most active form of vitamin E. Most promise seems related to causing plants to upregulate the biosynthetic pathway for vitamin E synthesis *(5)*. This achievement may be especially important because many studies show that supranatural amounts of vitamin E are beneficial, and because these amounts cannot be attained by consumption of conventional foods.

2.6. Golden Rice with Improved Nutrient Content

Billions of people in developing countries depend on rice as a food staple. Many of the same people suffer from vitamin A and iron deficiencies. Hence, the motivation to genetically modify rice was generated. To this end, Swiss scientists undertook research to introduce into rice the genetic capability of synthesizing β-carotene and of increased iron content (8). Because about 400 million people in the world suffer vitamin A deficiencies, and up to 3.7 billion people, particularly women, are iron deficient, development of this type of modified rice is of major humanitarian importance. Rice plants synthesize no β-carotene but do synthesize geranylgeranyl pyrophosphate, which can be converted to β-carotene with four additional enzymes. The Swiss researchers used daffodil and the bacterium *Erwinia uredovora* as the source of the four required genes and the plant-infecting microbe *Agrobacterium tumefaciens* to transfer the four genes into rice cells in culture. The result was rice plants that produce golden rice rich in β-carotene (8). About 300 g of this modified rice will meet the daily needs for vitamin A for an adult human.

The same scientists studied development of iron-enriched rice (8). This development required introduction of three genes. Normally, iron in rice is unavailable for absorption because of phytate. One gene introduced was for a heat-stable phytase, which improves iron availability. Introduction of the ferritin gene into rice doubled the iron content (8). The gene for a third protein, metallothionein-like protein, improves the absorption of iron from the human digestive tract. Consumption of modified rice with these three genes has great potential to decrease iron malnutrition throughout the world. Hybrid rice that contains both significant β-carotene and improved iron content has been developed. It is anticipated that this golden rice can be in commercial use in a few years.

3. USE OF BIOTECHNOLOGY TO IMPROVE FOOD PRODUCTION BY ANIMALS

For thousands of years, people have attempted to improve animal genetics through selection of animals with desired or superior phenotypes. Success depends on identifying traits and transmissibility of traits to offspring. Improvements are limited by naturally occurring variations and mutations within the species of interest. With the advent of recombinant DNA technology, a variety of new technologies became available that allowed the acceleration and refinement of genetic manipulation of animals.

Insertion of modified human gene constructs into livestock can be used to create "designer production animals" that are capable of enhancement of indigenous genes potentially can improve disease resistance and productivity of target animals. Furthermore, producing useful proteins, tissues, and organs for pharmaceutical and biomedical use is another future use of genetically modified animals. In general, scientists hope to produce animals that are larger, leaner, grow faster and more efficiently, produce more healthful foods, and are more resistant to diseases. These improvements may be made by development of transgenic animals, where a transgene (functional sequence of DNA) is integrated into the host genome. More recently, cloning of animals through the transfer of a nucleus, as opposed to single gene transfer, into enucleated oocytes capable of differentiating into an intact animal in surrogate mothers has opened new opportunities. Thus, generation of a large number of identical animals from a single donor with a superior genotype is possible. The following examples illustrate the breadth of applications of animal transgenesis for improved food and even pharmaceutical production *(1,9,10)*:

1. Meat animals, including fish, with increased copy numbers of genes for somatotropin or insulin-like growth factor for improved growth efficiency,
2. Food-producing animals with greater resistance to viral and bacterial diseases for improved productivity,
3. Lactating cattle with specific genes that increase efficiency of milk production,
4. Lactating animals with capability of secreting novel proteins into milk such as human albumin, α_1-antitrypsin, α-glucosidase, antibodies, antithrombin III, collagen, factor IX, fibrinogen, hemoglobin, lactoferrin, protein C, tissue plasminogen activator, and cystic fibrosis transmembrane conductance regulator (CTFR), and
5. Genetic modification of animals for use in human organ replacement.

3.1. Modification of Digestive Tract Microorganisms to Improve Efficiency of Food Production by Animals

An important application of biotechnology to animal agriculture is the genetic modification of microbes that inhabit the rumen and cecum of food animals. For example, development of a modified microbe population that could be maintained in the rumen and/or cecum and that increased lignin degradation in fibrous feeds would improve digestibility of dietary fibers *(11)*. Degradation of lignin in fibrous feeds would, in most cases, improve the degradation of cellulose and thus increase the quantity of useful products absorbed from a given quantity of consumed feed. Another application is the modification of the rumen microbial population so that a greater amount of microbial protein is synthesized from a given amount of dietary proteins. As a result, less of the feed protein would be degraded and excreted as urea in the urine. Genetic modifications for improvement of cellulose digestion and protein utilization by microbes merit great research emphasis because feed represents a major cost of food production by animals and because there is sufficient margin for improvement in digestibility of dietary fibers and proteins.

Recombinant phytase represents another unique application of biotechnology to animal agriculture. Depending on diet composition, a significant fraction of phosphate especially in the cereal component of the diet is linked covalently to inositol. This phosphate is unavailable to the nonruminant animal and thus is excreted into the feces. Incorporation of recombinant phytase into the diet results in the hydrolysis of phosphate from the inositol; this released phosphate then is available for absorption. The phytase has two pH optima; one is similar to the pH of the stomach, and the other is similar to that of the small intestine. Use of phytase has proven practical in regions of the world where the amount of fecal phosphate spread on farm fields as manure is limited by regulations based on environmental concerns.

3.2. Production of Low-Lactose Milk

To assist lactose-intolerant humans with consumption of dairy foods, lactose-free dairy products can be made by treatment of milk with β-galactosidase (lactase). The capability of expressing a lactose-hydrolyzing enzyme in the mammary gland of mice has been developed *(12)*. These transgenic female mice secreted lactase into milk that contained 50–85% less lactose and no changes in fat and protein concentrations. Thus, a milk with more desirable composition for lactose-intolerant humans can be developed through animal transgenesis.

3.3. Gene Farming with Cloned Animals

Sheep, cows, mice, and goats have been cloned by somatic cell nuclear transfer *(13–15)*. In the latest development, nuclei from quiescent fetal cells of goats were transferred into enucleated oocytes and the manipulated embryos were implanted into surrogate mothers *(16)*. The fetal cells were derived from a goat that had been mated to a transgenic male containing a human antithrombin transgene. One of the cloned offspring that began lactating produced milk with 3.7–5.8 g/L of antithrombin in her milk, which was similar to that of her female ancestors. Thus, cloned animals still synthesized a foreign protein at the expected level. This technology indicates a potential method to produce a herd of lactating animals from one transgenic animal for production of a useful pharmaceutical compound.

3.4. Use of Recombinant Somatotropin for Production of Dairy Foods

In 1937, scientists documented that injections of crude extracts of pituitary glands stimulated milk production by dairy cows. This initial discovery led to a classic study at Cornell University in which dairy cows produced about 40% more milk during a 188-d period when injected daily with purified bovine somatotropin *(17)*. Numerous follow-up studies at many research institutions demonstrated efficacy and safety of the technology to increase milk production with natural or recombinantly derived bovine somatotropin. The following list summarizes many of the findings of these studies *(18–20)*:

1. Milk production is increased,
2. Feed intake increases to compensate for increased milk production,
3. Amount of milk produced per unit of feed consumed increases,
4. Milk composition is not changed, and
5. Milk quality is not changed.

Milk produced by cows treated with recombinant bovine somatotropin was considered safe because *(21)*:

1. The hormone is a protein and is degraded during normal digestive processes,
2. The hormone is species specific and thus is inactive in humans,
3. Milk from treated cows contains normal concentrations of the hormone,
4. The hormone is inactivated by the commonly used pasteurization process, and
5. All animal-derived foods contain small amounts of natural somatotropin.

Monsanto Co. of St. Louis, MO, received Food and Drug Administration (FDA) approval in 1995 for commercialization of their product called Posilac, which is an injectable and slow release preparation of recombinant bovine somatotropin. In 1999, approximately a third of the dairy cows in the United States were treated with Posilac to improve profitability *(18)*. In a recent study of use of recombinant somatotropin in the northeastern United States, scientists concluded that this technology improves lactation yield and persistency and consistently over the 4-yr postapproval period with no effects on cow stayability and herd life *(18)*.

3.5. Use of Recombinant Somatotropin for Meat Production

In 1934, scientists noted that injections of pituitary gland extracts into rats stimulated growth and produced carcasses with more protein and less deposited fat. Hence, administration of exogenous somatotropin to meat-producing animals seemed to merit additional study. Subsequently, researchers demonstrated that injections of bovine somatotropin into growing beef cattle improved growth rate and slightly increased the lean-to-fat ratio of carcasses. Such improvements, however, have not yet proved economical, and thus commercial adoption of this technology has not occurred.

Similarly, injections of porcine somatotropin into young growing pigs caused marked increases in the lean-to-fat ratio of pig carcasses *(22)*. Efficiency of growth improved as well. Color of lean pork was slightly paler because of the treatment; firmness, juiciness, and flavor were not changed, but tenderness tended to be slightly decreased. Especially important for fat-conscious consumers, marbling or fat content of the pork was decreased markedly. To date, however, economics and injection protocol have not justified commercialization of administration of recombinant porcine somatotropin to growing pigs, even though the pork from treated pigs seems more desirable for human health.

Administration of recombinant somatotropin does not show promise in poultry meat production because no significant improvements in growth efficiency or carcass composition were observed.

4. SAFETY OF GENETICALLY MODIFIED FOODS

The concept of substantial equivalence has been used for approval of genetically modified foods by the FDA. In other words, if a genetically modified food can be characterized as substantially equivalent to its "natural" antecedent, it can be assumed to pose no new health risks to consumers and hence to be acceptable for commercial use. The concept of substantial equivalence was introduced in 1993 by the Organization for Economic Cooperation and Development and was endorsed by the Food and Agricultural Organization and the World Health Organization in 1996 *(23)*. Use of this concept was made for approval of glyphosate-tolerant soybeans. These genetically modified soybeans, although clearly different because of the newly acquired biochemical trait, are not different from their nonmodified counterparts in terms of amounts of protein, carbohydrates, vitamins and minerals, amino acids, fatty acids, fiber, ash, isoflavones, and lecithins. Thus, the modified soybeans were deemed substantially equivalent and acceptable. More recent debate has questioned the use and definition of this concept and encouraged the use of more biochemical and toxicological testing before commercial use is allowed. Of principal concern is the presence of foreign proteins in the modified foods that cause human allergies.

5. SUMMARY

Application of techniques of biotechnology have permitted the development of transgenic bacteria, plants, and animals that have a wide variety of new capacities. For example, new plant varieties have been developed that produce grains with more desirable composition for consumption by humans and animals and that are highly resistant to infectious diseases, insects, and adverse environmental conditions. Additionally, bacteria and yeast can be altered genetically to produce vaccines, dietary constituents, biologically active compounds such as insulin and somatotropin, and a variety of other protein products that are used directly by humans or are used in food production by animals. The only limits to what a microbe can be used to produce seems to be whether the corresponding specific gene can be isolated. Moreover, transgenic animals show promise of increased efficiency of production of foods and fiber and perhaps even of pharmaceutical compounds by the mammary gland of lactating transgenic animals. Scientific discoveries before modern biotechnology became available led to improved agricultural productivity and improved food composition. The use of biotechnology, however, has accelerated the rate of those improvements and will continue to do so in the future.

REFERENCES

1. Madden D. Food Biotechnology: An Introduction. ILSI Press, Washington, DC, 1995.
2. National Research Council. Design Foods. Animal Product Options in the Marketplace. National Academy Press, Washington, DC, 1988.

3. Ferber D. GM crops in the cross hairs. Science 1999; 286:1662–1666.
4. Thayer AM. Ag biotech food: risky or risk free? Chem Eng News, 1999 (November 1):11–20.
5. DellaPenna D. Nutritional genomics: Manipulating plant micronutrients to improve human health. Science 1999; 285:375–379.
6. Moffatt AS. Engineering plants to cope with metals. Science 1999; 285:369–370.
7. Broun P, Gettner S, Somerville C. Genetic engineering of plant lipids. Annu Rev Nutr 1999; 19:197–216.
8. Gura T. New genes boost rice nutrients. Science 1999; 285:994–995.
9. National Research Council. Agricultural Biotechnology: Strategies for National Competitiveness. National Academy Press, Washington, DC, 1988.
10. Schnieke AE. Human factor IX transgenic sheep produced by transfer of nuclei from transfected fetal fibroblasts. Science 1997; 278:2130–2133.
11. Russell JB, Wilson DB. Potential opportunities and problems for genetically altered rumen microorganisms. J Nutr 1988; 118:274–279.
12. Jost B, Vilotte JL, Duluc I, Rodeau JL, Freund JN. Production of low-lactose milk by ectopic expression of intestinal lactase in the mouse mammary gland. Nat Biotechnol 1999; 17:180–184.
13. Hammer RE, Pursel VG, Rexroad CE, Wall RJ, Bolt DJ, Ebert KM, et al. Production of transgenic rabbits, sheep, and pigs by microinjection. Nature 1985; 315:680–683.
14. Wilmut I, Schnieke E, McWhir J, Kind AJ, Colman A, Campbell KHS. Nuclear transfer in the production of transgenic farm animals. In: Murray JD, Anderson GB, Oberbauer AM, McGloughlin MM, eds. Transgenic Animals in Agriculture. CABI Publishing, New York, 1999, pp. 67–78.
15. Wilmut I. Viable offspring derived from fetal and adult mammalian cells. Nature 1997; 385:810–813.
16. Baguisi A. Production of goats by somatic cell nuclear transfer. Nat Biotechnol 1999; 17:456–461.
17. Bauman DE, Eppard PJ, DeGeeter MJ, Lanza GM. Response of high producing dairy cows to long-term treatment with pituitary somatotropin and recombinant somatotropin. J Dairy Sci 1985; 68:1352–1362.
18. Bauman DE, Everett RW, Weiland WH, Collier R J. Production responses to bovine somatotropin in Northeast dairy herds. J Dairy Sci 1999; 82:2564–2573.
19. McGuffy RK, Green HB, Easson RP, Ferguson TH. Lactation response of dairy cows receiving bovine somatotropin via daily injections or in a sustained-release vehicle. J Dairy Sci 1990; 73:763–771.
20. Soderholm CG, Otterby DE, Ehle FR, Linn JG, Hansen WR, Annerstad RJ. Effects of recombinant bovine somatotropin on milk production, body composition, and physiological parameters. J Dairy Sci 1988; 71:355–365.
21. Juskevich JC, Guyer CG. Bovine growth hormone: human food safety evaluation. Science 1990; 249:875–884.
22. Etherton TD, Wiggins J P, Chung C S, Evock C M, Rebhun J F, Walton PE. Stimulation of pig growth performance by porcine somatotropin and growth hormone releasing factor. J Anim Sci 1986; 63:1389–1399.
23. Millstone E, Brunner E, Mayer S. Beyond substantial equivalence. Nature 1999; 401:525–526.

19 Nutrition on the Internet

Tony Helman

1. INTRODUCTION

The Internet is the fastest growing communication medium in history. It has the potential to profoundly impact our commercial, personal, and professional lives. The health arena is no exception, and in this chapter, we examine some of the current and potential applications of the Internet in the world of nutrition.

2. WHAT IS THE INTERNET?

The Internet is a network that connects computers. There is nothing remarkable in this—most organizations with more than a handful of computers have a network. What makes the Internet unique are two things:

1. Size: Nobody knows for sure exactly how many computers are permanently connected to the Internet nor how many people have access to the Internet through those computers. Current industry estimates are that the total number of Internet users as of the end of 1999 is around 260 million worldwide, and that this number is doubling every 24 mo *(1a)*. Although the Internet has spread to cover many countries, access is still very much lopsided toward the developed world, with 80% of users being based in just 15 countries. In the United States, which is one of the world's most Internet-connected countries, it is estimated that over 40% of the population now have Internet access *(2)*.
2. Decentralized organization: Because of its origins as a communication medium for institutions engaged in military research, the Internet was deliberately organized to be free of central administration as much as possible (by diffusing control, it is more protected from deliberate attack or malfunction). Thus, there is no central controlling body to set standards of content or acceptable use.

From: *Nutritional Health: Strategies for Disease Prevention*
Edited by: T. Wilson and N. J. Temple © Humana Press Inc., Totowa, NJ

3. IMPLICATIONS OF THE INTERNET

Stemming directly from these two characteristics, the Internet provides in the broadest sense a brand new medium with three striking features: (1) distance-independent communication, (2) universal availability of information, and (3) immediate interactivity.

3.1. Distance-Independent Communication

The Internet is the first communications medium in history where the cost and ease of use is essentially independent of distance.

It is now possible for a person to send an e-mail (electronic mail) to another person almost instantaneously without any regard for (or indeed knowledge of) where or at what distance the person lives. Thus, for example, if I have read an interesting research paper in which the author's e-mail address is given (increasingly the case), I can contact the author with a question or comment and not unreasonably expect to hear back from him/her the next day.

E-mail also differs from the telephone/fax in two other ways. First, it does not matter whether the other person is at home or not (one can pick up one's e-mail from any Internet-connected computer anywhere in the world). This has helped to considerably speed up communication exchanges between itinerant academics!

E-mail technology is such that it is a simple matter to send the same message to large numbers of people at once. This has engendered a new form of communication called a *mailing list (*sometimes known as a discussion list) in which large numbers of people can discuss topics of mutual interest by sharing e-mails amongst the whole group. A closely related resource is the *newsgroup* in which messages are posted on a common "bulletin board," which must be specifically sought out when one wishes to read the messages.

3.2. "Universal" Availability of Information

Although "universal" in this context means "universal amongst those with Internet access," the ability of the Internet to make information available instantaneously across the globe is quite unparalleled in history.

The Internet has always allowed documents to be shared between computers on its network, and if I chose to update the content of my document, the new content will be instantly available to any reader who chooses to download it, wherever they may live.

But it is the development of *web sites* with their multimedia and interactive capacity which has moved the Internet to becoming a part of everyday life in countries with high levels of Internet use.

A web site is a collection of web pages or documents, each of which is written in a standard language (*html* and its more recent developments such as *vrml*), which allow rich multimedia and interactive capabilities, such as animated graphics, sound, and interactive input and responses, etc. *Hyperlinking* is a feature by which clicking on a highlighted word or image automatically takes the viewer to another section of the text, or another resource altogether. In this way, it is possible to weave an almost endless web of interconnected material from many different sites. Furthermore, the presentation of this rich environment takes place on the user's screen (and computer speakers in the case of audio files!) largely independent of what type of computer they have (e.g., PC, Macintosh, Unix).

A web site may contain anything from transcripts of the latest decisions of the US Supreme Court, to downloadable tracks from a hot band's new rock video and album, to an individual's philosophical musings.

Although nobody knows how many web sites and pages are on the Internet, it is believed to be at least several hundred million and growing at a rapid rate.

Writing a web site is now a relatively trivial technical exercise. As a result, the web has effectively democratized the flow of information. Anyone can put whatever they wish on the web. In essence, it is a gigantic library, with little or any organization. Even so, by using an appropriate *search engine* it is possible to read about almost anything. The only problem being, as mentioned before, is that there is nobody to vouch for the accuracy of the material. Just three relatively trivial uses for such an instantly editable, universally viewable library will suffice to illustrate the potential of the web. The author is a fan of the great English game of cricket. No matter where he travels, he is now able to tune into instant score updates complete with live commentary and video highlights of an important game as it takes place *(3)*. Before setting out on his travels, he can obtain a complete weather report for any possible location of interest *(4)*, as well as a check on that day's exchange rate between any two currencies *(5)*.

3.3. Immediate Interactivity

The Internet's true potential for interactivity is really only beginning to unfold. Two obvious examples: online share trading and interactive auction sites where a bidder and a seller may interact in real time from anywhere in the world.

4. NUTRITION APPLICATIONS

There are nutrition applications paralleling all of the foregoing features of the Internet. Broadly these can be divided into resources for health professionals and resources for the lay public.

This chapter focuses mainly on the former. At the same time, it is important to note that one of the more interesting aspects of the Internet is its democratization of information, which allows lay users to have much the same access to health professional resources as do health professionals.

4.1. E-Mail-Based Nutrition Applications

4.1.1. PRIVATE COMMUNICATION

Many biomedical journals now publish the e-mail address of the lead or contact author of their articles, thus facilitating private communication between readers and authors. This includes such prominent journals as the *British Medical Journal (6)*. Unfortunately, this practice is not particularly common among nutrition journals as yet. For example, the *American Journal of Clinical Nutrition (7)* used to publish author e-mail addresses, but currently does not do so.

4.1.2. MAILING LISTS AND NEWSGROUPS

There are a considerable number of nutrition-related mailing lists and newsgroups, allowing discussion among small to large numbers of like-minded individuals. These include lay or patient mailing lists for people suffering from or interested in such nutrition issues as weight problems *(8)*, eating disorders, diabetes, vegetarianism, and so forth. Topics of discussion can vary from patient support to the latest news on treatment, to alternative therapies, to philosophical debates. The easiest way to find such resources is through a web site dedicated to cataloging mailing lists *(9)*.

Mailing lists for nutrition professionals are also in plentiful supply. There is a certain level of turnover with new lists starting up, whereas other lists die a natural death through lack of interest; Table 1 highlights some of the most important and enduring of these.

4.1.3. NEWSLETTERS

There are some useful, free, one-way nutrition e-mail communications that mirror the traditional function of the printed newsletter. For the nonprofessional reader, *Nutrition News Focus* is a daily newsletter providing lay interpretation on current nutrition news as provided by a well-known US-based professor of nutrition *(10)*. For the nutrition or other health professional, the *Arbor Clinical Nutrition Update* is the Internet's most widely read nutrition communication. It contains weekly summaries of the latest clinical nutrition research, together with information on the best nutrition resources available on the Internet. Readership at the end of 1999 totaled more than 15,000 health professionals based in 150 countries *(11)*.

4.2. Web-Based Nutrition Applications

There are an enormous number of web sites concerned with nutrition. Entering "nutrition" as the search term into the general search engine Alta Vista *(12)* returns over 1.3 million listings (using the term "food" adds another 8.5 million!). It is impossible to say how many of these web sites are commercial (although it is clear from casual inspection that many are), how many represent the private musings of nonprofessional individuals, how many are targeted at a noncommercial lay audience, and how many are intended for nutrition professionals.

In the following sections, we examine some of the more useful categories of nutrition web sites from the health professional perspective. They can conveniently be broken down into portal sites, guides and search engines, institutional home pages, nutrition science (including research), dietetics, healthy diet, clinical nutrition, and food and food science (*see* Table 2).

4.2.1. PORTAL SITE, GUIDES, AND SEARCH ENGINES

One of the greatest problems in approaching the Internet is knowing where to find things. For this reason, some of the most popular web sites are those that tell the user what is available and present in such an organized manner that the desired information source can be found quickly. Such sites may operate as directories, search engines, or both. They are often the first port of call en route to finding the resource one actually wants, and are therefore often referred to as *portal sites*. Provided they are updated regularly, portal sites can be an invaluable resource for the novice and experienced user alike. Because of the rapidly changing nature of the subject, no printed publication will ever replace portal sites in providing current information on what is available on the Internet. The reader is advised to consult such portal sites for current and more detailed information to accompany the content of this chapter.

The *Arbor Nutrition Guide (11)* is the largest portal site specifically focused on resources for health professionals. It has over 3000 listings and covers the broad range of categories referred to before. It includes descriptions of the web sites listed and a search engine, and is updated regularly.

Perhaps the best of all the portal sites aimed at the lay public is the *Nutrition Navigator* site *(13)*. Produced by staff from the nutrition department at Tufts University, it has fewer listings than the Arbor site but provides an independent rating score for each of them, based on measures including how often the listings are updated. It also has a search engine, and has found widespread acceptance as a portal site.

Other portal sites have a more food and food science approach. For the lay audience, this includes the *Martindale "Virtual" Nutrition Center (14)*, whereas for nutrition professionals there are two useful web sites from Australia and the US National Agricultural Library *(15,16)*.

4.2.2. INSTITUTIONAL HOME PAGES

A *home page* refers to a web site focused on providing information about its owner. A large number of institutions relevant to nutrition professionals now have home pages on the Internet. This includes government organizations, universities, NGOs, book publishers, and many commercial bodies.

The usefulness of these institutional home pages varies enormously. In some cases, they have little more than descriptions of what the organization does and

Table 1
Some Mailing Lists for Nutrition Professionals[a]

Mailing list	Contact address	Purpose/ subscriber base	Started	Web page	Subscribers (@ 12/99)	Digest available	Level of activity[b]
NGONUT	Owner-ngonut @abdn.ac.uk	Those who work in nutrition programs in developing countries	1997	www.univ-lille1.fr/pfeda	525	No	Moderate
FNSPEC	Eversb@purdue.edu	Extension, nutrition professionals providing information to the public	1993	hermes.ecn.purdue.edu/ Links/fnspec_mg	800	No	Heavy
NUTNET	Majordomo @dietitians.net	Australian nutritionists	1995	www.daa.net/cgi-bin/lwgate/NUTNET-LIST%40dietitians.NET/ archives/	460	No	Heavy
PHNUTR-L	Larsson@u. washington.edu	Public health nutrition edu: 70/11/public/phnutr-l	1996	gopher://lists.u.washington.	600	Yes	Heavy
NUTR-MED	Nutrmed@ ozemail.com.au	Medical and nutrition professionals interested in primary care nutrition	1996	—	250	Yes	Moderate
NUTSCI	Owner-nutsci@hc-sc.gc.ca	Canadian food/ nutrition regulatory issues	1997	www.hc-sc.gc.ca/food-aliment/	425	No	Light
MEALTALK	Owner-mealtalk @nal.usda.gov	USDA School Meals Initiative for Healthy Children		www.nal.usda.gov:8001/ Discussion/index.html	900+	Yes	Heavy

Name	Subscription address	Purpose	Year	URL	Subscribers	Archived	Volume[b]
FOODSAFE	Croberts@nal.usda.gov	Professionals interested in food safety issues		www.nal.usda.gov/fnic/cgi-bin/mealtalk.pl	1200+	Yes	—
PEDI-RD	Susan-carlson@uiowa.edu	Neonatal and pediatric nutrition		www.uihc.uiowa.edu/pubinfo/pedi-rd.htm		—	—
FEEDING-CHILDREN	Eanderson@uidaho.edu	Information related to FeedingChildren	1996	—	80	—	—
DIET-EPI	Gblock@uclink2.berkeley.edu	Nutritional epidemiology research	1996	—	220	—	—
ASPENE	www.clinnutr.org/listserv/aspenet.html	Nutrition and metabolic support	1999	www.clinnutr.org/listserv/aspenet.html	Yes	Yes	Heavy

[a]Dash means information or feature not available.

[b]Light = < 1 messages/d; Moderate = 1–4 messages/d; Heavy = > 4 messages/d.

Table 2
Some Starting Points for Web Browsing

Category	Site	Web address	Comments
Portals, guides	Arbor Nutrition Guide	arborcom.com	For health professionals
	Tufts Nutrition Navigator	navigator.tufts.edu	For lay public
Home pages	USDA	www.usda.gov	Professional and lay resources
	Food and Nutrition Information Center	www.nalusda.gov:80/fnic	Professional and lay resources
	Health Canada	www.hc-sc.gc.ca/main/hppb/nutrition/	Especially food for lay resources
	ILSIrofessional and lay resources	www.ilsi.org	Food safety and general nutrition
Nutrition science	Am J Clin Nutr	www.ajcn.org	Nutrition specific
	British Medical Journal	www.bmj.com	General but with nutrition "collection"
Dietetics	American Dietetics Association	www.eatright.org	Professional and lay resources
	Dietitians of Canada	www.dietitians.ca	Professional and lay resources
	Dietetics Online	www.dietetics.com/	Dietetic professional issues
Clinical nutrition	ASPEN	www.clinnutr.org	Nutrition support
	Family physician nutrition articles	arborcom.com/frame/clinical.htm	Various topics
	HINS	www.hins.org	Pediatric
Food science	USDA food composition tables	www.nal.usda.gov /fnic/cgi-bin/nutsearch.pl	Individual food values
	Drive Thru Diet	www.bgsm.edu/nutrition/FFMainF.htm	Fast food chain foods
	You Are What You Eat	library.advanced.org/11163 /gather/cgi-bin/wookie.cgi/?id=5CMO	Dietary intake analysis

the names of personnel. In other cases, they carry information of more general nutrition interest, which can range from Extension (educational) newsletters to the actual content of courses as well as reports and lay education resources.

A few of the more interesting such institutional web sites with rich nutrition content include US Department of Agriculture (USDA) *(17)*, Health Canada *(18)*, United Nations Committee on Nutrition *(19)*, International Life Sciences Institute (ILSI) *(20)*, and US National Academy of Science *(21)*.

There are several web sites that provide reasonably comprehensive lists of the home pages of university nutrition and food science departments, both internationally *(22)* and within North America. These inform the user of those universities that have accredited nutrition science graduate or dietetic training programs *(23, 24)*.

4.2.3. Nutrition Science (Including Research)

The Internet has significantly enhanced access for those who wish to keep up with the latest in nutrition knowledge, including published research. Improvements have come about in both the ability to access this kind of information much more quickly after it is published, and the ability to filter and sort the vast amount of such information for what is relevant to the individual.

In this respect, nutrition science has benefited from developments in biomedical science generally. Various journal abstract services are now available on-line, many without charge. These include *Cancerlit*, a collection from the National Cancer Institute, and *Medline*, the journal abstract service of the National Library of Medicine, which provides references and abstracts from 4300 biomedical journals *(25)*. A wide variety of third-party providers has made Medline access freely available to Internet users in many guises, and it is possible to tailor the service to specific needs.

For example, *Infotrieve (26)* allows the user to register a specific Medline search and receive weekly e-mail updates of all new Medline entries matching that search. *Pubmed (27)*, which is the National Library of Medicine's own Internet Medline service, allows full Boolean queries of the complete range of Medline fields and can produce very large results going back many years. A simplified version from the same source is *Grateful Med (28)*, which also incorporates pre-Medline for rapid access to literature not yet incorporated into the main Medline index. *Biomednet (29)* has a literature search service that provides "intelligent Medline," combining the results of a normal Medline search with other resources some of which have been evaluated by independent assessors. "On-searching" is provided, which is the ability to search for articles similar to a selected article (based on MESH headings) or for articles by the same author. In some cases, these sites allow the user to order full-text articles, as well as viewing the abstracts, but this is normally a commercially charged add-on feature.

At the same time, individual journals have been making use of the Internet to expand the reach and scope of the printed journals. One of the best examples of this is the *British Medical Journal* with its *eBMJ* web site *(6)*. As each new issue of the journal is posted to eBMJ, at the same time if not a little before the printed version is available, on-line visitors have immediate access to the latest content. A number of articles are available to all visitors in full text, whereas most of the rest appears in abstract form with full text for subscribers. References cited within an eBMJ article are linked to the relevant original abstract within Medline. Many biomedical journals now allow e-mailed letters to the editor, but in eBMJ you can read all the letters pertaining to a particular topic and participate in a forum on the topic. The site also has a *Customised @lerts* feature, which sends emailed tables of contents on request for each new issue. This feature can be further customized by selecting from one or more of the 100 plus clinical categories into which journal content has been arranged. A search engine allows ready access to archived material, which is also grouped within "clinical collections" corresponding to the same clinical categories as the e-mail alerts. As *Nutrition* is one of those collections *(30)*, it is a simple matter to track nutrition-related content on what is one of the world's leading medical journals.

Although the *British Medical Journal* is perhaps the best implementation of an electronic biomedical journal site, a substantial number of nutrition journals have provided on-line sites that provide some combination of these features. More than 50 nutrition and 30 food science journals currently offer at least free on-line tables of contents. A comprehensive list of these is maintained on the *Arbor Nutrition Guide (31)*.

The *American Journal of Clinical Nutrition* web site *(7)* is a well-implemented example, providing abstracts of the current issues with archives back to 1996, as well as a search engine and e-mail table of contents. The *Journal of Nutrition (32)* offers an interesting twist to e-mail updates, offering alerts whenever another journal article cites the paper in question.

Exciting as these developments are, they are only the beginning. A recent trend is the prepublishing of research articles on the Internet prior to acceptance by the printed journal. This not only cuts down enormously on the time lag between submission of a paper and its availability to the health professional community, but it also allows the democratization of the peer review process.

The *Medical Journal of Australia (33)* was the first major medical journal to experiment with this concept, allowing any qualified viewer to submit peer review comments on articles that have been accepted in principle. The comments and the authors' responses to those comments are all publicly posted. In this way, it is hoped that the peer review process will become a more open and transparent one. Two web sites initiated toward the end of 1999, *Clinical Medicine NetPrints (34)* and *Biomedcentral (35)*, offer anyone who wishes the ability to put up a paper, whether or not it has been accepted by any particular journal. Both have excellent academic credentials, one being sponsored by the British Medical Journal and

Stanford University Libraries. Like eBMJ, it allows browsing by medical specialty, of which nutrition is one area.

The ultimate conclusion of Internet publishing may be journals that exist only on the Internet. However, although there are a scattering of such e-journals already, current trends suggest that Internet publishing is going to enhance rather than take over from the traditional hard copy journals.

From the lay perspective, there are many ways to keep up with recent developments in nutrition science in a less formal way. Commercial news agencies such as *Reuters (36)* and *CNN (37)* have health news web sites, both of which allow the user to specify a food and nutrition focus. For health professionals, several of the web sites established specifically for physicians run regular nutrition articles and case reviews, for example *Doctors Guide (38)*.

4.2.4. DIETETICS, HEALTHY DIET

There are a very large number of web sites containing information on healthy diet, dietary guidelines, recommended dietary intakes, and the like *(39)*. The *Food and Nutrition Information Center* of the US Department of Agriculture has one of the better collections on its web site *(40)*, including, for example, both the text and graphics of the US dietary guidelines, along with the report of the committee that produced them *(41)*, and the Recommended Dietary Allowances as produced by the National Academy of Sciences.

For lay information sheets, a good starting point is the *American Dietetic Association* web site, which has a large range of "Nutrition Fact Sheets" *(42)*. The International Food Information Council has a good collection of lay information, with material on food safety and on the general healthy diet *(43)*.

Dietitians have not been slow to take advantage of the Internet, both to promote their services commercially and to communicate among themselves. The *American Dietetic Association* web site *(44)* has a good deal of material about the dietetic profession, position statements, and a database of dietitians, which can be searched by location and specialty interest. *Dietitians of Canada* also has a well thought-out web site *(45)* with professional and lay resources. It is host to the home page of the *International Committee of Dietetic Associations (46)*, within which can be found a list of dietitians' associations around the world. Surprisingly few have web sites as of the date of writing.

Dietitians have also organized informal groupings to communicate via the Internet. *Dietetics Online* is the web site of "a worldwide networking organization of nutrition and dietetic professionals" *(47)*. First developed to provide information on and archives from a long-standing dietitians' bulletin board on the proprietary America Online service, it has grown to include recipes, marketplace information on dietetic-related products, job information, and a reference point for state dietetic associations and several dietitian special interest groups.

There are numerous sites belonging to individual dietitians, which generally feature some lay nutrition information along with advertisements for the owner's dietetic services. *Cyberdiet (48)* is a particularly good example of a web site originally set up by an individual dietitian, which has now become part of a larger Internet health network. *Ask the Dietitian (49)* is another of the best dietitian-authored web sites, with a particularly good Q&A section for the lay visitor.

4.2.5. Clinical Nutrition

There are many Internet resources of relevance to clinical nutritionists, but they are scattered amongst many web sites, including university medical school curricula and course notes, medical CME sites, and organizational home pages. Once again, a good portal site can help to locate what the user is seeking *(50)*.

The *American Society for Parenteral and Enteral Nutrition* web site is one of the better examples, providing news, clinical updates, and lay information on nutrition support *(51)*. The Arbor Nutrition Guide has a series of articles tailored for family physicians *(50)*.

Nutrition elements of specific diseases are often best covered by medical organizations concerned with those diseases. For example, useful nutrition resources are available at the *American Diabetes Association (52)*, *American Heart Association (53)*, *National Heart, Lung, and Blood Institute (54)*, *International Association of Physicians in AIDS Care (55)*, and *Canadian Pediatric Society (56)*. The *American Association of Clinical Endocrinologists* web site *(57)* has quite a bit of nutrition material related to osteoporosis and growth disorders, whereas the *Heinz Institute of Nutritional Sciences (HINS)* web site *(58)* has health professional material on pediatrics.

4.2.6. Food and Food Science

The interactive nature of the Internet is particularly suited to accessing food tables and other forms of nutrition software. The *USDA Nutrient Database* food composition data can be accessed through a simple search engine *(59)*, in which users can specify food and food quantity in several ways. *Cyberdiet* offers food label food composition data *(60)*; it is particularly suited to lay users. This site will also calculate a person's recommended dietary intake based on age, gender, anthropometric measures, and activity level *(61)*.

More specialized food composition sites include: *Drive Thru Diet (62)* from Wake Forest University, which provides nutritional information on foods from the seven largest fast-food chains in the United States, and *You Are What You Eat (63)*, an imaginative site originally designed by nutrition students offering nutrient and food label information, food counter and planner, and the ability to report intake data in relation to an individualized nutrient profile.

Other types of interactive nutrition calculators are available on-line, particularly for calculating body mass index *(64)*, energy requirements *(65)*, compliance with dietary pyramid recommendations *(66)*, and intake of various specific nutrients such as calcium *(67)*. For a complete list, *see* the Arbor Nutrition Guide *(68)*.

The food industry is well covered by web sites: generic, industry-wide, and those dealing with individual companies. The range and number of such sites is, however, larger than can be accommodated in this chapter; this is even more the case in relation to sites devoted to food and cooking. Once again, reference to a good nutrition portal site is recommended.

5. WHAT DOES IT MEAN?

What does all this mean to the nutrition professional and what of the future? The Internet has already boosted the accessibility of nutrition information and fostered communication between nutrition professionals to a degree that few would have anticipated even four or five years ago. The nutritionist who wants to keep up with the latest developments in their field has unprecedented opportunity to do so.

Knowledge has also been democratized—our patients and clients are increasingly likely to come to us with information they looked up on the Internet. Essentially, anyone with an inquiring mind and the determination to do so can now access the same information base as any health professional. To a large extent this is a good thing, but it is also important to remember that there is no quality control on the Internet. We will have to help our patients to learn to distinguish reliable science-based information from the unreliable non-science-based.

Quite how the Internet will develop over the next five years is hard to tell. It is likely that there will be a major growth in the degree of multimedia richness and interactivity in nutrition sites—both are relatively primitive in most current nutrition sites (compared to what is commonly seen in web sites dedicated to youth culture and media, for example).

We are likely to see an increasing number of interactive web-based nutrition courses available, both reputable and less reputable. Major web sites devoted to the ever-popular topic of weight loss are already in development, and we will soon feel their influence. Indeed, the Internet will ensure that the spread of the "latest diet"—whether related to weight loss or some other fad—will be faster than ever before. Those who give professional nutrition advice will therefore need to find ways of keeping up with these fads so as to wisely advise their patients and clients.

Whatever the direction will be, one thing is certain. With billions of dollars of investment funds pouring into it, and a potential market of hundreds of millions of people, this medium, which has developed so fast in such a short time, has only just begun to unfold its wings.

DISCLAIMER

1. The author is editor of one of the Internet nutrition resources mentioned in this chapter *(1)*.

2. The Internet is subject to rapid change. Although every effort has been made to ensure the information in this chapter is correct prior to publication (as of September 2000), it may no longer be so at the time of reading. Check one of the portal sites listed in this chapter for the most current information.

REFERENCES

1. www.arborcom.com <http://www.arborcom.com/> or mail to: update@arborcom.com
1a. cyberatlas.internet.com/big_picture/geographics/article/0,1323,5911_151151,00.html
2. www.c-i-a.com
3. www.cricket.org
4. weather.yahoo.com
5. quote.yahoo.com/m3?u
6. www.bmj.com
7. www.ajcn.org
8. news:alt.support.diet
9. tile.net/
10. www.nutritionnewsfocus.com
11. www.arborcom.com/updatescore.htm<http://www.arborcom.com/updatescore.htm>
12. www.altavista.com
13. navigator.tufts.edu/
14. www-sci.lib.uci.edu/~martindale/Nutrition.html
15. www.dfst.csiro.au/fdnet.htm
16. http://www.nal.usda.gov/fnic/etext/fnic.html
17. www.usda.gov/
18. www.hc-sc.gc.ca/main/hppb/nutrition/
19. www.unsystem.org/accscn/
20. www.ilsi.org/
21. www.nas.edu/
22. arborcom.com/frame/arb_n_hp.htm
23. www.faseb.org/asns/graddir/gradframe.html
24. www.eatright.org/caade/dpd.html
25. www.nlm.nih.gov/hinfo.html
26. www3.infotrieve.com
27. www.ncbi.nlm.nih.gov/PubMed/
28. 130.14.32.42/cgi-bin/startIGM?account=&password=
29. http://www.bmn.com
30. www.bmj.com/cgi/collection/nutrition_and_metabolism
31. arborcom.com/frame/arb_journals.htm
32. www.nutrition.org/
33. www.mja.com.au
34. clinmed.netprints.org
35. www.Biomedcentral.com/
36. www.reutershealth.com/
37. www.cnn.com/HEALTH/index.html
38. www.pslgroup.com/dg/nutritionnews.htm
39. arborcom.com/frame/arb_RDI.htm
40. www.nalusda.gov:80/fnic
41. www.nalusda.gov:80/fnic/Dietary/dgreport.html
42. www.eatright.org/nfs/

43. ificinfo.health.org/
44. www.eatright.org
45. www.dietitians.ca
46. www.dietitians.ca/icda/index.html
47. www.dietetics.com/
48. www.Cyberdiet.com
49. www.dietitian.com
50. arborcom.com/frame/clinical.htm
51. www.clinnutr.org/
52. www.diabetes.org/
53. www.amhrt.org
54. www.nhlbi.nih.gov/index.htm
55. www.iapac.org/
56. www.cps.ca
57. www.aace.com/
58. www.hins.org/
59. www.nal.usda.gov/fnic/cgi-bin/nut_search.pl
60. www.Cyberdiet.com/ni/htdocs/
61. www.Cyberdiet.com/profile/profile.html
62. www.bgsm.edu/nutrition/FFMainF.htm
63. library.advanced.org/11163/gather/cgi-bin/wookie.cgi/?id=5CM0
64. www.Cyberdiet.com/bmi/bmi.html
65. www.healthcalc.net/hcn/tools.htm
66. homearts.com/helpers/calculators/ddiary.htm
67. www.whymilk.com/trainer/
68. arborcom.com/frame/calculator.htm

20 Nutrition in the 21st Century

Ted Wilson and Norman J. Temple

1. THE BASIS OF NUTRITION KNOWLEDGE

As nutrition books go, this one is distinctly unusual in that it was written in one millenium and published in another. Perhaps, therefore, this is an excellent juncture to reflect on a century of tremendous advance and peer forward to a century of improved nutrition and health opportunities.

Much can be gained by looking back and learning from the past as to what types of nutrition investigations have been most fruitful. In our opinion, three types of study stand out: epidemiology, animal studies, and human intervention trials. Epidemiology includes both population comparisons as well as studies on individuals (prospective, case-control, and cross-sectional). Animal studies, and here we mean testing whether an aspect of diet or lifestyle directly affects risk of disease, are most often used to test hypotheses generated by epidemiology. Intervention trials typically follow from the two previous types of study and are rightly referred to as the "gold standard."

It cannot be stressed too strongly that conclusions, whether tentative or (more or less) definitive, must reflect the totality of the evidence. We can define a triad of evidence where ideally a conclusion is supported by evidence from all three types of study. Table 1 illustrates examples of these three types of study and their relationship to specific diseases.

It is important to bear in mind the value and limitations of epidemiology. This is well illustrated by the controversy in recent years concerning the efficacy of β-carotene as a preventive agent against cancer. The foundation of this hypothesis was epidemiological evidence, namely the negative association between nutrient intake and the risk of various types of cancer (1). However, intervention trials failed to demonstrate any reduction in cancer risk after supplementation with β-carotene (2). In actuality, what the epidemiological evidence showed was association, not causation. A better interpretation of the

From: *Nutritional Health: Strategies for Disease Prevention*
Edited by: T. Wilson and N. J. Temple © Humana Press Inc., Totowa, NJ

Table 1
Triad of Evidence for Diet-Disease Relationships

Relationship	Epidemiological	Animal studies	Intervention studies	Overall evidence
Sodium-blood pressure	XX	XX	XX	XX
Saturated fat-hypercholesterolemia	XX	XX	XXX	XXX
β-carotene-cancer	XX	X	O	X
Fat-breast cancer	X	XX	—	X
Selenium-cancer	XX	XXX	XX	XX
Fat-obesity	XX	XXX	XX	XX

Single X indicates weak evidence; XX indicates fairly strong evidence; XXX indicates convincing evidence. An O indicates evidence against. A dash indicates absence of evidence (either for or against). Evidence refers to whether a causal association exists, not to the strength of the association.

evidence is that fruit and vegetables prevent cancer and that any substance commonly present in these foods will also manifest such an association (3,4). The apparently spurious association between β-carotene and cancer is a common problem in epidemiology.

2. STUDIES OF DISEASE MECHANISMS

Although the foregoing types of study have contributed the bulk of our practical knowledge, most resources, in fact, do not go to that type of research. The lions' share goes instead to studies of disease mechanisms (5–7). This unbalanced distribution of resources has delayed vital discoveries in the area of how nutrition can prevent disease.

Different types of research can be divided into two groups: "simple research," which includes the three types outlined previously; and "complex research," which includes most studies on disease mechanisms. Complex research most often leads not to light at the end of the tunnel but to more tunnel where the light should be. The words "simple" and "complex" refer to the degree of complexity in translating observations into practical knowledge that can be applied to problems of human health. We can illustrate this principle with the following examples.

There has been much debate in the last few years regarding the role of salt in hypertension and the efficacy of a low-salt diet as a treatment for the condition. This was reviewed in Chapter 4 by Weinberger. The critical evidence that has helped resolve this question is direct studies of the relationship between salt intake and blood pressure, both those done epidemiologically and those done by intervention studies. By contrast, the great number of studies of disease mechanisms, such as those attempting to comprehend the interaction between salt, hormone levels, and kidney function, have contributed little to the debate.

Returning to the question of β-carotene and the prevention of cancer, it is difficult to find any evidence of where research into disease mechanisms, such as studies of carcinogen metabolism and of oncogenes, have illuminated the problem and thereby paved the way for effective changes in nutrition habits. The same may be said of the relationship between selenium and cancer risk. Although complex research has told us little of value, international correlation studies, animal experiments, and an intervention study have indicated that the nutrient is a potent anticarcinogen (2,8).

Another example that illustrates how simple research has given information of superior value is provided by studies of n-3 fats. Evidence from epidemiological and intervention studies indicate that these lipids may protect against common heart disease (CHD) (Chapter 13 by de Deckere). By contrast, the extensive body of evidence from complex research that attempts to elucidate how these lipids affect metabolism, although expensive, has done little to answer the question as to whether an increased intake of n-3 fats prevents CHD.

The central aim of research into disease mechanisms is to understand the detailed functioning of the body. This is sometimes disparagingly referred to as "reductionism" as it assumes that the whole is no more than the sum of the parts. But it may well be that nutrients and phytochemicals often induce their health-protecting effects by extremely complex interactions. For this reason, it is likely that studying substance-disease interactions one at the time may fail to show the whole picture. Perhaps instead of asking: "Do supplements of β-carotene prevent cancer and how do they work?" we should be asking: "Do vegetables prevent cancer?"

3. THE GREAT LEAP FORWARD

In nutrition and the medical sciences, as much as anywhere else in science, we occasionally see a great leap forward when an investigator with especially well developed powers of insight grapples with a problem and sees things that were under everyone's nose but were otherwise out of sight.

An excellent example of such a person is the late Denis Burkitt, who one of us (NT) had the great fortune to know and collaborate with (9). Burkitt carried out an epidemiological study in Africa into the geographical distribution of a type of cancer common in children. This cancer is now known as Burkitt's lymphoma. Although the cancer was there for anyone to see, it was Burkitt who put one and one together. Quite remarkably, he did this using the resources available in Africa in the 1950s on a grant worth under $1000 in today's money. This work led to the identification of the Epstein-Barr virus. In collaboration with Hugh Trowell and others, Burkitt later went on to establish the vital importance to health of dietary fiber and, hand in hand with this, developed the concept of Western disease (10). Again, this was done using little more than great perceptive powers and a shoestring budget.

Is the age of the great leap forward behind us? We doubt that very much. Buried in the next section, perhaps, are the seeds of one or two great leaps forward.

4. CHALLENGES AHEAD

Rather than making any bold predictions it may be useful to give the following quote:

> So much precise research has been done in the laboratory and so many precise surveys have been made that we know all we need to know about the food requirements of the people....The position is perfectly clear-cut [with respect to Britain].

These prophetic words were penned by Drummond and Wilbraham in *The Englishman's Food,* which was published in 1939. Jack Drummond was a major nutrition authority in the 1920s and 1930s and coined the term "vitamin." It would be foolhardy to believe that we can be any more accurate today in our predictions.

In this closing section of the book, we highlight 11 problem areas that we feel constitute some of the key challenges in nutrition science in the coming years and decades.

4.1. Nutrients and Disease Prevention

As discussed earlier, consumption of fruits and vegetables has a strong protective association with various types of cancer. We still do not know which substances in these foods are responsible for the anticarcinogenic action. Although most attention has hitherto been directed to β-carotene, other substances likely play more important roles, especially phytochemicals (*see* Chapter 5 by Clifford and McDonald). One class of possibly anticarcinogenic phytochemicals is soy isoflavones. The phytoestrogenic action of these substances and how they may be protective against breast cancer (and CHD) is explored in Chapter 6 by Wilson and Murphy. Similarities between these phytoestrogens and pharmacological estrogen agonists continue to blur the differences between foods and drugs. With a better understanding of the anticarcinogenic potential of such substances as phytochemicals, folate, and selenium, it should be possible to produce a supplement that provides an effective, safe, and cheap way to prevent a great many cases of cancer.

Vitamin C has a negative association with various conditions, including cataracts (11), asthma (12), and loss of pulmonary function (13). As in the case of β-carotene and cancer, it is critically important to bear in mind that what these data really reveal is not that vitamin C protects against these conditions, but rather that ascorbate-rich fruit and vegetables do. As with cancer, therefore, once the responsible substances have been identified, we can better understand how to enrich our dietary intake, perhaps using supplements, so as to prevent these conditions.

A nutrient that merits further investigation is vitamin E. There is evidence that it may have some prophylactic effectiveness against cancer and CHD (3). These benefits are generally seen only at intakes several times higher than the RDA. These levels cannot be achieved through food consumption alone. This suggests that vitamin E is acting as a nutraceutical rather than as a vitamin. We have growing evidence that optimal dietary intake (especially vitamin E) may enhance immune function and thereby reduce the burden of infectious disease *(14)*. Clarification of these relationships may be of enormous value, especially to the elderly and malnourished and to populations at high risk of infectious disease.

4.2. Optimal Intake of Nutrients

Information that has emerged in recent years challenges our concepts of nutrient requirements. Although the details are still hazy, it is becoming increasingly clear that many substances have disease-preventing actions in ways that do not fit into the classic model of nutrient/deficiency disease. In some cases, these substances are nutrients, notably vitamin E and selenium, but are apparently most effective at intakes far above what is required for preventing deficiency diseases. In other cases, the phytochemicals, there is no requirement, as the substances are not nutrients in the classic sense; possible examples of this are particular carotenoids and flavonoids. Chapter 4 by Weinberger and Chapter 3 by Heaney indicate that this concept applies to potassium and calcium by virtue of their hypotensive action.

In a previous work, one of us (NT) argued that it is short sighted to define recommended nutrient intakes narrowly in terms of preventing deficiency diseases *(15)*. For various nutrients, we can more accurately speak of three levels of intake. A low intake is clearly deficient by any definition and will produce clinical symptoms or, at least, subclinical deficiency. A somewhat higher intake will prevent deficiency symptoms but will not fully protect health; it is best described as a suboptimal intake. A yet greater intake is required for maximal health preservation: an optimal intake. In the case of the phytochemicals, of course, we cannot talk of deficiency, although there does appear to be an optimal intake. Taking vitamin E as an example, a daily intake of under 5 mg is deficient, 10 mg (the US RDA) is suboptimal, whereas an optimal intake (assuming the previously cited evidence is correct) is between 50 and 500 mg.

The reason for these different levels of requirement stems from the relationship between the nutrient or phytochemical and the cause of the disease. With classic deficiency diseases, such as scurvy, the disease is solely due to lack of the nutrient. As a result, one or more specific biochemical pathways fail to operate normally. But with diseases prevented by relatively high doses of nutrients and phytochemicals, the true cause is a factor, such as tobacco, which the protective substances can counter to some extent. However, they typically do this in ways where the required dose is much higher than that pertaining to the prevention of a deficiency disease.

Just as the discovery of the relationship between nutrients and deficiency diseases necessitated the establishment of the concept of recommended nutrient requirement, so the foregoing arguments suggest the necessity of a new concept based on optimal intake. In this regard, it matters little whether the substance in question is a nutrient or not. Gey's proposed term, recommended optimum intake, closely corresponds to the aforementioned concept (16).

4.3. Nutrition and Aging

Many features associated with aging—for instance, atherosclerosis, impaired immune function, declining respiratory function, decreasing lens opacity (leading to cataract), and increasing blood pressure—are all associated with diet, and therefore preventable to a greater or lesser extent. Recent evidence suggests that age-related cognitive decline and memory loss may also come into this category (17). Indeed, optimal nutrition may be acting not so much by a different mechanism in each of these conditions but by a common pathway. Oxidative stress is the mechanism that first springs to mind, but the supporting evidence is far from overwhelming (3; see Chapter 7 by Temple and Machner).

4.4. Diet and Fetal Programming

This has been a contentious issue for decades (see Chapter 16 by Barker and Godfrey). Determining its importance with respect to the development of obesity, CHD, diabetes, cancer, and other diseases in adults remains a challenge. More work is clearly needed to clarify the ideal fetal and infant diet for the prevention of these diseases in adulthood.

4.5. Diet and CHD

The relationship between diet and CHD cannot help but appear as a confusing picture. There are several areas of potential importance which require further investigation before we can formulate an overall strategy for the prevention of this ongoing pandemic. These areas include homocysteine (see Chapter 8 by Woodside and Young), high doses of vitamin E (discussed previously), n-3 fatty acids (see Chapter 13 by de Deckere), and determining the maximum safe intake of saturated fat and *trans* fatty acids (see Chapter 9 by Clarke and Frost).

4.6. Diet and Obesity

The chapter by Richards and colleagues authoritatively reviews our present position with regard to obesity. Four centuries ago, William Shakespeare wrote: "They are as sick that surfeit with too much as they that starve with nothing" (*Merchant of Venice*). Despite decades of intensive research, effective dietary therapy for the condition remains as out of reach as it was two-thirds of a century ago when Somerset Maugham wrote what is arguably the finest picture painted of the pain and frustration of weight loss in his story *The Three Fat Women of Antibes*. Here, in more ways than one, "An ounce of prevention is worth a pound of cure." The area of prevention and treatment of obesity will hopefully see ongoing progress.

4.7. The Ideal Diet

Central to any discussion on the subjects of CHD is the debate regarding the ideal level of fat, saturated fat, and dietary fiber. This also has major implications in regard to obesity, diabetes, and colon cancer. It has often been suggested that the ideal diet is one based largely on low-fat plant foods with little or no meat. Research may well prove that this is the best means to incorporate into the diet the optimal quantities of fruit, vegetables, and perhaps soy foods. We should also keep our minds open to the possibility that there is no ideal diet for a population, but rather unique nutritional needs of the individual.

4.8. Future Nutritional Contributions from Two Opposites: Herbal Medicine and Bioengineering

As discussed in Chapter 15 by Craig, traditional medicine continues to predominate in less developed regions of the world. In the next millenium, we can expect to see continued developments in these low-technology supplements and this will lead to promotion of health in the developed regions of the world. Our scientific understanding of herbal medicine and nutraceuticals remains in its infancy; clearly some provide reproducible health benefits and others are useless. Their nutritional significance remains hazy at present. Herbals that can be incorporated into our diet and do prevent diseases will become important given their generally low cost.

Nutritional impacts of high-technology changes have been taking place since the days of Norman Borlaug and his "Green Revolution." The impact of biotechnology was discussed in Chapter 18 by Beitz. Genetically modified crops and livestock have become fairly common in the United States, although they are as yet poorly accepted elsewhere. The risks and benefits of the use of these technologies to increase yields comes with risks that are still poorly understood and risks that may yet to be appreciated. Until there is a much better understanding of the nutritional benefits/risks, the use of this technology is likely to remain controversial.

4.9. Dietary Assessment

An ongoing problem in nutritional epidemiology is the quality of dietary assessment (see Chapter 17 by Margetts). So many of the controversies in the area of nutrition and disease emanate from inaccuracies in measuring people's dietary intake. Well-known examples include sodium/blood pressure, energy intake/obesity, and fat intake/breast cancer.

4.10. Nutrition, Health Promotion, and Government Policy

All the foregoing research is worth little if people cannot be persuaded to actually follow dietary advice. One approach is that discussed in Chapter 1

Coventry University

by Jacobson, i.e., how a private organization can be highly effective at promoting healthier diets. Chapter 2 by Temple and Nestle discusses a crucial area for investigation, i.e., the limitations of health promotion interventions and why government policy may prove to be a more effective vehicle of change. Clearly, this whole area offers great challenges and cries out for radical new ideas.

4.11. The Internet and Nutrition Information

We are now entering the information age. Given the widespread access to Internet web sites, as discussed in Chapter 19 by Helman, our access to nutrition information will undoubtedly grow rapidly. In the 21st century, the long time gaps between data collection, writing, publishing, and the reading of articles will undoubtedly shrink. Answers in an instant will be the norm in the future.

FINAL NOTE

To paraphrase Churchill, advances in the field of nutrition science in recent years represent not the beginning of the end but, perhaps, the end of the beginning. In the opinion of the editors, we are ready to move from the *hors d'oeuvres* to the main course.

ACKNOWLEDGMENT

The work in this chapter done by NT was carried out at the CDL Programme, Medical Research Council, Cape Town, South Africa.

REFERENCES

1. Temple NJ, Basu TK. Does beta-carotene prevent cancer? Nutr Res 1988; 8:685–701.
2. Greenwald P, McDonald SS. Antioxidants and the prevention of cancer. In: Basu TK, Temple NJ, Garg ML, eds. Antioxidants in Human Health and Disease. CAB International, Wallingford, UK, 1999, pp. 217–234.
3. Temple, NJ. Antioxidants and disease: more questions than answers. Nutr Res 2000; 449–459.
4. Wilson T. Whole foods, antioxidants and health. In: Basu TK, Temple NJ, Garg ML, eds. Antioxidants in Human Health and Disease. CAB International, Wallingford, UK, 1999; 141–150.
5. Temple NJ, Burkitt DB. The war on cancer—failure of therapy and research. J R Soc Med 1991; 84:95–98.
6. Temple NJ. Simplicity—the key to fruitful medical research. Med Hypotheses 1985; 17:139–145.
7. Temple NJ. Medical research. A complex problem. In: Temple NJ, Burkitt DB, eds. Western Diseases: their Dietary Prevention and Reversibility. Humana Press, Totowa, NJ, 1994, pp. 419–436.
8. Clark LC, Combs GF, Turnbull BW, Slate EH, Chalker DK, Chow J, et al. Effects of selenium supplementation for cancer prevention in patients with carcinoma of the skin. JAMA 1996; 276:1957–1963.
9. Nelson CL, Temple NJ. Tribute to Denis Burkitt. J Med Biogr 1994, 2:180–183.

10. Burkitt DP. The emergence of a concept. In: Temple NJ, Burkitt DB, eds. Western diseases: their Dietary Prevention and Reversibility. Humana Press, Totowa, NJ, 1994, pp. 1–13.

11. Taylor A, Jacques P, Epstein E. Antioxidant status and risk for cataract. In: Basu TK, Temple NJ, Garg ML, eds. Antioxidants in Human Health and Disease. CAB International, Wallingford, UK, 1999, pp. 271–284.

12. Young IS, Roxborough HE, Woodside JV. Antioxidants and respiratory disease. In: Basu TK, Temple NJ, Garg ML, eds. Antioxidants in Human Health and Disease. CAB International, Wallingford, UK, 1999, pp. 293–311.

13. Hu G, Zhang X, Chen J, Peto R, Campbell TC, Cassano PA. Dietary vitamin C intake and lung function in rural China. Am J Epidemiol 1998; 148:594–599.

14. Bendich A. Immunological role of antioxidant vitamins. In: Basu TK, Temple NJ, Garg ML, eds. Antioxidants in Human Health and Disease. CAB International, Wallingford, UK, 1999, pp. 27–41.

15. Temple N.J. Vitamins and minerals in cancer, hypertension, and other diseases. In: Temple NJ, Burkitt DP, eds. Western Diseases: their Dietary Prevention and Reversibility. Humana Press, Totowa, NJ, 1994, pp. 209–235.

16. Gey KF. Ten-year retrospective on the antioxidant hypothesis of arteriosclerosis: threshold plasma levels of antioxidant micronutrients related to minimal cardiovascular risk. J Nutr Biochem 1995; 6:206–236.

17. Perrig WJ, Perrig P, Stahelin HB. The influence of antioxidants on cognitive decline in the elderly. In: Basu TK, Temple NJ, Garg ML, eds. Antioxidants in Human Health and Disease. CAB International, Wallingford, UK, 1999, pp. 335–350.

INDEX

About the Editors

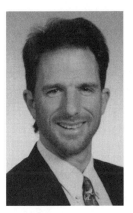

Dr. Ted Wilson teaches nutrition in the Department of Health Education at the University of Wisconsin-La Crosse, and is a Research Scientist in the Department of Exercise and Sport Science at the University of Wisconsin-La Crosse in collaboration with the Cardiac Rehabilitation Program. His primary interest is to find ways to use better nutrition to improve our quality of life. His were the first published studies on the cardiovascular disease prevention effects of cranberry juice on low-density lipoprotein oxidation, arterial vasodilation, and platelet aggregation. He has also performed research that evaluates how creatine, tea, food supplements, and soy phytoestrogens affect cardiovascular disease and cancer risk factors.

Dr. Norman J. Temple teaches nutrition at Athabasca University in Alberta, Canada, and develops distance education courses in nutrition and health. Dr. Temple's specialty is diet in relation to disease, particularly the influence of dietary factors in heart disease and cancer. *Nutritional Health: Strategies for Disease Prevention* is his fourth book on diet, health, and disease. He is coeditor with Denis Burkitt of *Western Diseases: Their Dietary Prevention and Reversibility* (Humana Press, 1994), which continued and extended Burkitt's pioneering work on the role of dietary fiber in Western diseases. Other publications include *Health for the New Century,* and *Ethics, Medical Research and Medicine,* a book on medical ethics to be published in 2001.

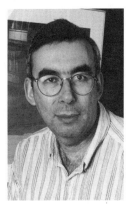

About the Series Editors

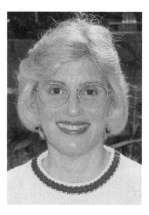

Dr. Bendich is Associate Director, New Product Research at GlaxoSmithKline, where she is responsible for leading research initiatives for products that include TUMS, Os-Cal and Geritol, as well as other nutrient-containing dietary supplements marketed in and outside the US. Prior to joining SmithKline Beecham, Dr. Bendich was Assistant Director of Clinical Nutrition at Roche where she participated in many of the groundbreaking clinical studies involving antioxidants and folic acid.

Dr. Bendich is an internationally recognized authority on antioxidants, nutrition and immunity and pregnancy outcomes, vitamin safety and the cost-effectiveness of vitamin/mineral supplementation. Author of over 100 scientific papers, editor of seven books, including *Preventive Nutrition: The Comprehensive Guide For Health Professionals* and Series Editor of *Nutrition and Health* for Humana Press, Dr. Bendich also serves as Associate Editor for *Nutrition: The International Journal* and is a member of the Board of Directors of the American College of Nutrition. Dr. Bendich was recently a recipient of the Burroughs Wellcome Visiting Professorship in Basic Medical Sciences, 2000–2001, and holds academic appointments as Adjunct Professor at Columbia University, UMDNJ, and Rutgers University.

Dr. Richard J. Deckelbaum is the Robert R. Williams Professor of Nutrition and a Professor of Pediatrics at Columbia University, where he serves as Director of the Institute of Human Nutrition and Director of Pediatric Gastroenterology and Nutrition. He also founded the Children's Cardiovascular Health Center at Columbia Presbyterian Medical Center.

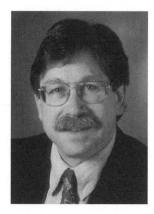

Dr. Deckelbaum's primary research interests concern human plasma lipoproteins, the metabolism of intravenous lipid emulsions, and the cellular effects of dietary fats and free fatty acids. His work has contributed to better understanding of mechanisms whereby human lipoproteins are structurally remodeled in the plasma compartment, factors modulating receptor-lipoprotein interactions, and nutrient-gene interactions.

In 1996, Dr. Deckelbaum conceived and initiated the first M.D. Program in International Health and Medicine as a collaboration with colleagues at Israel's Ben Gurion University of the Negev and Columbia University.

Author of over 200 articles, reviews, and chapters, Dr. Deckelbaum has served on numerous national task forces, as well as review boards for nutrition and clinical research. He chaired a 1997 national conference on *Preventive Nutrition: Pediatrics to Geriatrics* and served as a member of the United States Department of Agriculture and Health and Human Services Advisory Committee for Dietary Guidelines for the year 2000. He currently chairs the International March of Dimes Task Force on Nutrition and Optimal Human Development.